The Diagnosis of Psychosis

The Diagnosis of Psychosis

Rudolf N. Cardinal
Edward T. Bullmore
Behavioural and Clinical Neuroscience Institute and Brain Mapping Unit
Department of Psychiatry, University of Cambridge
Addenbrooke's Hospital, Cambridge, UK
Cambridgeshire and Peterborough NHS Foundation Trust
Fulbourn Hospital, Cambridge Road, Fulbourn, Cambridge, UK

CAMBRIDGE
UNIVERSITY PRESS

CAMBRIDGE UNIVERSITY PRESS
Cambridge, New York, Melbourne, Madrid, Cape Town,
Singapore, São Paulo, Delhi, Tokyo, Mexico City

Cambridge University Press
The Edinburgh Building, Cambridge CB2 8RU, UK

Published in the United States of America by Cambridge University Press, New York

www.cambridge.org
Information on this title: www.cambridge.org/9780521164849

First published by Cambridge University Press 2011

Printed in the United Kingdom at the University Press, Cambridge

A catalogue record for this publication is available from the British Library

Library of Congress Cataloguing in Publication data
Cardinal, Rudolf N.
The diagnosis of psychosis / Rudolf Cardinal, Edward Bullmore.
p. cm.
ISBN 978-0-521-16484-9 (pbk.)
1. Psychoses–Diagnosis. 2. Physicians (General practice) I. Bullmore, Edward T. II. Title.
RC512.C356 2011
616.89–dc22 2010051717

ISBN 978-0-521-16484-9 Paperback

To Hannah, Thorn, and Phoebe, and to the staff and patients of CAMEO

Contents

Detailed table of contents

Section 2: A clinical approach to the diagnosis of psychosis

Preface

Psychosis is one of the syndromes at the heart of psychiatry. Any patient who develops psychosis is likely to be referred to a psychiatrist, whether from primary care, at the point of admission to a psychiatric unit, or by other hospital physicians. Naturally, patients, carers, and other physicians expect psychiatrists to be expert in the diagnosis of psychosis, regardless of its cause, just as (for example) they expect respiratory physicians to be expert in the diagnosis of breathlessness, even if the cause is not primary respiratory disease.

Thus, psychiatrists frequently meet patients exhibiting psychotic symptoms and signs. Classificatory systems within psychiatry (such as the World Health Organization's *ICD-10 Classification of Mental and Behavioural Disorders* and the American Psychiatric Association's *Diagnostic and Statistical Manual of Mental Disorders*) lay heavy emphasis on primary psychiatric disease, acknowledging with broad brush strokes that psychosis can be the result of other conditions but giving relatively little guidance on exactly what those conditions are, or how to diagnose them. Some psychiatric textbooks give a short list of relevant organic disorders, but these are often not comprehensive or oriented towards the diagnosis of psychosis, while reference works in neurology, general medicine, and sometimes psychiatry provide great detail on individual diseases without always making it easy for the psychiatrist to compile a relevant differential diagnosis for a psychotic patient. For the trainee psychiatrist, who may not have had extensive training in general medicine or neurology, this can make it difficult to acquire the mental templates that allow a diagnosis of all types of psychosis.

This state of affairs also makes for a potential gap between psychiatry and other branches of medicine. If a psychiatrist suspects a secondary psychosis, it might be optimistic to refer to a physician from another specialty (such as general internal medicine) asking "is there an organic cause?" This requires the non-psychiatrist to know the differential diagnosis of psychosis. A response from the general physician of "none that I know" may therefore be less helpful than was hoped. Psychiatrists should not rely on non-specialists to exclude secondary psychosis. Likewise, if a general physician asks a psychiatrist to diagnose a psychotic patient, it may well be because that physician cannot find a cause or suspects a primary psychiatric disease. Replying that the cause is "organic" or "delirium" is not a diagnosis, and leaves the general physician little better off; they need a more specific diagnosis. Finally, there is sometimes concern among patients and their carers about missed secondary causes of psychosis (whether this be because of stigma, concern about physical health, or their thoughts about prognosis and treatment), and a good knowledge of the differential diagnosis of psychosis makes this less likely.

In Section 1 of this book, we aim to provide a comprehensive account of the causes of psychosis, be it primary psychosis, with no clearly identified biological aetiology, or secondary psychosis, in which psychosis is a symptom and sign of another identified disease. Because our aim is to be comprehensive, we recognize that we are likely to have failed in this, and also that we may have included some conditions the causal role of which in producing psychosis is not established beyond all doubt. For primary psychoses, we describe the disease characteristics and psychiatric diagnostic criteria. For secondary psychoses, we describe the causative condition, and suggest an approach to diagnosis. Our descriptions are brief in order to keep this book short, but we aim to give sufficient detail that the psychiatrist is able to recognize each condition's characteristic constellation of features, have an idea of how often psychosis is seen in that condition and under what circumstances, and know what is required to achieve a firm diagnosis.

In Section 2 of this book, we describe an approach to diagnosis, giving formal diagnostic criteria and flowcharts to aid the diagnosis of primary psychosis, and pointers towards the diagnosis of secondary psychosis.

We hope this book will be of use to the trainee psychiatrist acquiring the knowledge necessary to practise independently, and as a convenient reference work for senior psychiatrists and others interested in psychosis. We suggest that Section 1 may be useful for acquiring background knowledge, and subsequently as a reference section, while Section 2 may be useful when faced with a patient whose psychosis is of uncertain aetiology.

Acknowledgements

We thank the staff and patients of CAMEO, a clinical service in Cambridge for patients with a first episode of psychosis. We thank also David Dodwell, Emilio Fernández-Egea, Paul Fletcher, Carol Gregory, Jeremy Hall, Catherine Hatfield, Ehab Hegazi, Peter Jones, Belinda Lennox, Graham Lennox, Graham Murray, Martin Stefan, Zahoor Syed, Petrus de Vries, Cathy Walsh, Mai Wong, and Asif Zia for helpful discussion. Any errors or omissions are, of course, our own.

RNC was supported by an academic clinical fellowship from the UK NHS National Institute of Health Research. The work was conducted within the Department of Psychiatry, University of Cambridge, and the University of Cambridge Behavioural and Clinical Neuroscience Institute (funded by the UK Medical Research Council and the Wellcome Trust). We thank all those who supported this work.

Abbreviations and symbols

[X]	concentration of X
▶	indicates a topic covered in more detail elsewhere in this text
2-DPMP	2-diphenylmethylpiperidine
4-MMC	4-methylmethcathinone
5-HT	5-hydroxytryptamine (serotonin)
a.k.a.	also known as
ABG	arterial blood gas
ACE	angiotensin converting enzyme
ACE-R	Addenbrooke's Cognitive Evaluation, revised
ACh	acetylcholine
AChR	acetylcholine receptor
ACTH	adrenocorticotrophic hormone
ADEM	acute disseminated encephalomyelitis
ADH	antidiuretic hormone (arginine vasopressin; vasopressin)
ADHD	attention-deficit/hyperactivity disorder
ADP	adenosine diphosphate
AGD	argyrophilic grain disease
AIDS	acquired immunodeficiency syndrome
ALA	δ-aminolevulinic acid (a.k.a. 5-aminolevulinate, 5-aminolaevulinate)
ALA-D	5-aminolaevulinate dehydratase
ALD	adrenoleukodystrophy
alkP	alkaline phosphatase
ALS	amyotrophic lateral sclerosis (= MND)
ALT	alanine aminotransferase
AlzD	Alzheimer's disease
AMT	Abbreviated Mental Test
ANA	antinuclear antibody
ANCA	antineutrophil cytoplasmic antibody
ANNA	antineuronal nuclear antibody
aPL	antiphospholipid antibody
ApoE	apolipoprotein E
APP	amyloid precursor protein
APS	antiphospholipid syndrome
ARF6	ADP-ribosylation factor 6
ASO	antistreptolysin O
AST	aspartate aminotransferase
ATP	adenosine triphosphate
ATPase	adenosine triphosphatase
AV	atrioventricular
AZT	azidothymidine
BACNS	benign angiopathy of the central nervous system
BFT	"bone function" tests (corrected calcium, phosphate, alkaline phosphatase)

BG	basal ganglia
BGC	basal ganglia calcification
BLIPS	brief limited intermittent psychotic symptoms
BP	blood pressure
BPRS	Brief Psychiatric Rating Scale
CAARMS	Comprehensive Assessment of At-Risk Mental State
CADASIL	cerebral autosomal dominant arteriopathy with subcortical infarcts and leukoencephalopathy
CAG	cytosine, adenine, guanine
CBGD	corticobasalganglionic degeneration
Cbl	cobalamin metabolism defect
CD	cluster of differentiation
ChAc	autosomal recessive chorea–acanthocytosis
CI	confidence interval
CJD	Creutzfeldt–Jakob disease
CK	creatinine (phospho)kinase
CLN	ceroid lipofuscinosis, neuronal
CMV	cytomegalovirus
CNS	central nervous system
CO	carbon monoxide
COHb	carboxyhaemoglobin
COMT	catechol-*O*-methyltransferase
CPAP	continuous positive airway pressure
CRF	corticotrophin-releasing factor (a.k.a. corticotrophin-releasing hormone)
CRMP	collapsin response mediator protein
CRMP-5	collapsin response mediator protein 5, the main antigen recognized by CV2 antibodies
CRP	C-reactive protein
CSF	cerebrospinal fluid
CT	computerized/computed tomography
CVA	cerebrovascular accident (stroke)
CVST	cerebral venous and sinus thrombosis
CXR	chest X-ray (radiograph)
DA	dopamine
DAT	dopamine transporter
DCR-10	*ICD-10 Classification of Mental and Behavioural Disorders: Diagnostic criteria for research*
DHEAS	dehydroepiandrosterone sulphate
DILE	drug-induced lupus erythematosus
dl	decilitre
DLB	dementia with Lewy bodies (Lewy-body dementia)
DMT	dimethyltryptamine
DNA	deoxyribonucleic acid
DNAse	deoxyribonuclease
DOET	dimethoxyethylamphetamine
DOM	dimethoxymethylamphetamine
DRPLA	dentatorubropallidoluysian atrophy

dsDNA	double-stranded DNA
DSM-IV[-TR]	*Diagnostic and Statistical Manual of Mental Disorders*, 4th edition [text revision]
DVT	deep-vein thrombosis
DWI	diffusion-weighted imaging
ECG	electrocardiogram
EDTA	ethylenediaminetetraacetic acid
EEG	electroencephalogram
EFA6A	exchange factor for ARF6
ELISA	enzyme-linked immunosorbent assay
ESR	erythrocyte sedimentation rate
FBC	full blood count: WBC and differential, Hb and Hct, platelet count; MCV, MCH and MCHC
FDG-PET	fluorodeoxyglucose positron emission tomography
FENIB	familial encephalopathy with neuroserpin inclusion bodies
FFI	fatal familial insomnia
FISH	fluorescent *in situ* hybridization
fl	femtolitres
FLAIR	fluid-attenuated inversion recovery (as an MRI technique)
FSH	follicle-stimulating hormone
FTD	frontotemporal dementia
FTDP17	frontotemporal dementia and parkinsonism linked to chromosome 17, a set of tau protein mutations
FTLD	frontotemporal lobar degeneration
g	gram
G6PD	glucose-6-phosphate dehydrogenase
GABA	γ-aminobutyric acid
GAD	glutamic acid decarboxylase
GBL	γ-butyrolactone
GCA	giant cell arteritis
GCS	Glasgow Coma Scale
GFR	glomerular filtration rate
GH	growth hormone
GHB	γ-hydroxybutyric acid
GI	gastrointestinal
GSS	Gerstmann–Sträussler–Scheinker disease
h	hour
Hb	haemoglobin concentration
HCG	human chorionic gonadotrophin
Hct	haematocrit
HD	Huntington's disease
HDL2	Huntington's disease-like 2
HERNS	hereditary endotheliopathy with retinopathy, nephropathy, and stroke
HHV-6	human herpesvirus 6
HIV	human immunodeficiency virus
HLA	human lymphocyte antigen
HSV	herpes simplex virus

HUS	haemolytic–uraemic syndrome
i.m.	intramuscular(ly)
i.v.	intravenous(ly)
ICD-10	*World Health Organization International Classification of Diseases*, 10th revision (specifically, the *ICD-10 Classification of Mental and Behavioural Disorders*)
Ig	immunoglobulin
INR	international normalized ratio (of prothrombin time to normal prothrombin time)
l	litre
La	not an abbreviation; a small nuclear RNA protein; also known as Sjögren's syndrome antigen B (SS-B)
LDH	lactate dehydrogenase
L-DOPA	3,4-dihydroxy-L-phenylalanine
LFT	"liver function" tests: albumin, ALT, alkaline phosphatase, bilirubin
LH	luteinizing hormone
LHRH	luteinizing-hormone-releasing hormone
LP	lumbar puncture
LSD	lysergic acid diethylamide
mAChR	muscarinic acetylcholine receptor
MAO	monoamine oxidase
MAOI	monoamine oxidase inhibitor
MC	malignant catatonia
MCH	mean cell (corpuscular) haemoglobin
MCHC	mean cell (corpuscular) haemoglobin concentration
MCV	mean cell (corpuscular) volume
MDMA	methylenedioxymethamphetamine ("Ecstasy")
MELAS	mitochondrial myopathy, encephalopathy, lactic acidosis, and stroke-like episodes
Mg	magnesium
mGluR1	metabotropic glutamate receptor 1
MI	myocardial infarction
MIM	Mendelian Inheritance in Man
MLD	metachromatic leukodystrophy
mM	millimolar (millimoles per litre; mmol/l)
MMSE	Mini-Mental State Examination
MND	motor neuron disease (= ALS)
MPA	microscopic polyangiitis
MPO	myeloperoxidase
MR	magnetic resonance
MRA	magnetic resonance angiography
MRI	magnetic resonance imaging
MRS	magnetic resonance spectroscopy
MRV	magnetic resonance venography
MS	multiple sclerosis
MSA	multiple system atrophy
MSH	melanocyte-stimulating hormone

MTHF	methyltetrahydrofolate
MTHFR	methylenetetrahydrofolate reductase
N	North
NA	noradrenaline (norepinephrine)
NAD	nicotinamide adenine dinucleotide
NADP	nicotinamide adenine dinucleotide phosphate
NAIM	non-vasculitic autoimmune inflammatory meningoencephalitis
NASBA	nucleic acid sequence-based amplification
NBIA	neurodegeneration with brain iron accumulation
NCL	neuronal ceroid lipofuscinosis
NICE	United Kingdom National Institute for Health and Clinical Excellence
NMDA	*N*-methyl-D-aspartate
$NMDA_R$	NMDA receptor
NMS	neuroleptic malignant syndrome
NPH	normal-pressure hydrocephalus
NPSLE	neuropsychiatric systemic lupus erythematosus
NR2	subunit 2 of the NMDA glutamate receptor
NSAID	non-steroidal anti-inflammatory drug
NSS	neurological "soft" signs
OCD	obsessive–compulsive disorder
OH	obesity hypoventilation
OMIM	Online Mendelian Inheritance in Man
OSA	obstructive sleep apnoea
OTC	ornithine transcarbamylase
$P(A \mid B)$	probability of A, given B
PACNS	primary angiitis of the central nervous system
$PaCO_2$	partial pressure (arterial) of carbon dioxide
PAN	polyarteritis nodosa
PANDAS	paediatric autoimmune neuropsychiatric disorders associated with streptococcal infections
PANSS	Positive and Negative Syndrome Scale
PaO_2	partial pressure (arterial) of oxygen
PBG	porphobilinogen
PCA	Purkinje-cell cytoplasmic antibody
PCO_2	partial pressure of carbon dioxide
PCP	phencyclidine; 1-(1-phenylcyclohexyl)piperidine
PCR	polymerase chain reaction
PD	Parkinson's disease
PDALS	Parkinsonism–dementia–amyotrophic lateral sclerosis complex
PE	pulmonary embolus
PET	positron emission tomography
PIP	syndrome of psychosis, intermittent hyponatraemia, and polydipsia
PKAN	pantothenate kinase-associated neurodegeneration
PKU	phenylketonuria
PLE	paraneoplastic limbic encephalitis
PLOSL	polycystic lipomembranous osteodysplasia with sclerosing leukoencephalopathy

PLP	pyridoxal 5′-phosphate
PMID	PubMed identification number (http://www.pubmed.com)
PML	progressive multifocal leukoencephalopathy
PNS	peripheral nervous system
PPI	proton pump inhibitor
PR3	proteinase 3
PRES	posterior reversible encephalopathy syndrome
PrP	prion protein
PSP	progressive supranuclear palsy
PTH	parathyroid hormone
PTHrP	parathyroid-hormone-related peptide
PTSD	post-traumatic stress disorder
q.v.	*quod vide* (which see)
REM	rapid eye movement
RhF	rheumatoid factor (antibodies against the Fc [fragment crystallizable] portion of immunoglobulin G)
RNA	ribonucleic acid
RNP	ribonuclear protein
Ro	not an abbreviation; a small nuclear RNA protein; also known as Sjögren's syndrome antigen A (SS-A)
rT3	reverse T3
s	second
S	South
SANS	Scale for the Assessment of Negative Symptoms
SAPS	Scale for the Assessment of Positive Symptoms
SCA	spinocerebellar ataxia
SCL-90-R	Symptom Checklist-90-Revised [questionnaire]
SD	standard deviation
SIADH	syndrome of inappropriate ADH secretion
SLE	systemic lupus erythematosus
Sm	Smith antigen, a ribonucleoprotein
SOD	superoxide dismutase
SPECT	single photon emission computed tomography
SPGR	spoiled gradient-recalled (images) (in MRI)
SpO_2	saturation percentage of oxygen in blood by pulse oximetry
SREAT	steroid-responsive encephalopathy associated with autoimmune thyroiditis
SS	Sjögren's syndrome
SSADH	succinic semialdehyde dehydrogenase
ssDNA	single-stranded DNA
SSPE	subacute sclerosing panencephalitis
SSRI	selective serotonin reuptake inhibitor
Sv	Sievert
T1	spin–lattice (T1) relaxation on MRI
T1WI	T1-weighted images
T2	spin–spin (T2) relaxation on MRI
T2WI	T2-weighted images

T3	3,5,3′-triiodothyronine
T4	thyroxine; levothyroxine
TFT	thyroid function tests (TSH ± T4/T3)
THC	Δ9-tetrahydrocannabinol
TIA	transient ischaemic attack
TLE	temporal lobe epilepsy
TMA	trimethoxyamphetamine
TNF	tumour necrosis factor
TPHA	*Treponema pallidum* haemagglutination assay
TPO	thyroid peroxidase
TRH	thyrotropin-releasing hormone
TSH	thyroid-stimulating hormone (a.k.a. thyrotropin)
TTP	thrombotic thrombocytopenic purpura
U	unit
U&E	urea and electrolytes (sodium, potassium, urea, creatinine)
UHR	Ultra High Risk (for the development of psychosis)
URL	uniform resource locator
USA	United States of America
UTI	urinary tract infection
VCFS	velocardiofacial syndrome
vCJD	variant Creutzfeldt–Jakob disease
VDRL	Venereal Disease Research Laboratory
VGKC	voltage-gated potassium channel
viz.	*videlicet* (that is to say)
VLCFA	very long chain fatty acids
VT	ventricular tachycardia
VWM	vanishing white matter leukoencephalopathy
VZV	varicella zoster virus
WBC	white blood cell (leukocyte)
WD	Witson's disease
WG	Wegener's granulomatosis
μM	micromolar (micromoles per litre; μmol/l)

Section 1

The causes of psychosis

Chapter 1 Introduction

We aim in this book to provide a review of all conditions known to cause psychotic symptoms, along with an approach to their diagnosis.

1.1 The definitions of psychosis

Psychosis originally meant any kind of disordered mental state [1], and subsequently a severe mental disorder involving loss of contact with reality [2, 3]. Nowadays it may be defined (1) narrowly as the presence of delusions and/or hallucinations without insight, or (2) more broadly to include delusions and/or hallucinations with insight into their hallucinatory nature, or (3) more broadly still to include disordered thought or speech, or (4) yet more broadly to include severe behavioural abnormalities including behavioural disorganization, gross excitement and overactivity, or psychomotor retardation and catatonia [4, 5]. To add to the ambiguity, some classificatory systems vary the definition of psychosis according to the condition being diagnosed. For example, in DSM-IV-TR, thought disorder, disorganized behaviour, and catatonia are considered "psychotic" for the purposes of the diagnosis of schizophrenia, but not for psychotic disorders caused by a general medical condition [5], and for substance-induced psychotic disorders, DSM-IV excludes hallucinations with insight and uses definition 1 [5]. The ICD-10 uses definition 4 [4].

Recent neurobiologically led views of psychosis emphasize the occurrence of abnormal salience phenomena (the perception of sensory input as having unusual significance) [6] and abnormal associative learning [7], particularly in early psychosis, along with imbalances in bottom-up versus top-down sensory processing and a disrupted sense of agency regarding representations produced by the brain [213, 1302, 1303]. There is growing appreciation that delusional and hallucinatory experiences represent a continuum [8], and that the position on this continuum is functionally important [9]; this dimensional perspective is not one taken by current formal categorical diagnostic systems [4, 5, 10].

1.2 Scope and threshold for inclusion

Here we seek to review the known causes of psychosis and the methods by which they may be diagnosed, and we cast the net broadly. These conditions include the primary psychiatric psychoses, such as schizophrenia – conditions in which psychosis arises without a clearly defined biological aetiology – but these are all diagnoses of exclusion [4, 5, 10]. The known secondary causes of psychosis are numerous, and we describe our methods for gathering them below (Chapter 2 ▶). (We use "secondary" in preference to "organic" when referring to conditions whose biological aetiology is clear, holding it self-evident that all psychoses, like all mental states, arise from biological processes. The exceptions are where we quote others' criteria or definitions directly.) Indeed, psychosis has been called the "fever" of severe mental illness: serious but non-specific [11]. Given that many causes are rare, there is a frequent clinical dilemma: to what extent should an individual patient be investigated for unusual secondary causes of psychosis before a primary psychiatric diagnosis is given? Here we seek to provide enough information to give clinicians useful templates for the causes of psychosis, since expert diagnosis rests in part on pattern recognition based on mental templates of diseases [12, 13]. We indicate cross-references to other chapters of the book with the symbol ▶.

1.3 Emphasis on non-psychiatric phenotype in diagnosing secondary psychosis, and on psychopathology in diagnosing primary psychosis

There may be clinical psychiatric features of the secondary causes of psychosis that are striking or characteristic. However, unless these are particularly unusual, an attempt has been made to avoid describing "typical" psychiatric presentations of these conditions, since there is no evidence that reliable exclusion of most of the medical and neurological conditions presented here can be made based on mental state, and there is very considerable overlap in phenomenology between primary and secondary psychoses [14–17]. This includes when Schneider's first-rank symptoms [18, 19] are present [16, 20]. As Asher noted [21], commenting on the variety of mental changes in hypothyroid psychosis, "No physician would attempt to diagnose lobar pneumonia or typhoid by the delirium they may produce, and likewise in myxoedema it is the disease which is the characteristic feature, not its mental manifestations." Similarly, a clinician's mind is most likely to pick a diagnosis that fits a disease pattern he or she is familiar with [12, 13], and in the situation where two diagnostic schemes compete – the hunt for secondary causes of psychosis and the descriptive classification when none is found [4, 5, 10] – the recognition of "typical" psychiatric patterns of disease may hinder the hunt for features in the history, examination, or initial investigations that give a clue to a secondary cause.

However, recognition of features that are not characteristic of primary psychiatric disease (such as clouding of consciousness, focal neurological abnormality, evidence of an inflammatory response, or systemic disease) is clearly an important clue to the presence of secondary psychosis. Likewise, atypical age of onset (over 35 years), lack of prior episodes of psychosis, lack of an expected family history, focal symptoms (e.g. unilateral hallucinations), non-auditory hallucinations, catatonia, coexisting deficit syndromes (delirium, dementia, aphasia, amnesia, etc.), and an atypical clinical course or atypical response to treatment should heighten suspicion [5, 16, 22]. If information from tests of known sensitivity and specificity is available, this can be combined with prior probability to estimate disease probability directly [23].

Despite our lack of emphasis on detailed psychopathology for the diagnosis of secondary psychosis, the pattern of psychiatric symptoms in psychosis is clearly salient and clinically relevant for management. We therefore refer occasionally to schizophrenia-like or schizophreniform psychosis, defined in relation to the symptoms of schizophrenia (even when the psychosis in question is secondary to another cause), and likewise to affective psychosis, for psychosis occurring in the context of significant mood disturbance such as depression or mania (again, regardless of aetiology).

1.4 Two useful approaches to the diagnosis of psychosis

A key point is this: there are two ways to think clinically about the causes of psychosis, and the psychiatrist must use both. (1) Medical causal thinking is exemplified as follows: "Hypothyroidism can cause virtually any psychotic symptom. Does this patient have features of hypothyroidism?" (2) Psychiatric classificatory thinking is exemplified as follows: "This patient's psychosis includes Schneider's first-rank symptoms, which suggest schizophrenia, but severe depression immediately preceded the psychosis, so this is probably depressive psychosis."

1.5 Arrangement of this book

This book is organized into two sections:

Section 1 covers the disorders that cause psychosis. It gives disease characteristics, the frequency of psychosis in patients with that disease where this is known, and key investigations or diagnostic criteria. Psychotogenic conditions are organized here in somewhat arbitrary categories, and there may be overlap (e.g. between neurodegenerative and metabolic diseases).

Section 2 deals with the diagnostic approach to a patient with psychosis, covering key points from the history, mental state examination, physical examination, and initial investigations, together with information regarding potential specialist investigations that may be required. It also provides decision trees for primary causes of psychosis and diagnostic criteria derived from the ICD-10 and DSM-IV classificatory systems.

For reasons of space, we will not discuss the treatment of specific causes of psychosis, and will assume referral to a clinician with expertise in the management of the condition where that is not a psychiatrist.

Chapter 2 Methods

The breadth of information covered did not allow for a systematic review of all possible primary sources (a PubMed search for 'psychosis OR delusion OR hallucination OR "thought disorder" OR schizophrenia' alone yielded in excess of 122 000 articles in December 2008). To obtain a list of known causes of psychosis, we conducted systematic reviews of the following:

- ICD-10 [4, 10], DSM-IV-TR [5], and the proposals for DSM-V [24];
- textbooks and reference works of medicine, neurology, psychiatry, and therapeutics [15, 20, 22, 25–33];
- a systematic review of physical illness in schizophrenia [34], a review of genetic disorders producing schizophreniform psychosis [35], and other reviews of "organic" or secondary psychosis [16, 17, 36];
- the Online Mendelian Inheritance in Man (OMIM) database [37]; we used the OMIM search terms '(psychosis) OR (psychoses) OR (psychot*) OR (hallucinat*) OR ("thought disorder") OR (delusion*) OR (schizophren*)' (search date 8 June 2008) and 'cataton*' (search date 24 October 2008), citations being given as MIM reference numbers;
- the US Agency for Toxic Substances and Disease Registry (http://www.atsdr.cdc.gov/);
- and the RxList drug information database [38]. We searched RxList using Google with the search term 'psychosis OR psychotic OR delusion OR delusions OR hallucination OR hallucinations OR catatonic OR catatonia OR "thought disorder" "drug information" site:www.rxlist.com more:for_health_professionals' and the 'filter = 0' option (search date 26 October 2008).

We also searched the PubMed (http://www.pubmed.com/) and Google (http://www.google.com/) databases non-systematically.

We then hand-reviewed each condition obtained, adding to the list of causes iteratively, and included all conditions where clear case reports or better evidence supported an association with psychosis. These methods have the potential for two kinds of error: the omission of psychotogenic conditions, and the inclusion of conditions whose causal role in producing psychosis is not established beyond all doubt. Because our aim was to be comprehensive, we tried to err on the side of over-inclusion rather than under-inclusion, but attempted to give brief details indicating the level of evidence for a causal role in psychosis, where this is known.

Chapter 3

Delirium

Delirium (Latin *delirare* = "out of the furrow") [39] is defined as a disturbance of consciousness that is accompanied by a change in cognition that cannot be better accounted for by a pre-existing or evolving dementia; the disturbance develops over a short period of time, usually hours to days, and tends to fluctuate during the course of the day; and there is evidence from the history, physical examination, or laboratory tests that the delirium is a direct physiological consequence of a general medical condition, substance intoxication or withdrawal, use of a medication, or toxin exposure, or a combination of these factors [5]. Attention is impaired. Cognitive impairments include memory, orientation, and language disturbances. Disturbance of the sleep–wake cycle is common, with variations in activity from lethargy or stupor to hyperactivity. There may be psychotic disturbances including hallucinations and delusions. Emotional disturbances may be evident, including anxiety, fear, depression, irritability, anger, euphoria, and apathy; these may lead to behavioural disturbances, including aggression. Generally, matters are worse at night and when stimulation and environmental cues are lacking [5]. Physical findings depend on the cause. Diagnosis is clinical, although the EEG typically shows generalized slowing [5]. Delirium is extremely common, occurring in 14–56% of elderly patients who are hospitalized; it is associated with high (22–76%) mortality. The underlying mechanisms are not known in detail and are likely multifactorial [40]. Psychosis in delirium has historically been referred to as "toxic psychosis".

3.1 Causes

Multiple causes are often identified. Age is a risk factor for delirium, and dementia is a very strong risk factor (raising the risk 2–3-fold) [40], likely reflecting decreased "brain reserve". Other strong risk factors include low serum albumin [41]. The direct causes of delirium are legion. Among the most common are infections, which can act via multiple mechanisms such as fever, hypoxia (pneumonia), hyperammonaemia (urinary tract infection with urease-secreting bacteria), direct CNS infection (meningoencephalitis), and septic encephalopathy, such as that induced by Gram-negative bacterial lipopolysaccharide [42, 43]. Some infections are historically famed for their ability to cause psychotic delirium, such as typhus (Chapter 8.1.9 ▶) [44]. Other causes include hypoglycaemia (Chapter 12.3 ▶), hyperthermia itself, hypotension, posterior reversible encephalopathy syndrome (Chapter 6.4 ▶) (associated with severe hypertension, chemotherapeutic and immunomodulatory drugs, and others), myocardial infarction, severe heart failure, alcohol or sedative withdrawal, drugs (including anticholinergics, sedatives, antiparkinsonian drugs, centrally acting antihypertensives, and corticosteroids; Chapter 15.1 ▶), a range of metabolic abnormalities

(Chapters 9, 10, 12 ▶), structural brain lesions and CVAs (Chapter 6.1, Chapter 6.7 ▶) including fat embolism and multiple cholesterol emboli, sensory deprivation and sleep deprivation (Chapters 16, 17 ▶), faecal impaction, and urinary retention. Postoperative states are also frequent causes, with rates of delirium of up to 42% following orthopaedic surgery, and a syndrome of "pump psychosis" described following surgery involving cardiac bypass (to which cerebral hypoperfusion and microemboli may both contribute), but with rates of 4.4% even following cataract surgery. Rare but obvious causes of delirium include altitude sickness [20, 22, 25, 40, 45–48].

A substantial number of other disorders that may cause delirium as well as isolated psychosis are discussed in the rest of this book.

3.2 Exclusion

Consistently normal cognitive status excludes delirium. Failing that, the combination of the following simple tests makes delirium much less likely as a cause of psychosis, *but does not exclude it*:

(1) Normal GCS (15).
(2) Normal general, cardiovascular, respiratory, neurological, and abdominal (including rectal) examination.
(3) Adequate cerebral oxygen delivery, to exclude hypoxic encephalopathy (Chapter 12.1 ▶). Assuming normal cerebrovascular circulation and excepting unusual poisoning syndromes (e.g. carbon monoxide, cyanide), this is simply indexed by:
  (a) Normal SpO_2 (94–98%, respiratory failure <90%) or, if available, normal PaO_2 (10.9–15.2 kPa at sea level, respiratory failure <8 kPa) [49]. If arterial blood gas measurement is undertaken, a normal $PaCO_2$ (4.6–6.1 kPa) also excludes hypercapnic encephalopathy (Chapter 12.2 ▶); a venous PCO_2 <6 kPa also eliminates the possibility of arterial hypercapnia [49].
  (b) Adequate blood pressure (mean arterial pressure ≥70 mmHg or systolic BP ≥90 mmHg). Absence of severe hypertension (i.e. systolic BP <220 mmHg and diastolic BP <120 mmHg) also excludes hypertensive encephalopathy (Chapter 6.4 ▶) [50].
  (c) Adequate haemoglobin (normal range: male 13–18 g/dl, female 11–17 g/dl; substantial anaemia <8 g/dl).
(4) Normal venous or capillary glucose (3.5–9 mM) (see Chapter 12.3 ▶).
(5) Normal sodium (135–145 mM), potassium (3.4–5.0 mM), and corrected calcium (2.1–2.5 mM) (see Chapter 12.5 ▶).
(6) Normal pH (arterial 7.35–7.45, more approximately indexed by venous pH, which is lower, or venous bicarbonate 22–30 mM) (see Chapter 12.2 ▶).
(7) Probable absence of neurotoxins induced by renal or hepatic failure:
  (a) normal urea (≤7.5 mM) and creatinine (normal <125 μM), but note that overt uraemic encephalopathy typically requires substantial renal failure (Chapter 12.4.1 ▶);
  (b) normal bilirubin (≤17 μM) and normal INR (≤1.5) (see Chapter 12.4.2 ▶).
(8) Normal body temperature (tympanic 35.4–37.8 °C) [51].

(9) Absence of significant inflammatory state:
  (a) normal CRP ($\leq$6 mg/l, with >100 mg/l being considerably elevated);
  (b) normal ESR (the normal range varies with age and sex but is $\leq$7 mm/h in men under 50 and $\leq$15 mm/h in women over 50, with >100 mm/h being very high);
  (c) normal leukocyte (4–11 $\times$ 10^9/l) and neutrophil (2–7.5 $\times$ 10^9/l) counts.

(10) Absence of evidence of poisoning (prescribed drug, recreational drug, or other) from the history, examination, and toxicological screening (see Chapter 15 ▶).

Chapter 4

Neurodevelopmental disorders and chromosomal abnormalities

4.1 Velocardiofacial syndrome

DiGeorge syndrome comprises abnormalities of the parathyroid glands, absence or hypoplasia of the thymus, and cardiac abnormalities such as pulmonary atresia and tetralogy of Fallot. Many patients have learning disability and/or schizophrenia. **Velocardiofacial syndrome** comprises similar cardiac abnormalities along with palatal abnormalities (from velopharyngeal incompetence to cleft palate, often with hypernasal speech), a characteristic facies (with hypoplastic nasal wings or alae nasae leading to a bulbous nasal tip and prominent nasal root, sometimes wide-spaced eyes [orbital hypertelorism], a long and narrow face with flat cheeks, narrow palpebral fissures, a small mouth, receding chin [micrognathia], and small cupped ears), long slender digits, and learning difficulty. There are further related clinical syndromes, representing a broad phenotype sometimes called **22q11 deletion** syndrome or **CATCH-22** (cardiac defects, abnormal facies, thymic hypoplasia, cleft palate, and hypocalcaemia), and all are caused by deletions or microdeletions at chromosome 22q11. These are usually sporadic but may be autosomal dominant [17, 26, 52–55] (MIM 188400). The phenotype is quite variable; for example, most but not all (74%) of those with the commonest deletion have congenital heart disease, whilst 27% have cleft palate [56]. The hypocalcaemia may be severe enough to become symptomatic, but it may also resolve in early childhood [57] (MIM 188400). It is the most common human deletion syndrome, occurring in at least 1:6000 births [58].

Velocardiofacial syndrome is one of the strongest known risk factors for psychosis and schizophrenia. In one survey of adults with VCFS, 30% had a psychotic disorder, with 24% fulfilling criteria for schizophrenia; 12% had non-psychotic major depression [59]. In another series, 64% met criteria for a bipolar spectrum disorder, some with psychosis, with a mean age of onset of 12 years [54]; see also [17]. Psychosis with 22q11.2 deletion may occur with only very minor physical features of VCFS [60], or with only learning disability [61]. Schizophrenic patients with at least one prominent physical manifestation of VCFS have a 22q11 deletion rate of 20%, while 60% of those with two features have the deletion [53]. The mean age of onset of psychosis for adults subsequently diagnosed with VCFS is 19.6 years (SD 4.6) [62]. In one series of patients with very early onset schizophrenia, 6.4% had VCFS [63].

The reason for the development of psychosis in VCFS is debated, but near to genes whose loss causes the physical abnormalities (MIM 188400) is the COMT gene [64]. The association between the well-described COMT rs165688 Val/Met polymorphism and schizophrenia is variable [65], but another polymorphism (rs165599) has emerged as a clear schizophrenia susceptibility gene in a genetically homogeneous group, if one of modest effect [66]; the allele frequency also varies with sex. In turn, the COMT effect may interact with sex and cannabis use [67, 68]. In patients with 22q11 deletion, COMT genotype in the intact chromosome predicts the development of psychosis, with the allele that has less activity for dopamine catabolism conferring higher risk [69, 70]. Other nearby genes on chromosome 22q are also of interest, such as the apolipoprotein L group proteins, which are upregulated in the prefrontal cortex in schizophrenia [71].

Diagnosis is cytogenetic, typically using fluorescent *in situ* hybridization (FISH) to identify the 22q11 deletion. Any adult with a congenital cardiovascular malformation and a psychiatric disorder should be evaluated for VCFS [72].

4.2 Trisomy 21

As discussed below, trisomy 21 (**Down's syndrome**) is a very strong risk factor for Alzheimer's disease (Chapter 5.1 ▶), which is a major cause of psychosis. Trisomy 21 is easily recognized morphologically, causing epicanthic folds, a flat nasal bridge, muscle hypotonia, a single palmar crease, white (Brushfield) spots on the iris, a small oral cavity and protruding tongue, a short neck, and joint laxity. Rates of congenital heart disease, intestinal malabsorption, infections, hypothyroidism, and autoimmunity are increased, among others [73] (MIM 190685). Seizures are also common, increasing in frequency with age, with simple or complex partial seizures being more common in adults [20].

4.3 Other chromosomal abnormalities

Familial **translocations involving chromosome 1q42** have been described that affect the DISC1 gene and are associated with schizophrenia and affective disorders [74–76]. **XXY (Klinefelter's syndrome)** and **XXX (triple X)** karyotypes are associated with increased rates of symptoms of schizophrenia, by a factor of about 3 [35, 77–80], and schizophrenia is potentially also associated with the much rarer **XXYY** [81] and (the usually mosaic) **trisomy 8** [82]. It is unclear whether XYY karyotype increases the risk [79, 83]. In children, karyotyping has been recommended as a routine investigation for psychosis [79].

Klinefelter's syndrome (affecting 1:500–1:1000 men) may be subtle physically, but affected men are hypogonadal, with eunuchoid body proportions, sparse or absent secondary sexual hair, decreased muscle mass, feminine distribution of adipose tissue, gynaecomastia, small testes and penis, diminished libido, and predisposition to osteoporosis [84, 85].

Triple X (karyotype 47, XXX) is the most common female chromosomal abnormality, occurring in 1:1000 female births. Most are mildly affected or asymptomatic. The phenotype may include tall stature, epicanthal folds, hypotonia, and clinodactyly (fingers angulated in the plane of the palm, typically curvature of the fifth finger towards the other fingers [86]). There may also be seizures, renal and genitourinary abnormalities, and ovarian failure. Attentional deficits and mood disorders occur with increased frequency. Magnetic resonance imaging may show white matter hyperintensities [87].

48, XXYY sex chromosome aneuploidy occurs in 1:17 000–50 000 male births. Affected males are often tall, with eunuchoid features (long legs, sparse body hair, small external genitalia), hypergonadotrophic hypogonadism, and gynaecomastia. There is increased risk of peripheral vascular disease. The typical IQ range is 60–80 [85].

Trisomy 8 mosaicism is a relatively common chromosomal abnormality (1:25 000–1:50 000 births) with a 5:1 male predilection. It is associated with approximately normal life expectancy, skeletal abnormalities (e.g. spinal deformity, hypoplastic patella, digit contractures), absence of the corpus callosum, developmental delay (particularly in language), a high and prominent forehead, broad-based nose, full lips, micrognathia, and a long slender trunk (sometimes misrecognized as Marfan's syndrome). About 25% have congenital heart defects, 10% have cleft palate, and about half have renal malformations. Affected children typically begin to walk on their toes [88].

Fragile X is a trinucleotide repeat expansion disease of the X chromosome that causes moderate to severe mental retardation and is associated with autism in males. It occurs in 1:2000 males. The male phenotype also includes macroorchidism and distinct facial features (long face, large ears, prominent jaw) (MIM 300624). Skeletal abnormalities (e.g. flat feet, joint laxity, scoliosis) are also common. Heterozygote female carriers have a milder phenotype and most have normal intelligence; premature ovarian failure is common. In addition to case reports of males with schizoaffective disorder and females with schizophrenia [89, 90], associations have been demonstrated between female carrier status and schizoaffective and affective disorders [89] and schizotypal features [91], though see [1328].

Turner's syndrome (45, X karyotype) occurs in ~1:2000 female live births. It causes short stature, gonadal dysgenesis, and distinct somatic features (cubitus valgus, widely spaced nipples, webbed neck), and usually presents in teenage years with failure to develop secondary sexual characteristics at puberty. There may be cardiovascular abnormalities (bicuspid aortic valve, coarctation of the aorta, hypertension), structural kidney abnormalities, and endocrine abnormalities (hypothyroidism, glucose intolerance, and the consequences of gonadal dysgenesis). This karyotype (usually in mosaic form, 45X/46XX) is over-represented in people with schizophrenia, occurring ~3 times more frequently than in the general population [33, 92, 93].

4.4 Agenesis of the corpus callosum

Partial or complete agenesis of the corpus callosum is associated with several heritable and acquired disorders of white matter development (including intrauterine infection and toxin exposure). Psychiatric disturbance in patients with agenesis of the corpus callosum is psychotic in at least half, and agenesis of the corpus callosum is increased in frequency in schizophrenia, and in other disorders associated with psychosis, including Andermann's syndrome, Apert's syndrome, and velocardiofacial syndrome (Chapter 4.1 ►) [94]. In contrast, callosal disorders acquired in adulthood (such as Marchiafava–Bignami disease, a necrotic myelinosis of the corpus callosum seen in alcoholics and suspected to be related to nutritional deficiency [95]) are not commonly associated with psychosis [94].

Agenesis of the corpus callosum with peripheral neuropathy, or **Andermann's syndrome**, is an autosomal recessive condition associated with mild facial dysmorphic features (e.g. hypertelorism, short nose, broad nasal root), learning disability, and seizures, in addition to those features obvious from its name. The neuropathy is sensorimotor (MIM 218000). Psychotic episodes may occur [96, 97].

Acrocephalosyndactyly (including **Apert's syndrome**, **Saethre–Chotzen syndrome**) is characterized by skull abnormalities including craniosynostosis, acrocephaly, syndactyly of the hands and feet, and CNS abnormalities (including ventriculomegaly or hydrocephalus, agenesis of the corpus callosum, and limbic abnormalities), and is sometimes associated with psychosis [98] (MIM 101400).

4.5 Prader–Willi syndrome

Prader–Willi syndrome is a genetically imprinted disorder, usually due to deletion of the paternal copy of genes on chromosome 15q, or maternal uniparental disomy, in which both copies of chromosome 15 come from the mother. Its birth incidence is 1:22 000. Affected babies are morphologically and behaviourally abnormal and become strikingly obese in childhood. The phenotype includes hypotonia at birth, difficulty feeding in early life followed by marked hyperphagia, mild learning disability, small hands and feet, dysmorphic face (narrow head, almond-shaped eyes, and a narrow or tented upper lip), hypogonadism, short stature, mood swings, obsessional behaviour, and skin-picking. About 75% have depigmentation relative to the familial background. Many have growth hormone deficiency, and a significant proportion develop hypertension and impaired glucose tolerance. Ventriculomegaly is universal. In early adulthood, ~28% develop a severe affective disorder with psychotic symptoms; this is more common with maternal uniparental disomy than with deletion (MIM 176270) [17, 20, 99–101].

4.6 Phenylketonuria

Phenylketonuria (PKU) is an autosomal recessive deficiency of phenylalananine hydroxylase, which catalyses the hydroxylation of phenylalanine to tyrosine. In PKU, hyperphenylalaninemia causes neurotoxicity and impaired postnatal cognitive development. It affects about 1 in 10 000 infants in European populations (MIM 261600). It is screened for by the neonatal Guthrie test. It causes mental retardation but psychosis is rare, though a few cases have been reported [94]. Untreated, it also causes a mouse-like odour, light pigmentation, abnormalities of gait and posture, epilepsy, and eczema (MIM 261600). In one study, stopping a phenylalanine-free diet did not provoke psychosis [102].

4.7 X-linked mental retardation syndromes

Mutations in the p21-activated kinase-3 (**PAK3**) gene cause a variable spectrum of mental retardation, sometimes borderline to mild, and can cause features of schizophrenia (MIM 300558). An X-linked condition in males comprising mental retardation, bipolar disorder with psychosis, parkinsonian features, pyramidal signs, and macroorchidism (**PPM-X**) has been described and mapped to Xq28 [103] (MIM 300055). **Coffin–Lowry syndrome** is characterized by skeletal malformations, growth retardation, hearing deficit, paroxysmal movement disorders, and cognitive impairment in affected males and some carrier females; it may be associated with depressive psychosis (MIM 303600). Other X-linked disorders causing psychosis with marfanoid features (e.g. tall stature, arachnodactyly, pectus excavatum/carinatum, high palate, flat feet) have been diagnosed as schizophrenia (MIM 300646, 300298) and **Lujan–Fryns syndrome** (characterized by marfanoid features with autistic spectrum disorder, shyness, and hyperactivity; MIM 309520) can also include psychotic symptoms including schizophreniform psychosis [104].

4.8 Other rare genetic conditions presenting early in life

Bardet–Biedl syndrome (formerly **Laurence–Moon–Biedl–Bardet syndrome**) is a disorder of cilia characterized primarily by retinitis pigmentosa, obesity, hypogonadism, polydactyly or syndactyly, and mental retardation, often with renal dysfunction (OMIM 209900). Schizophreniform psychosis has occasionally been reported [105, 106].

Darier–White disease (keratosis follicularis) is an autosomal dominant skin disorder with a frequency of 1:55 000, characterized by warty papules and plaques in seborrhoeic areas, and nail abnormalities. It has been associated with psychosis and affective disorders (MIM 124200).

Diabetes insipidus and mellitus with optic atrophy and deafness (DIDMOAD), or **Wolfram's syndrome**, is autosomal recessive (chromosome 4), though similar conditions also have autosomal dominant and mitochondrial inheritance patterns. Its prevalence is 1:770 000 live births. The defining characteristics are diabetes mellitus and bilateral optic atrophy. Diabetes insipidus, deafness, neurogenic bladder, and other neurological manifestations are frequent. Psychiatric illness occurs in most sufferers. Heterozygotes have an approximately 8-fold increase in the risk of hospitalization for psychiatric illness or suicide, and 16% of one series of homozygotes had paranoid delusions, auditory or visual hallucinations, or psychotic behaviour, with psychiatric manifestations in 60% overall [107, 108] (MIM 222300).

Lafora disease is progressive myoclonic epilepsy in which rapid and severe mental deterioration, often with psychosis, ensues rapidly after disease onset at the age of ~15 (MIM 254780). In addition to myoclonus and generalized seizures, occipital seizures (characterized by transient blindness and visual hallucinations) are often seen [33].

Landau–Kleffner syndrome is characterized by aphasia and epilepsy developing in young children (MIM 245570); occasionally, psychotic features have been observed [109].

Myoclonic dystonia is characterized by dystonia, often with tremor or jerky movements resembling myoclonus, and sometimes with a dramatic improvement in response to alcohol. The onset is usually in the first or second decade. It is associated with depression, and in some families with obsessive–compulsive disorder, substance abuse, anxiety disorders, and psychosis (MIM 159900).

Norrie disease is an X-linked recessive disorder characterized by early childhood blindness. Approximately 50% of patients show progressive mental disorder, often with psychosis; and about 33% develop sensorineural deafness in the second decade. Diagnosis is genetic (MIM 310600).

Oculocutaneous albinism has been associated with schizophrenia within families [35, 110, 111]. There is a defect of melanin synthesis, with decreased pigment in hair, skin, and eyes, and other ophthalmological abnormalities (MIM 203100). See also Prader–Willi syndrome (Chapter 4.5 ▶).

Sjögren–Larsson syndrome is a rare autosomal recessive deficiency of fatty aldehyde dehydrogenase, causing congenital ichthyosis (hyperkeratosis) with diplegia or quadriplegia, mental retardation, and frequently seizures (MIM 270200) [112]. There are case reports of associations with psychosis [113, 114].

Succinic semialdehyde dehydrogenase deficiency (gamma-hydroxybutyric aciduria). Deficiency of succinic semialdehyde dehydrogenase (SSADH) causes failure of normal GABA catabolism, urinary excretion of gamma-hydroxybutyric acid (GHB), and a variable neurological picture. This can include developmental delay, abnormal eye movements, hyporeflexia and hypotonia, seizures, EEG abnormalities, and psychosis including hallucinations. Developmental delay appears to be the most common presentation. The disease is probably autosomal recessive. Diagnosis is by urinary analysis, though as GHB is volatile, standard organic acid assays may miss the deficiency (MIM 271980). Psychosis is not a common feature [115], though hyperactivity and aggressiveness are common. Psychotic symptoms have been suggested to occur in 13% of adult patients [116]. (For exogenous GHB, see also recreational drugs, Chapter 15.3 ▶.)

4.9 Other rare neurodevelopmental disorders

Neurocutaneous melanosis is a developmental disorder of neuroectoderm characterized by large or multiple congenital melanocytic naevi and benign or malignant melanocytic tumours of the leptomeninges. Most patients exhibit neurological manifestations in childhood due to intracranial mass lesions or obstructed arachnoid villi, such as raised intracranial pressure, hydrocephalus, spinal cord compression, and seizures; there is often reduced intelligence. If there is a large naevus, it is typically central and posterior (head, neck, back, buttocks), often with smaller satellite naevi. Neurocutaneous melanosis has been associated with acute and chronic psychosis in adults [117, 118]. Diffuse contrast enhancement of the meninges is seen on imaging; the pre-contrast MRI may or may not show the melanin [47].

Chapter 5

Neurodegenerative disorders

5.1 Alzheimer's disease

Dementia is the commonest cause of psychosis in the elderly [119], and Alzheimer's disease (AlzD) is the most common cause of dementia, with a prevalence of >14% at age 65 and >40% at age 80. Pathologically, it is characterized by neurofibrillary tangles composed of tau protein, and neuritic (or senile) plaques of β-amyloid protein. Cortical atrophy is progressive and is particularly marked in the medial temporal lobe, disconnecting the hippocampus from its major afferent and efferent pathways. More than 90% of cases are sporadic and occur after the age of 60; <10% of cases are familial, of which some forms may occur as early as the third decade. Aside from age, the strongest risk factor is apolipoprotein E (ApoE) ε4 genotype: the lifetime risk of AlzD is 9% with no ApoE ε4 alleles, 29% with one copy, and 83% with two. Other risk factors (such as head injury) are less clearly established. The amyloid component, β-amyloid protein, is a cleavage product of amyloid precursor protein (APP), encoded on chromosome 21, and some familial forms of AlzD are associated with mutations in the APP gene (MIM 104300). Trisomy 21 is also a strong risk factor for AlzD, with nearly all patients over 40 having histological evidence of AlzD [28, 120].

AlzD typically presents with amnesia, sometimes monosymptomatically as mild cognitive impairment. It evolves to a cortical dementia syndrome. Definite diagnosis is by histology. Probable diagnosis is defined by progressive dementia in at least two cognitive domains, including memory, in the absence of an alternative cause and without atypical features such as focal sensorimotor abnormalities, sudden onset, or seizures or gait disorder early in the course. Early anosmia/hyposmia is common (85–90%) [28]. Advanced disease may include insomnia, incontinence, verbal or physical outbursts, sexual disorders, weight loss, increased muscle tone, abnormal gait, and seizures. Depression commonly complicates AlzD, as do illusions, but psychosis may also occur or be the presenting feature, most commonly with paranoid delusions and delusions of theft but sometimes with complex hallucinations; misidentification is also common [28, 33]. Psychosis occurs in 41% of those with AlzD (median figure from a series of studies) with delusions in 36% and hallucinations in 18% (visual 19%, auditory 9%, again as medians), with increasing incidence in the first 3 years of observation and then a plateau [121]. Susceptibility genes for psychosis in AlzD have been described, including COMT and serotonin transporter promoter polymorphisms [122, 123], and patients with AlzD who develop psychosis are more likely to be female and older with more severe and long-standing disease [124]. The presence of psychosis in AlzD is associated with greater cognitive impairment and more rapid decline [15].

Diagnosis is by clinical and cognitive assessment and exclusion of other causes. Magnetic resonance imaging is helpful, particularly in excluding vascular dementia, but may also show medial temporal or generalized atrophy in AlzD. Functional neuroimaging (e.g. PET, SPECT) may show bilateral temporoparietal and posterior cingulate hypometabolism and hypoperfusion, but is not usually necessary for diagnosis [28]. Formal clinical diagnostic criteria exist [33, 125].

Early-onset Alzheimer's disease is associated with **presenilin-1** mutations, whose phenotype also includes spastic paraparesis, myoclonus, parkinsonism, cerebellar degeneration, and multiple white matter lesions on MRI. Psychosis in this context, particularly with a family history, should prompt consideration of genetic testing (MIM 104311, 607822). **Presenilin-2** mutations are also a cause of early-onset AlzD, sometimes with parkinsonism (MIM 600759). Presenilin mutations may be associated with dilated cardiomyopathy (MIM 600759). AlzD with **APP gene mutations** may also be associated with multiple white-matter infarcts (MIM 104300).

5.2 Vascular dementia

Vascular dementia is discussed with cerebrovascular disease (Chapter 6.1 ▶).

5.3 Parkinson's disease and "Parkinson's plus" syndromes

Parkinson's disease (PD) is caused by loss of dopaminergic neurons from the substantia nigra. It has a prevalence of 1% in the over-60s, with a male:female ratio of 1.5:1 [126]. Psychosis occurs in 20–40% of patients with PD, predominantly but not exclusively as a drug side effect. Hallucinations (with illusions) are the most common psychotic symptom and are usually visual [15, 17, 33, 127–130]. In one 6-year study, 62% of patients had hallucinations by the end of the study [20, 131]. Depression is very common in PD but it is not clear that psychosis and depression co-occur more often than expected by chance [132]. Dopaminergic drugs (along with MAO and COMT inhibitors) are a common aggravating or precipitating factor, as are anticholinergics. Independent risk factors for psychosis include old age, prolonged disease duration and severity, cognitive impairment, depression, and sleep disorders [33, 127, 128]. Before levodopa was introduced, visual hallucinations were also reported in PD, but at a lower frequency of about 5% [127].

The cardinal features of PD are resting tremor, rigidity, bradykinesia, and postural instability (the last occurring much later). The onset is usually asymmetric. Diagnosis is clinical, based on two of the three early cardinal signs. Magnetic resonance imaging may be useful to exclude disorders such as multiple infarcts (Chapter 6.1 ▶), hydrocephalus (Chapter 6.6, Chapter 6.7 ▶), or Wilson's disease (Chapter 10.4 ▶), and PET/SPECT imaging of the dopamine transporter (DAT) may be useful where there is diagnostic doubt [126]. Hyposmia/anosmia occur early [28].

There is clinical overlap with the "Parkinson's plus" syndromes, in which parkinsonism occurs together with other neurological features such as dementia, early postural instability, psychosis, eye signs, pyramidal tract signs, cerebellar dysfunction, and autonomic dysfunction (e.g. postural hypotension, incontinence). Most are progressive and fatal. These syndromes include **multiple system atrophy** (multisystem atrophy, MSA; with a mix of autonomic and urinary dysfunction, cerebellar dysfunction, and corticospinal dysfunction), **progressive supranuclear palsy** (PSP; see below), **parkinsonism–dementia–amyotrophic**

lateral sclerosis complex (PDALS), **corticobasal ganglionic degeneration** (CBGD), and **dementia with Lewy bodies** (DLB; see below, Chapter 5.4 ▶) [133–135].

Of these, PSP and DLB involve prominent neuropsychiatric symptoms, and are sometimes initially misdiagnosed as primary psychiatric disease [136]. **PSP** is a tau protein disorder characterized by bradykinesia, rigidity, dysarthria, dysphagia, and dementia (like idiopathic PD), but tremor is rare, severe postural instability is usual, and there is supranuclear ophthalmoplegia often causing vertical gaze paralysis. There may be midbrain atrophy with dilation of the third ventricle and interpeduncular cistern [47]. Schizophreniform psychosis may appear early and in one series psychosis occurred in 18% [33]. Dementia with Lewy bodies is described below.

Some forms of Parkinson's disease are familial (e.g. MIM 168601), and very rarely, forms of parkinsonism with dementia and psychosis may present in childhood (e.g. **Kufor–Rakeb syndrome**; MIM 606693). See also FTDP17 (Chapter 5.5 ▶).

5.4 Dementia with Lewy bodies

In DLB, also known as diffuse Lewy body disease, dementia and psychotic symptoms are prominent. Both PD and DLB are alpha-synucleinopathies characterized by Lewy bodies. Hallucinations are prominent in DLB; the presence of hallucinations in unmedicated patients with parkinsonism makes DLB the likelier diagnosis [127]. Auditory hallucinations and delusions occur but are less common than visual hallucinations, which are often complex, well formed, and without insight [20]. The major clinical criteria for DLB are (1) visual hallucinations, (2) fluctuating cognition, and (3) spontaneous motor features of parkinsonism. One of these criteria is required to diagnose possible DLB, and two are needed for a diagnosis of probable DLB [137, 138]. The minor criteria include repeated falls, syncope, transient loss of consciousness, neuroleptic sensitivity, systematized delusions (which are common), and hallucinations in other modalities (auditory, olfactory, tactile). Clinical features also include apathy, anxiety, autonomic dysfunction, and REM sleep disorders [138]. Hallucinations and delusions occurring early in the course of a dementia syndrome strongly suggest DLB [33]. The distinction between DLB and dementia occurring in Parkinson's disease (**Parkinson's disease dementia**, which occurs in 15–30% of patients with Parkinson's disease) is made based on an arbitrary cut-off: onset of dementia within 12 months of parkinsonism qualifies as DLB, and if the parkinsonism predates the dementia by more than this, the disease is termed Parkinson's disease dementia [126, 138].

5.5 Asymmetric cortical degeneration syndromes, including frontotemporal dementia and Pick's disease

A further group of dementias produce asymmetric cortical degeneration. The traditional clinical classification was in four main categories: progressive aphasia, progressive perceptual–motor syndromes (including posterior cortical atrophy), progressive frontal/frontotemporal dementia syndromes, and progressive bitemporal syndromes. Since then, histological classification has blurred the boundaries. Many are "tauopathies", associated with cytoskeletal abnormalities related to the microtubule-associated protein tau. The two main histological types are prominent microvacuolar change without specific histological features (frontal lobe degeneration type) and **Pick's disease**; the latter is lobar atrophy, typically involving frontal and anterior temporal lobes, with severe astrocytic gliosis, usually with swollen chromatolytic neurons and intraneuronal inclusions (Pick bodies) [28, 139].

There are three prototypical syndromes of **frontotemporal lobar degeneration (FTLD)**. The first is **frontotemporal dementia (FTD)**, affecting primarily the frontal lobes. Frontotemporal dementia is characterized by personality change, with inertia and loss of volition (abulia) or social disinhibition and distractibility, together with emotional blunting, reduced speech, and loss of insight, with relatively preserved memory. There are "dysexecutive" cognitive deficits, i.e. deficits in attention, planning, abstraction, and problem solving. The other two FTLD syndromes are progressive non-fluent aphasia (asymmetrically affecting the left frontotemporal lobes, and causing effortful and error-ridden speech production with relatively preserved comprehension) and semantic dementia (bilateral temporal degeneration, causing a severe impairment in naming and word comprehension with associative agnosia, the inability to recognize the meaning of visual stimuli) [139].

The diagnostic criteria for FTD [139] are as follows. The *clinical profile* is of character change and disordered social conduct, dominating initially and throughout the disease course, with intact or relatively well preserved perception, spatial skills, praxis, and memory. The *core diagnostic features*, all of which are required, are: (A) insidious onset and gradual progression; (B) early decline in social interpersonal conduct; (C) early impairment in regulation of personal conduct; (D) early emotional blunting; and (E) early loss of insight. *Supportive diagnostic features*, which are not required but which add weight to the diagnosis, are a behavioural disorder (decline in personal hygiene and grooming, mental rigidity and inflexibility, distractibility and impersistence, hyperorality and dietary changes, perseveration and stereotyped behaviour, utilization behaviour); speech and language changes (altered speech output either as aspontaneity and economy of speech or pressure of speech, stereotypy of speech, echolalia, perseveration, mutism); physical signs (primitive reflexes, incontinence, akathisia/rigidity/tremor, low and labile blood pressure); and supportive findings from investigations (neuropsychological testing showing significant impairment on frontal lobe tests in the absence of severe amnesia, aphasia, or perceptuospatial disorder; a normal EEG despite clinically evident dementia; structural and/or functional brain imaging showing a predominantly frontal and/or anterior temporal abnormality).

Psychosis has been described in FTD, but is significantly less common than in AlzD [140, 141], with frequencies of 13–14% in some series [142]. Frontotemporal dementia can present in the young (aged 19–64) with schizophrenia-like psychosis as its early stage; psychosis is the presenting problem in approximately 6% [142, 143].

Diagnosis of the asymmetric cortical degeneration syndromes is usually clinical and neuropsychological, supported by structural ± functional brain imaging [28, 139]. However, identified mutations in the tau gene on chromosome 17 can cause **FTD with parkinsonism (FTDP17)** [144], and other mutations are also associated with FTD (MIM 600274). In some such families, schizophrenia-like psychosis may be the presenting feature in the fifth or sixth decade, followed later by severe dementia [145]. Frontotemporal dementia may associate with ALS/MND (Chapter 5.6 ▶) [142].

Subcortical gliosis (Neumann type) is a rare autosomal dominant early dementia that resembles Pick's disease clinically but is characterized by cortical fibrillary astrocytosis; it may present with psychotic depression (MIM 221820).

5.6 Motor neuron disease

Motor neuron disease (MND, or **amyotrophic lateral sclerosis**, ALS) is characterized by loss of spinal anterior horn α-motor neurons ("lower motor neurons") and primary motor cortex pyramidal cells ("upper motor neurons"). It presents classically with a mixture of upper motor neuron signs (weakness, increased tone, hyperreflexia) and lower motor neuron signs (weakness, flaccidity, hyporeflexia, atrophy, fasciculation) accordingly. Amyotrophic lateral sclerosis may be associated with frontotemporal dementia (Chapter 5.5 ▶), with or without parkinsonism, as the **ALS–dementia complex**, though this is rare [28, 33]. Amyotrophic lateral sclerosis, dementia, and psychosis have been described in a familial form [146]. Thalamic dementia (Chapter 5.15 ▶) with ALS exhibiting early psychotic symptoms has also been reported. Rates of ALS are increased in relatives of Ashkenazi Jewish schizophrenics [147]. Amyotrophic lateral sclerosis and psychosis are both features of hexosaminidase deficiency (Chapter 10.5.3 ▶) [148].

A further link to psychosis has been suggested through vulnerability to oxidative stress. Amyotrophic lateral sclerosis can be caused by mutations in genes encoding the cytoplasmic copper/zinc superoxide dismutase (SOD1) [28], while mitochondrial superoxide dismutase (SOD2) polymorphisms may be associated with vulnerability to methamphetamine psychosis (Chapter 15.3 ▶) [149] and schizophrenia (Chapter 21.1 ▶) [150]. Both SOD1 and SOD2 levels are altered in the frontal cortex of treated schizophrenics [151], and erythrocyte SOD activity and (more consistently) other biomarkers of mitochondrial oxidative phosphorylation and lipid peroxidation are altered in drug-naïve patients with first-episode psychosis [151, 152].

5.7 Huntington's disease

Huntington's disease (HD) is an autosomal dominant inherited disorder characterized by a trinucleotide cytosine–adenine–guanine (CAG) repeat expansion in the HD gene and loss of striatal GABAergic medium spiny neurons [153]. Clinically it is a progressive movement disorder with prominent psychiatric symptoms and cognitive dysfunction leading to dementia. Its prevalence is usually given as approximately 5 per 100 000 [154], though recently it has been suggested that this is an underestimate, with the true frequency being at least 12.4 per 100 000 [155]. Psychosis is variously estimated to occur in 3–25% of patients with Huntington's disease [17, 153, 156–159]; this is fewer than for obsessive-compulsive symptoms (10–52%) and mood changes, which are predominantly of depressed mood (33–69%, with major depression in 29% in one study), anxiety (34–61%), irritability (38–73%), and apathy (33–76%) [156]. Psychosis is more frequently characterised by delusions, typically persecutory, than by hallucinations [20]. Usually, psychosis occurs after the onset of chorea, but individuals and families have been described in which psychosis predated chorea [157, 160, 161]. There is no association between sex or CAG trinucleotide repeat number and psychiatric phenotype [162], but a family history of psychosis in HD is a predictor of psychosis and a higher number of CAG repeats is associated with earlier psychosis as well as earlier neurological symptoms [163]. Huntington's disease can present in juveniles with psychosis (MIM 143100).

The most common onset of HD is with involuntary movements or rigidity. The next most common primary presentation is with mental state changes, most commonly irritability, low mood, impulsivity, and antisocial behaviour. Family history is key to diagnosis. Early chorea often appears as facial twitching, or twitching and writhing of the extremities. There may be depression and impaired cognitive ability [154]. Olfactory impairment is also an early feature (e.g. [164–166]). Computerized tomography or MRI may show evidence of caudate atrophy. Definitive diagnosis is genetic [154], though a few cases may be due to mutations other than in the usual gene (MIM 603218).

For non-acute chorea with psychosis, see also DRPLA (Chapter 5.8 ▶), SCA type 17 (Chapter 5.9 ▶), neuroacanthocytosis (Chapter 5.10 ▶), BGC (Chapter 5.11 ▶), PKAN (Chapter 5.12 ▶), neuroferritinopathy (Chapter 5.13 ▶), WD (Chapter 10.4 ▶), SLE (Chapter 13.1.1 ▶).

5.8 Dentatorubropallidoluysian atrophy

Dentatorubropallidoluysian atrophy (DRPLA) is an autosomal dominant trinucleotide repeat expansion disease that resembles Huntington's disease, and causes a variable combination of movement disorders (chorea, myoclonus, dystonia, or parkinsonism), cerebellar ataxia, epilepsy, psychosis, and dementia [167, 168]. Psychosis may be the presenting feature [20]. It is most common in Japan, but rare even there (prevalence 2–4 per million) and very rare elsewhere, though it has been reported in Europe [169]. **Haw River syndrome** is the equivalent condition observed in the USA [170]. The term "Luysian body" or "body of Luys" is a synonym for the subthalamic nucleus [171]. EEG slowing is seen in ~80% of patients, with epileptiform patterns and photoparoxysmal responses also being common. Magnetic resonance imaging may show atrophy of the superior cerebellar peduncles and high-intensity lesions in the pallidum on T2-weighted imaging (T2WI) [28]. Diagnosis is genetic [172].

5.9 Spinocerebellar ataxia

The spinocerebellar ataxias (SCA) are a group of autosomal dominant neurodegenerative diseases characterized by ataxia with various combinations of pyramidal, extrapyramidal, and sensory signs [173]. Diagnosis is usually genetic. Many are known to be trinucleotide repeat expansion diseases, and the trinucleotide repeat expansion at 13q21 that is responsible for SCA type 8 may be over-represented in patients with major psychosis diagnosed as having bipolar affective disorder or schizophrenia [174, 175]. Delusions have been seen in SCA type 3 (MIM 109150). Spinocerebellar ataxia type 17, which differs from all the others in that its phenotype and inheritance pattern resembles HD, can also cause psychiatric features (in 75% in one series, including personality change, depression, delusions, and hallucinations; MIM 607136). **Friedreich's ataxia**, usually classified separately, is an autosomal recessive form of spinocerebellar ataxia in which psychosis may develop in late stages [17, 25, 29, 33, 176].

5.10 Neuroacanthocytosis

Neuroacanthocytosis is an umbrella term for a rare group of disorders characterized by acanthocytosis (red blood cells having a spiky or thorny appearance) and neurological dysfunction, which can include movement disorders (including chorea, parkinsonism, and ataxia), personality change, cognitive deterioration, seizures (temporal lobe epilepsy may be the presenting feature), peripheral neuropathy, myopathy, psychosis, OCD, Tourette's syndrome, and depression [177–186]. Self-mutilating lip and tongue biting is uncommon but distinctive [20]. Psychiatric features are common and schizophrenia-like psychosis may be the presenting feature. The clinical picture is very like HD (Chapter 5.7 ▶), except early dementia is not as common.

The defect is likely in cell membrane regulation. It can be autosomal recessive, autosomal dominant, or X-linked. The most common form is the autosomal recessive form (**autosomal recessive chorea–acanthocytosis, ChAc**), in which basal ganglia degeneration is a consistent feature (particularly in the caudate and putamen, and to a lesser extent in the globus pallidus and substantia nigra). The onset of neurological symptoms is normally in the patient's 20s. The X-linked form, **McLeod syndrome**, is also associated with cardiomyopathy and haemolytic anaemia. The most typical presentation is with abnormal orofacial movements and gait instability in young adulthood. Other forms of neuroacanthocytosis include **Huntington's disease-like 2 (HDL2)** and pantothenate kinase-associated neurodegeneration (PKAN; Chapter 5.12 ▶).

Creatinine (phospho)kinase levels are usually raised. Acanthocytosis is common but not universal, and may come and go, and may increase with time. Acanthocytosis >3% is abnormal and the level is usually 10–30% in ChAc and McLeod syndrome (the differential includes liver disease, splenectomy, and haemolytic anaemia). Acanthocytes are less frequent in HDL2 (occurring in about 10% of patients, with normal CK levels) and PKAN. Magnetic resonance imaging often shows caudate atrophy but the "eye of the tiger" sign is seen in PKAN. Genetic testing is possible for some forms of neuroacanthocytosis [33, 177, 178, 183, 184, 186, 187] (MIM 200150).

Some forms of acanthocytosis are lipoprotein disorders (e.g. abetalipoproteinaemia) and their neurological features are chiefly spinocerebellar [33, 187]; these days, the term neuroacanthocytosis is reserved for those disorders affecting the basal ganglia [186].

5.11 Basal ganglia calcification

Idiopathic basal ganglia calcification (BGC) may be sporadic or familial. It is sometimes termed **Fahr's disease** (MIM 213600) or **bilateral striopallidodentate calcinosis** [33]. It affects principally the globus pallidus. Neurological features include parkinsonism or choreoathetosis, subcortical dementia, and others including paralysis, stroke-like events, headache, vertigo, seizures, and syncope [153]. Basal ganglia calcification is common (0.93% of head CT scans) [153]. It may be asymptomatic, though mild neuropsychological abnormalities are detectable in patients with BGC as a group [188]. About 40% of patients with symptomatic BGC present with psychiatric features, including schizophreniform psychosis, cognitive change, and mood disorders [153, 159] (MIM 213600). It appears that disease with early adult onset (aged 20–40) is more likely to present with psychosis, whereas late-onset disease is more likely to present with dementia and a movement disorder [153, 189], but even in the elderly, BGC is associated with psychotic symptoms [190]. Basal ganglia calcification before the age of 50 requires further investigation [153].

Basal ganglia calcification may also be due to pseudohypoparathyroidism (insensitivity to PTH) and chronic hypoparathyroidism (Chapter 9.5 ▶) [191, 192], and is associated with infections including neuropsychiatric brucellosis (Chapter 8.1.7 ▶) [193]. It is also associated with trisomy 21 (Chapter 4.2 ▶), trisomy 5, mitochondrial encephalopathies (Chapter 10.6 ▶), CNS lupus (Chapter 13.1.1 ▶), tuberous sclerosis (Chapter 6.10 ▶), early-onset Alzheimer's disease (Chapter 5.1 ▶), motor neuron disease (Chapter 5.6 ▶), myotonic muscular dystrophy, anticonvulsants [153], and a number of other conditions [17, 33].

5.12 Pantothenate kinase-associated neurodegeneration

Pantothenate kinase-associated neurodegeneration (PKAN; **Hallervorden–Spatz disease; neurodegeneration with brain iron accumulation 1, NBIA1**) is a rare disorder characterized by abnormal iron accumulation in the globus pallidus and substantia nigra pars reticulata. It may be sporadic or familial with autosomal recessive inheritance, due to mutation in the pantothenate kinase-2 gene (MIM 234200). It is characterized by progressive dementia, extrapyramidal signs (e.g. rigidity, dystonia, choreoathetosis), and corticospinal signs (e.g. spasticity, hyperreflexia). Seizures and retinitis pigmentosa may also be observed [194]. Ataxia is rare [195]. Acanthocytosis (Chapter 5.10 ▶) occurs in ≥8% of those with classic disease [196]. It may present with depression [197] and may cause florid psychosis [198] though this is uncommon [20]. Disease onset is usually in adolescence and patients typically die after 10–12 years [199]. Magnetic resonance imaging typically shows bilateral T2WI hyperintensity with surrounding hypointensity in the globus pallidus ("eye of the tiger" sign).

A similar iron-accumulating disease, **NBIA2**, can also result from mutations in the PLA2G6 phospholipase A2 gene (MIM 610217) [33].

5.13 Neuroferritinopathy

Neuroferritinopathy is a rare autosomal dominant disorder characterized by an adult-onset progressive movement disorder (chorea or dystonia) with evidence of excess brain iron accumulation on MRI, particularly in the basal ganglia (and in advanced cases, cystic brain degeneration). The imaging findings may be very similar to those in PKAN (Chapter 5.12 ▶). The mean age of onset is 40 years, with a range from early teenage years to the sixth decade. There may be marked asymmetry of the movement disorder. Cognitive impairment may occur and progress, as can dysphagia, but cognitive impairment is less common than in PKAN. Serum ferritin may be low or normal (more commonly low in males). Psychotic episodes are not a typical feature but have been reported, including early in the disease course, with one individual presenting with paranoid psychosis. The differential diagnosis of basal ganglia abnormalities on MRI also includes mitochondrial disease (Chapter 10.6 ▶) [200, 201].

5.14 Argyrophilic grain disease

Argyrophilic grains, named for their strong uptake of silver-based stains, accumulate progressively with age in many cognitively normal elderly people (~30% of those aged 70–80), but argyrophilic grain disease (AGD) has also been suggested to be a primary cause of up to 5% of dementia [202]. Argyrophilic grain disease is a tauopathy. Argyrophilic grains accumulate in the medial temporal lobe (hippocampus, subiculum, entorhinal and adjacent cortex, amygdala), orbitofrontal cortex, insula, and hypothalamus; in later stages they may be more widespread. Their importance is debated since patients with histological AGD and clinically apparent dementia commonly have other co-occurrent neuropathology, including AlzD, Pick's disease, PSP, CBGD, alpha-synucleinopathies (DLB, PD dementia, MSA), and sometimes CJD. The presence of AGD appears to act as an additive factor, worsening the effects of a given load of AlzD pathology [202].

Argyrophilic grain disease may begin with mild amnestic cognitive impairment, progressing to cognitive decline with loss of episodic memory and overt dementia. Personality change and behavioural disturbance (including aggression) is common, as are mood disturbances including dysphoria and apathy. Delusions are not infrequent and hallucinations may occur. Sometimes AGD presents with frontotemporal dementia, but this is rare [202].

Argyrophilic grain disease is currently a histological diagnosis; there are no clinical characteristics or non-histological tests to distinguish it from AlzD [202].

5.15 Thalamic degeneration

Selective thalamic degeneration (**thalamic dementia**) in the absence of a known cause (such as CJD) is very rare. It can begin at any age from adolescence onwards, and have subacute or very gradual onset. It is characterized clinically by dementia in all cases, variably accompanied by apathy, somnolence, emaciation, or myoclonus. In one case the dementia was preceded by psychotic features and subsequently accompanied by motor neuron disease; pathologically, the thalamic degeneration was most marked in the mediodorsal nucleus [20, 203].

5.16 Other rare genetic conditions presenting late in life

Familial British/Danish dementia (psychosis heredopathia) is a syndrome caused by mutations of the ITM2B gene on chromosome 13. It is characterized by early cataracts (before the age of 30), followed by hearing loss 10–20 years later, cerebellar ataxia in the fifth decade, and paranoid psychosis and dementia 10 years later. It is a severe, diffuse encephalopathy with amyloid angiopathy and amyloid deposition (MIM 117300, 176500). Related hereditary forms of cerebral amyloid angiopathy causing recurrent cerebral haemorrhage (MIM 605714) have not been associated directly with psychosis. Another, as yet unknown, disorder can cause congenital cataract and psychosis and dementia with onset in the fifth decade (MIM 607674).

Hereditary endotheliopathy with retinopathy, nephropathy, and stroke (HERNS) is a syndrome with a clinical presentation resembling CADASIL (Chapter 6.1 ▶). It was described in a Chinese–American family and has autosomal dominant inheritance. There was universal retinopathy, frequent migraine, stroke-like episodes and dementia, with variable renal insufficiency and proteinuria, subcortical lesions, and psychiatric disturbance (in which paranoia was mentioned by the authors but psychosis has not been clearly characterized) [204]. It appears to be due to a mutation in the TREX1 exonuclease gene involved in DNA repair (MIM 606609).

Leptomeningeal amyloidosis is a rare form of autosomal dominant amyloidosis limited to the CNS and eyes, causing dementia, seizures, strokes, visual deterioration, and coma. Symptoms begin in adulthood and can include hallucinations (MIM 105210).

Pelizaeus–Merzbacher disease is a sudanophilic leukodystrophy. There is an infantile X-linked recessive form that is a hypomyelinative leukodystrophy characterized by nystagmus, spastic quadriplegia, ataxia, and developmental delay (MIM 312080) [28]. However, there is also a late-onset autosomal dominant form (adult-onset autosomal dominant demyelinating leukodystrophy, MIM 169500), in which neurological dysfunction begins in the fourth or fifth decade. Psychosis can be among the presenting features [205]. Neurological features include cerebellar dysfunction, pyramidal signs, autonomic dysfunction, and dementia. Imaging studies show progressive cortical and subcortical white matter abnormalities (MIM 169500).

Polycystic lipomembranous osteodysplasia with sclerosing leukoencephalopathy (PLOSL), also called **Nasu–Hakola disease, brain–bone–fat disease**, or **membranous lipodystrophy**, is an autosomal recessive condition characterized by dementia, sometimes with psychosis progressing to dementia, and bone cysts in the wrists and ankles (sometimes with associated fractures), with onset in the third decade (MIM 221770, 604142) [17, 94].

Chapter 6

Focal neurological disease

6.1 Cerebrovascular disease

Vascular dementia is the second most common cause of dementia in Europe and the USA [206]. Cognitive impairment may be caused by infarcts, haemorrhage, and diffuse hypoxia and ischaemia. The two major subtypes of vascular dementia are those with multiple large-artery territory infarcts, with stepwise progression, and small-vessel cerebrovascular disease caused by arteriosclerosis or by cerebral amyloid angiopathy [28]. Small-vessel disease produces two major syndromes, lacunar disease and Binswanger's disease (a.k.a. subcortical leukoencephalopathy; subacute arteriosclerotic encephalopathy). **Lacunar infarcts** are due to small-vessel occlusion and produce small parenchymal cavities, typically in the internal capsule, deep grey nuclei, and white matter. **Binswanger's disease** is associated with fibrohyalinosis of small arteries and fibrinoid necrosis of larger vessels, and produces diffuse white-matter disease [28, 206]. A mixture of vascular dementia and Alzheimer's disease commonly exists.

In one study, the one-month prevalence of psychosis in vascular dementia was 46% (delusions 36%, delusional misidentification 23%, visual hallucinations 22%, and auditory hallucinations 8%) [207]; see also [17].

Diagnosis is clinical and by neuroimaging, ideally MRI [208]; research diagnostic criteria also exist [209]. If embolic infarcts are suspected, a cause should be sought.

Psychosis after isolated **CVA (ischaemic stroke, intracerebral haemorrhagic stroke, subarachnoid haemorrhage)** is rarer [15, 17]. One study found an in-hospital incidence of delusional ideation in 4% of patients admitted for strokes, with onset within a few days and an average duration of 13 days; all had right hemisphere strokes, mostly posterior temporoparietal [210]. Frontal lobe syndrome with psychosis has been described following pontomesencephalic infarction [211]. Complex visual hallucinations have long been known to follow some rostral brainstem lesions (**peduncular hallucinosis**), most commonly in the midbrain close to the level of the raphé nuclei [17, 25, 212, 213]; auditory hallucinosis has also followed brainstem lesions in the pontine tegmentum [213], and likewise visual hallucinosis ("Pick's visions") [20]. Lesions causing peduncular hallucinosis are often, but not always, vascular [212, 214], involving branches of the basilar artery. Acute posterior cerebral artery infarcts have caused severe agitation mistaken for primary psychiatric disease [215], but also visual hallucinosis as visual cortex and/or thalamus is infarcted [212]. Hallucinations and delusions have also followed damage to the caudate or putamen [216, 217], paramedian thalamus [218, 219], and otherwise "silent" right hemisphere infarcts [33, 220, 221]. Hallucinations can occur in scotomas caused by occipital lobe damage [213]. Transient ischaemic attacks (TIAs) can produce similar brief hallucinations [25]. Psychosis is also a highly atypical presentation of subarachnoid haemorrhage, likely due to hydrocephalus (Chapter 6.7 ▶) [222], and occasionally patients with chronic **subdural haemorrhage (haematoma)** are suspected to have a psychotic prodrome [223] or develop psychotic depression [224].

Some psychotic symptoms following focal brain damage can be interpreted more clearly than usual in terms of the function of the damaged region; these include several hallucinatory syndromes (as above) but also anosognosia (lack of awareness of disability, e.g. of hemiparesis or blindness), in which delusions may be contributed to by lack of awareness and confabulation [36, 225, 226].

Some specific causes of ischaemic stroke are worth noting. **Cerebral autosomal dominant arteriopathy with subcortical lacunar infarcts and leukoencephalopathy (CADASIL)** is a heritable cause of multiple strokes with young onset (aged 30–50) and white-matter dementia; it also causes migraine (in ~30% of cases), pseudobulbar palsy, spastic quadriparesis, and depression (~20%) [227–230]. The arteriopathy is neither atherosclerotic nor amyloid [28]. CADASIL may cause psychosis, sometimes over a long period before the nature of the condition becomes apparent [231]. The initial presentation is psychiatric in up to 15% of cases [232]. In other studies, psychosis is particularly associated with multiple subfrontal white matter infarcts [233]. The prevalence of CADASIL is unknown, as it was only recognized as a distinct clinical entity with a specific gene mutation in the early 1990s, but is at least 2 per 100 000 [234]. See also HERNS (Chapter 5.16 ▶).

Moyamoya disease is a non-inflammatory progressive stenosis of the intracranial internal carotid arteries [28]. Collateral channels (moyamoya vessels) form, and give rise to the name, which means "puff of smoke" in Japanese and refers to the appearance of the collateral vessels on angiography. It is a very rare cause of large-vessel stenosis, except in Japan where the annual incidence is ~0.5 per 100 000 [235]. Pathologically, there is endothelial hyperplasia and fibrosis with intimal thickening. Children under 15 usually present with transient hemiparesis, headache, seizures, or other focal neurological deficits, often precipitated by exercise or hyperventilation. Adults typically present with intracranial haemorrhages, often in the thalamus, basal ganglia or deep white matter but sometimes as subarachnoid haemorrhage [28]. There is a case report of moyamoya presenting with psychosis in adolescence [236]. Diagnosis is by cerebral angiography [28].

Thromboangiitis obliterans (Buerger's disease) is a non-atherosclerotic panarteritis of small and medium-sized arteries and veins, causing thrombosis. It is strongly associated with tobacco smoking and the male:female ratio is 3:1. Typically, it presents with peripheral ischaemia with pain, ulceration, and gangrene, but it can involve cerebral vessels, causing transient ischaemia and infarcts, sometimes with seizures and migrainous headaches [25, 237]. It can also cause schizophreniform psychosis [238]. One set of diagnostic criteria are: (1) age <45 years; (2) current or recent history of tobacco use; (3) distal extremity ischaemia (claudication, rest pain, ischaemic ulcers, or ulcers) documented by non-invasive vascular testing; (4) exclusion of autoimmune diseases, hypercoagulable states, and diabetes mellitus; (5) exclusion of a proximal source of emboli by echocardiography and arteriography; (6) consistent arteriographic findings in the clinically involved and non-involved limbs. An alternative point-scoring system allows the probability of diagnosis to be assessed. Inflammatory markers are not raised [237].

Mitochondrial myopathy, encephalopathy, lactic acidosis, and stroke-like episodes (MELAS) (Chapter 10.6 ▶) can likewise cause CVAs and psychosis [239], as can hypercoagulable states including antiphospholipid syndrome (Chapter 13.1.2 ▶), and infectious and autoimmune vasculitides (Chapter 13 inc. Chapter 13.2.5 ▶) [33].

In general, initial diagnosis of small infarcts and leukoencephalopathy is best done by MRI, followed by investigations as to the cause. Since atherosclerosis is rare in those under 40, brain ischaemia in this age group has an extensive differential diagnosis, covered elsewhere [28]. For diagnosis of MELAS, see Chapter 10.6 ▶. CADASIL may be diagnosed genetically, with ~65% of cases being accounted for by mutations in exons 3 and 4 of the notch gene [227] (MIM 125310), and/or by skin biopsy with electron microscopy showing granular osmiophilic material in vascular smooth muscle [232, 240].

Uncommonly, a cerebrovascular accident is due to **cerebral venous and sinus thrombosis** (CVST); this is also recognized as a cause of psychosis [241]. Cerebral venous and sinus thrombosis may be spontaneous, associated with pregnancy or the oral contraceptive pill, due to hereditary thrombophilia, or triggered by local factors including mass lesions and spread from cranial infections. The presentation is varied, depending on the site and extent of the veins and/or sinuses thrombosed. Headache is very common (75–95% of cases); it can be of any severity, and usually precedes other features. The onset is usually subacute, over days or even weeks (as the thrombotic process progresses), though occasionally sudden-onset headache occurs. Seizures are much more common with CVST than with arterial stroke, and occur in 35–50% of all patients, and 76% of peripartum CVST. Focal neurological findings (including focal seizures) are common. Sometimes the presentation is with a subacute encephalopathy with mental state changes. Definitive diagnosis is by CT venography, MRI with MRV, or invasive angiography [241].

Cerebral vasculitis is discussed elsewhere (Chapter 13 ▶).

6.2 Epilepsy

Epilepsy is a chronic disorder characterized by a spontaneous tendency for recurrent seizures. It affects ~0.65% of the population, and in two thirds of cases the aetiology is not identified [28]. The lifetime risk of at least one afebrile seizure is much higher, at ~6%. The lifetime prevalence of psychosis amongst epileptic patients is 7–12% [22]. The relative risk of people with a history of epilepsy receiving a diagnosis of schizophrenia is 2.48, and 2.93 for schizophrenia-like psychosis more broadly defined [242] (see also [17] for a review of the putative risk factors and pathophysiology).

6.2.1 Classification of seizures

Seizures are divided into *focal (partial)* and *generalized*, depending on whether the initial neuronal activation is in a limited population of neurons in one hemisphere or across both hemispheres.

Focal seizures are subdivided into *simple partial seizures*, in which consciousness is preserved; *complex partial seizures*, in which consciousness is impaired, either from the onset or subsequently, and there may also be automatisms; and *secondarily generalized seizures*, in which a focal seizure evolves to a generalized seizure.

Generalized seizures may be convulsive (with motor features) or non-convulsive. They are subdivided into *absence seizures*, in which activity is interrupted and the patient may stare blankly for a while (once termed petit mal seizures); *myoclonic seizures*, characterized by myoclonic jerks; *clonic seizures*, in which repetitive clonic jerks occur; *tonic seizures*, in which muscle tone is violently increased; *tonic–clonic seizures*, or grand mal fits, the most common generalized seizure, in which a tonic component gives way to clonic convulsions; and *atonic seizures*, in which all muscle tone is lost (if brief, this is known as a drop attack).

The classification is partly clinical and partly based on EEG features; thus, a seizure that manifests as staring and loss of awareness might be an absence seizure, if generalized spike-and-wave complexes are seen on the EEG, or a complex partial seizure, if there are focal epileptiform discharges [28, 243].

Seizures may be preceded by a *prodrome* of non-specific mood changes or a sense of unease, lasting hours to days [29].

Status epilepticus is a medical emergency in which continuous seizure activity (clinical or electrical) occurs, or repetitive seizures occur without full interictal neurological recovery. It is classified as generalized or partial, and convulsive or non-convulsive. Operationally, generalized convulsive status epilepticus is defined as ≥5 minutes of continuous seizures, or two or more discrete seizures between which there is incomplete recovery of consciousness [244]. The clinical signs may mute with time ("subtle" status) despite seizures continuing. It requires rapid resuscitation, including exclusion of hypoglycaemia, and treatment with oxygen, glucose, thiamine, and sufficient sedation to terminate the seizure [28, 49].

Differentiation of epilepsy from *psychogenic seizures* may be difficult, and is based on atypical clinical features (such as less stereotyped and less synchronized motor activity seen in psychogenic seizures) and EEG monitoring, sometimes with seizure provocation measures. Demonstrating elevated serum prolactin 10–20 minutes after an attack (falling again by ~1 hour) supports the diagnosis of epilepsy; however, it is also raised following syncope, and a normal prolactin does not exclude an epileptic seizure [28, 245].

6.2.2 Psychosis and epilepsy

Psychosis can occur as a result of epilepsy as an ictal, postictal, or interictal phenomenon. In ictal psychosis, the psychotic symptoms depend on the site of the seizure, as follows.

Temporal lobe epilepsy (TLE). Temporal lobe epilepsy accounts for nearly two-thirds of focal epilepsy with onset in adolescence and adulthood [28], and ~75% of focal seizures [29]. It may begin in the neocortex, but more commonly (~80%) begins in medial temporal lobe structures, the amygdala or hippocampus. Stress, sleep deprivation, and menstruation are common provoking factors [28]. "Medial" TLE symptoms include visceral sensations (epigastric aura, which occurs in up to 50% of patients), fear, anxiety, ecstasy, olfactory disturbance, depersonalization, derealization, déjà vu, prescience, and thought disorder [25, 28, 29, 33]. "Neocortical" TLE symptoms include auditory hallucinations and complex visual phenomena including misperceptions and hallucinations, sometimes Lilliputian [22, 28, 29]. The aura may show a characteristic "march" (e.g. moving consistently from an epigastric sensation to gustatory hallucinations to forced thinking) [33]. Olfactory symptoms, including hallucinations of foul odours, are particularly characteristic of uncinate seizures; the uncus (part of the primary olfactory area) receives afferents from the olfactory bulb [28]. There may also be gustatory hallucinations [17]. Complex partial seizures are characterized by behavioural arrest, staring, automatisms, and sometimes contralateral dystonic posturing. Seizures typically last 30–120 s [28]. There is typically postictal confusion, and language disturbance following dominant hemisphere seizures. Status epilepticus is rare, and the neurological examination is usually normal [28].

Medial temporal sclerosis (hippocampal sclerosis) may be seen on MRI. Pathologically, this corresponds to marked hippocampal granule cell loss, following which reactive synaptogenesis produces an epileptic focus [28]; its aetiology is unclear but it predisposes to seizures [47]. Hippocampal sclerosis is also associated with a history of childhood febrile convulsions, though the direction of causality is unclear [33]. Developmental abnormalities such as hamartomas may also cause focal epilepsy, as may other focal lesions (e.g. infection, neoplasms, vascular malformation, cortical dysplasia, scarring following meningoencephalitis or trauma, cerebrovascular accident). The interictal EEG may show temporal slowing and spikes or sharp waves (as for any epileptogenic focus), accentuated during non-REM sleep. The abnormalities may be bilateral. Scalp electrodes may miss TLE, and additional temporal scalp electrodes or sphenoidal electrodes (wires inserted under local anaesthesia through the cheek) improve the diagnostic yield [28]. Subtle focal lesions may cause epilepsy, and high-field MRI, leaving no gaps between image "slices", may be necessary to find them [246, 247].

Frontal lobe epilepsy. Frontal lobe seizures tend to have a more abrupt onset and shorter duration than TLE, with less postictal confusion, but a higher incidence of status epilepticus [28]. Seizures arising from the orbitofrontal or cingulate cortex may be clinically indistinguishable from TLE, producing staring, automatisms (sometimes complex, such as clapping, stamping, singing, and sexual manipulation), and autonomic and affective symptoms [28, 29]. There may be speech disturbance, thought disorder, and forced thinking (recurrent intrusive thoughts or ideas or crowding of thoughts) or forced actions [22]. Operculum seizures produce salivation, mastication, speech arrest, laryngeal symptoms, autonomic changes, and gustatory or epigastric disturbances [28]. Posterior frontal lobe seizures (e.g. motor cortex) produce the expected motor consequences.

Parietal lobe epilepsy accounts for ~5% of partial seizures. Symptoms may include lateralized somatosensory symptoms (tactile hallucinations, tingling, numbness, sense of movement), vertigo, visual distortions, visual hallucinations, and abnormal epigastric or head sensations [28, 29, 212].

Occipital lobe epilepsy accounts for ~3% of partial seizures, and causes elementary visual hallucinations that may be limited to the contralateral hemifield, sensations of eye movement, blinking, and temporary blindness. It may be difficult to distinguish from migraine [28, 29].

Ictal psychosis, therefore, includes hallucinations, thought disorder, and behavioural disturbances such as automatisms resulting from ongoing seizures, including non-convulsive status epilepticus. Most partial seizures last under 3 minutes, so troublesome psychosis as a result of these is rare [248]. In contrast to this is non-convulsive status epilepticus, the main types of which are absence status and complex partial status. Non-convulsive status may cause confusion and psychosis, with a fluctuating level of consciousness that may be accompanied by episodic hallucinations, marked mood changes, bizarre behaviour, and complex automatisms. The onset may be sudden or gradual, and it may last from minutes to months. It may be misdiagnosed as "primary" psychiatric disease, but requires early diagnosis with EEG and rapid termination of seizure activity, like other forms of status epilepticus, as prolonged complex partial status may sometimes lead to persistent intellectual deficit [29, 249].

Postictal psychosis. Postictal psychosis comprises 25–30% of the psychoses associated with epilepsy [250]; it is seen in 6–10% of epilepsy patients undergoing inpatient monitoring for consideration of neurosurgery [250] and 2–7.8% of epilepsy patients overall [248].

The conventional diagnostic criteria [251] are (1) psychosis developing within 1 week of a seizure; (2) psychosis lasting ≥15 hours and <2 months; (3) mental state characterized by delirium, or delusions or hallucinations in clear consciousness; (4) no evidence of (a) a history of treatment with antipsychotics or psychosis within the past 3 months, (b) antiepileptic drug toxicity, (c) an EEG demonstrating non-convulsive status epilepticus, or (d) a recent history of head trauma or alcohol/drug intoxication or withdrawal, other than benzodiazepines used for epilepsy [250].

Typically, the patient is psychiatrically well until a cluster of seizures. After an initial postictal period of confusion and lethargy (which may last a few hours, and be accompanied by EEG slow-wave changes) [29], the patient improves (the lucid interval, of between 2 hours and a week, which is not typical of other postictal phenomena). Subsequently, psychosis develops and lasts days to weeks (in one study, a mean duration of 3.5 days with a range of 16 hours to 18 days); it may feature thought disorder, auditory and visual hallucinations, delusions, suspiciousness, mania or depression, and aggression. Mild confusion and delirium are often seen. It is more common after partial than generalized epilepsy. It may represent a "rebound" phenomenon following postictal depression of activity; of note, benzodiazepine withdrawal can also induce psychosis in patients with epilepsy. In comparison with those with chronic interictal psychosis (see below), visual hallucinations, grandiose and religious delusions, pressured speech, and illusions of familiarity are more common in postictal psychosis [33, 250]. The EEG may show diffuse background slowing or interictal epileptiform abnormalities, which are typical in any case of postictal EEGs [33].

Some classify postictal confusional psychoses as fugues or twilight states. Fugues are prolonged episodes of wandering, altered behaviour, amnesia, and impaired consciousness; they last hours to days and the EEG can be normal. They are hypothesized to be dissociative states provoked by the seizure [29]. Twilight states are characterized by abnormal perceptual and affective experiences, and are associated with cognitive impairment, delusions, hallucinations, and perseveration. They have been hypothesized to be due to ongoing non-convulsive paroxysmal activity, but the mechanism is controversial [29].

Other peri-ictal psychosis. In some cases, reproducible psychotic symptoms may precede overt seizures; it is not always clear whether this is a non-seizure prodrome or ictal psychosis progressing to a generalized seizure [250].

Chronic interictal psychosis. A long history of uncontrolled seizures can lead to chronic psychosis in 3–5% of patients, typically after temporal lobe epilepsy. It may begin with a slow onset of delusions and hallucinations; thought disorder is uncommon. In comparison to postictal psychosis, there is often less of an affective component [29, 248]. In some series, schizophrenia-like illness accompanied temporal lobe epilepsy in 7–23% of patients, usually with a long delay (on average 14 years from the onset of epilepsy to the onset of the psychosis) [16]. It is unclear if the epilepsy predisposes to psychosis, or a developmental abnormality predisposes to both [29]. One set of operational criteria for interictal psychosis is: (1) the psychosis develops after the onset of epilepsy; (2) the psychotic episodes occur with no distinct antecedent seizures when the patient is seizure free or between habitual seizures; (3) the psychotic episodes last 24 hours or more in a state of clear consciousness [252]. It has been suggested that postictal psychosis lasting more than a month should be reclassified as interictal psychosis, though this is debated [17].

"Forced normalization" is a controversial concept that refers to mental state changes (including psychosis) in association with normalization of the EEG in patients with epilepsy. Since this often occurs after an effective antiepileptic drug is added, it may represent psychosis as a side-effect of these drugs (Chapter 15.1 ▶) [248], though there is a case report of schizophreniform psychosis with onset following successful control of epilepsy through vagal nerve stimulation [253]. See [17] for further discussion and suggested diagnostic criteria. **"Alternating psychosis"** is a similar term referring to psychosis in the context of a reduction in seizure frequency [254], and the term **"brief interictal psychosis"** is also sometimes used, while **"bimodal psychosis"** refers to the occurrence of both postictal psychosis and brief interictal psychosis [see 17].

Psychosis following neurosurgery for epilepsy. New-onset psychosis following epilepsy surgery has been variously estimated to occur in <1–28.5% of patients, typically transient postoperative psychosis [248], but see also [17].

6.2.3 EEG features of relevance and underlying causes

Common EEG abnormalities are discussed elsewhere [22, 29]. The EEG hallmark of a seizure disorder is a spike, sharp wave, and/or spike-and-wave discharge, be it generalized, hemispheric, or focal. (Spike discharges are potentials with sharp countours lasting <80 ms, whereas sharp waves last 80–200 ms.) However, many other EEG abnormalities have been associated with seizures, and patients with epilepsy can have normal interictal EEGs [22, 28]. Standard techniques for provoking evidence of a seizure disorder include hyperventilation, photic stimulation, and sleep [22]. A single routine EEG will be normal in 20–30% of patients with epilepsy, and epilepsy remains a clinical diagnosis [25].

Seizures are a common feature of a wide range of other neurological disorders, as discussed elsewhere in Section 1, and a search for an underlying cause should be made.

6.3 Migraine

Migraine occurs in 18% of women, 6% of men, and 4% of children; it usually begins in the first three decades of life, with maximum prevalence in the fifth decade. Most sufferers have a family history of migraine [28]. Its exact pathophysiology is uncertain. However, fortification spectrum aura (described below) corresponds to an event moving across the cortex at 2–3 mm/minute; it is associated with cortical spreading depression of electrical activity and hyperaemia, followed by spreading oligaemia. Headache probably arises from a change in central pain modulation plus activation of meningeal and vascular nociceptors. Trigger factors include psychological stress, anxiety, exercise, fatigue, sexual activity, high altitude, bright lights or glare, odours, change in sleep patterns, menstruation, changes in weather or temperature, missing meals, some foods, and alcohol [28, 255].

Migraine attacks have up to four phases: the prodrome (occurring hours or days before the headache), aura (immediately preceding the headache), headache, and postdrome [28]. Rarely, the aura accompanies or follows the headache [28]. The migrainous aura may be misdiagnosed as primary psychiatric psychosis [256]. In a series of patients hospitalized with migraine, 6% had complex visual or auditory hallucinations, and delirium and severe mood changes were also common [25]. Very rarely, the visual hallucinatory phenomena from the aura persist for months to years [257].

Prodrome symptoms may include depression, hyperactivity, euphoria, talkativeness, irritability, drowsiness or feeling tired and weary (72%), restlessness, photophobia, difficulty concentrating (51%), phonophobia, dysphasia, hyperosmia, yawning, stiff neck (50%), food cravings, cold feelings, anorexia, sluggishness, diarrhoea or constipation, thirst, urination, and fluid retention [28].

The aura, if present, develops over 5–20 minutes and usually lasts <60 minutes. The most frequent aura is visual. Elementary visual disturbances are most common, including scotomas, photopsia (flashes) and other phosphenes, specks, geometric forms, shimmering, or undulations (a differential diagnosis is occipital epilepsy; see Chapter 6.2 ▶). More complicated visual hallucinations include fortification spectra (nearly diagnostic of migraine), in which an arc of scintillating lights migrates across the visual field, often with a zigzag or flashing edge. There may be visual distortions including metamorphopsia (a change in the shape of perceived objects), micropsia, macropsia, zoom vision, or mosaic vision. Paraesthesiae are the next most common aura (typically migrating from the hand up to the face over >5 minutes). More complex symptoms may include other perceptual disturbances, speech and language disturbance, subjectively altered states of consciousness including déjà and jamais vu, and complex hallucinatory or dreamlike states [17, 28]. Motor symptoms are rare but define *hemiplegic migraine* [28]. Very rarely, hemiplegic migraine may progress to *migraine coma*, and prominent and prolonged hallucinations have been reported during recovery from this [212, 258].

The headache is usually unilateral, throbbing, moderate to severe in intensity, and aggravated by physical activity; it lasts 4–72 hours. It is often associated with anorexia, nausea (90%), and vomiting (33%). There is sensory hyperexcitability and sufferers seek a dark, quiet room. Blurred vision, nasal stuffiness, diarrhoea, polyuria, pallor, or sweating may occur. There may be localized oedema or tenderness of the scalp or neck [28].

In the postdrome, patients often feel tired and "washed out", and may have mood disturbances [28].

The diagnostic criteria for migraine with aura (classic migraine) are at least three of: (1) one or more fully reversible aura symptoms; (2) at least one aura symptom over >4 minutes or two or more symptoms occurring in succession; (3) no single aura symptom lasts >60 minutes; (4) headache follows aura with a symptom-free interval of <60 minutes, or begins before or simultaneously with the aura. The criteria for migraine without aura are at least five attacks fulfilling all of the following: (A) headache lasting 4–72 hours (untreated or unsuccessfully treated); (B) the headache has at least two of the following characteristics: (B1) unilateral, (B2) pulsating, (B3) moderate or severe pain, (B4) aggravation by or causing avoidance of routine physical activity; (C) during the headache, there is at least one of: (C1) nausea and/or vomiting, (C2) photophobia and phonophobia; (D) the condition is not attributed to another disorder [28].

If performed, the EEG is usually normal, but focal or generalized slowing may be seen (especially during or immediately after an attack), but epileptiform transients may also be seen [28, 212]. Severe migraine is also associated with increased CSF protein and cell counts [28].

Basilar migraine involves a visual aura, then brainstem signs (ataxia, vertigo, tinnitus, diplopia, nausea, vomiting, dysarthria, bilateral paraesthesiae, and altered consciousness and cognition, which may include gradual loss of consciousness), then severe headache [25, 28]. *Confusional migraine* involves headache accompanied by inattention and distractibility. *Familial hemiplegic migraine* is an autosomal dominant calcium channel disorder; attacks may be triggered by minor head injury and may be accompanied by coma and hallucinations [259]. Rarely, intense vasospasm in migraine may cause stroke (*migrainous infarction*) [28].

Familial hemiplegic migraine has been described in which the migraine was associated with paranoid psychosis, anxiety, and auditory/visual hallucinations, with cerebellar ataxia also a feature (MIM 141500). The combination of migraine and psychosis should also raise the possibilities of CADASIL (Chapter 6.1 ▶), MELAS (Chapter 10.6 ▶), and ornithine transcarbamylase deficiency (see Chapter 10.1 ▶); the latter may resemble confusional migraine with hallucinations in children and young adults [28]. Migraines are also common in antiphospholipid syndrome (Chapter 13.1.2 ▶).

Very rarely, **cluster headaches** (recurrent unilateral orbital, periorbital, or temporal headaches with ipsilateral local autonomic changes) can have features of a migrainous aura including simple hallucinatory phenomena [17, 260, 261].

6.4 Hypertensive encephalopathy and posterior reversible encephalopathy syndrome

Posterior reversible encephalopathy syndrome (PRES) is a state of brain vasogenic oedema in the setting of neurotoxicity, which is normally fully reversible. It is also known as **reversible posterior leukoencephalopathy**. It was first described in the context of severe hypertension (hypertensive encephalopathy), eclampsia, and transplantation (solid organ and bone marrow) and the use of immunosuppressive drugs (e.g. cyclosporin, tacrolimus). It has subsequently been noted in the context of autoimmune disease (e.g. SLE [Chapter 13.1.1 ▶], systemic sclerosis [Chapter 13.1.4 ▶], Wegener's granulomatosis [Chapter 13.2.4 ▶], PAN [Chapter 13.2.3 ▶], and perhaps Hashimoto's encephalopathy [Chapter 14.1 ▶]), infection with sepsis and shock, chemotherapy for cancer, thrombotic thrombocytopenic purpura (Chapter 13.7 ▶), renal disease (Chapter 12.4.1 ▶), acute porphyria (Chapter 10.2 ▶), and potentially a number of other conditions [262–265]. It was originally thought that hypertension exceeded the autoregulatory pressures in the cerebral vasculature and caused hyperperfusion, but in ~25% of cases of PRES, hypertension is absent, and in many others hypertension is milder (with mean arterial pressure not exceeding the 150–160 mmHg autoregulation threshold). Alternative theories involve endothelial injury, vasoconstriction, and hypoperfusion; there is doubt as to the cause [262, 266].

Clinical features are typically of headache, nausea, altered vision (including visual loss, visual hallucinations, and neglect), paralysis, and cognitive changes including confusion. These may develop rapidly or over days. Generalized seizures are common and coma may follow [262–264].

It is diagnosed by finding characteristic oedema on CT or MRI imaging; this is symmetric and may be widespread but typically affects the parietal and occipital lobes the most, hence the "posterior" designation. The oedema is most marked at vascular watershed regions [262].

6.5 Head injury (traumatic brain injury)

Acutely, psychosis may occur during the recovery from unconsciousness immediately following head injury (**"acute post-traumatic psychosis"**) [25, 33], with delusional misidentification perhaps being especially common [33]. Subsequently, there are many reports of psychosis following head injury [15, 25, 29, 267] but generally poor evidence for a causal association, even if other psychiatric morbidity is frequent following significant head injury [33]. A systematic review in 2005 found little evidence that head injury was a cause of subsequent psychosis [268]. Since then, a large Swedish case–control study, examining all patients in a cohort of >785 000 with an admission for schizophrenia or non-affective psychosis, found that prior head injury leading to hospital admission represented a significant but small risk factor (odds ratio 1.37) for non-schizophrenic, non-affective psychoses [269], but not for schizophrenia, though the authors were unable to exclude the possibility that a general liability to trauma was responsible for this association. There is stronger evidence that head injury is a risk factor for post-traumatic stress disorder and depression [270, 271], and a link with dementia is debated [272]. Nonetheless, if epilepsy develops following closed head injury, temporal lobe epilepsy (Chapter 6.2 ▶) (a cause of psychosis) is the commonest form [25], though see also [17] for further discussion.

However, repeated brain injury (as seen in boxing) also predisposes to **chronic traumatic encephalopathy (dementia pugilistica; "punch-drunk" syndrome)**, in which dementia may be accompanied by cerebellar, pyramidal, and extrapyramidal motor signs. The dementia may also be accompanied by psychotic features such as delusions. Histologically, it resembles Alzheimer's disease [25, 28, 29, 273].

6.6 Normal-pressure hydrocephalus

Hydrocephalus may be divided into *communicating* hydrocephalus, in which the ventricles communicate normally with the subarachnoid space but CSF production exceeds absorption (usually due to insufficient absorption), and *non-communicating (obstructive)* hydrocephalus, in which the path from ventricles to subarachnoid space is obstructed [274]. Normal-pressure hydrocephalus is a form of communicating hydrocephalus, but one in which the ventricles become enlarged but not the subarachnoid space; the distended ventricles distort the corona radiata and periventricular structures [275]. The annual incidence of idiopathic NPH is approximately 0.2–2:100 000 [33]. It is a misnomer in that the actual CSF pressure may be high-normal, intermittently high, or initially high and returning to normal following ventricular enlargement [275].

Clinically, NPH is characterized by the triad of *dementia*, *urinary incontinence*, and *gait abnormalities* [275]. There is often memory loss and bradyphrenia. Urinary urgency and frequency may precede incontinence, and faecal incontinence may also occur. The gait is often broad-based, slow, and shuffling; there may be parkinsonian features (e.g. tremor, bradykinesia). Less commonly, NPH can present with psychosis in the absence of the classic triad, or with psychosis predominating [17, 33, 276, 277]. Initial diagnosis is clinical and by structural brain imaging [275].

6.7 Intracranial mass lesions (tumours) and obstructive hydrocephalus

Case reports of psychosis in temporal association with primary or metastatic brain tumours (see also Chapter 7 ▶) are legion, with a causative role supported by remission following resection in many cases [25]. Involvement of sensory cortex is an obvious potential mechanism for hallucinations (e.g. [17, 28]). Tumours of the frontal lobe, temporal lobe, and diencephalon are over-represented in patients presenting with psychotic symptoms [15, 17, 278]. Neuropsychiatric presentations including psychosis have also been observed with posterior fossa tumours, posterior fossa structural abnormalities such as megacisterna magna and the Dandy–Walker malformation [25, 279], ventricular tumours [280, 281], pituitary adenomas (including adenomas not causing Cushing's disease) [282–284], and, returning to the diencephalon, hypothalamic hamartomas [285] (though these are also associated with severe epilepsy [Chapter 6.2 ▶]). In some cases obstructive hydrocephalus and raised intracranial pressure appear to play a role [286–288]. See also CVAs (Chapter 6.1 ▶).

Diagnosis is by history, clinical examination, and structural imaging (CT or MRI) [25, 28]. The localizing features of tumours will not be reiterated here, but red-flag symptoms include new-onset seizures, new-onset or progressive headache (particularly if it is persistent, non-migrainous, nocturnal, present on waking, or worsened positionally or by a Valsalva manoeuvre), nausea and vomiting, visual changes (decrease in acuity, field loss, or diplopia), unilateral hearing loss, tinnitus, vertigo, focal weakness or somatosensory changes, gait disturbance, incoordination, ataxia, and dysarthria [22]. Intravenous contrast enhances the ability of CT and MRI to detect tumours [22].

6.8 Multiple sclerosis

Multiple sclerosis (MS) is an idiopathic inflammatory CNS demyelinating disorder characterized by multiple demyelinated lesions discrete in time and space [289, 290]. Initially, there is recovery and remyelination, though this is not durable, and subsequent chronic neurodegeneration may ensue [290]. It is most common in northern European races. The prevalence is approximately 1:1000 people in Canada but has wide geographical variation [291]. The clinical presentation is varied and depends on the site of the lesion(s), which most commonly involve the optic nerve and periventricular white matter of the cerebellum, brainstem, basal ganglia, and spinal cord.

Features include sensory loss (e.g. paraesthesiae), motor symptoms (e.g. spasticity), autonomic symptoms (e.g. bladder, bowel, sexual), cerebellar symptoms (e.g. dysarthria, ataxia, tremor), constitutional symptoms (e.g. fatigue [70% of cases], dizziness), cognitive symptoms (e.g. poor attention, concentration, memory, judgement), mood symptoms (most commonly depression, occurring in 25–50% of cases), and eye symptoms (33% of cases, e.g. diplopia) [289, 292]. Optic neuritis is the initial presentation in 15% of cases, causing acute onset of blurring and decreased visual acuity in one eye, reduction in colour perception, and sometimes eye discomfort, phosphenes precipitated by movement, or deterioration of vision with exercise, hot meals, or baths. Acute transverse myelitis is another presentation, with acute partial loss of motor, sensory, and autonomic function below the level of the spinal cord lesion. Less common presentations include aphasia or dysphasia, hemianopia (hemianopsia), seizures (5%), isolated cranial nerve lesions, and acute disseminated encephalitis (sometimes fatal; see also ADEM [Chapter 8.7.3 ▶]) [289].

Examination findings match the lesion pattern. Eye findings may include reduced visual acuity, optic atrophy (though retrobulbar optic neuritis is invisible on fundoscopy), internuclear ophthalmoplegia, and a relative afferent pupillary defect [289]. Internuclear ophthalmoplegia, Lhermitte's symptom (an electric sensation running down the limbs or spine on neck flexion), and the Uhthoff phenomenon (worsening of symptoms when body temperature rises, as with a hot bath or exercise) are relatively specific [20, 290]. Diagnosis is by clinical assessment, MRI, and often LP [289]; a formal diagnostic pathway is given in [293].

Individual demyelinating lesions typically have subacute onset (days to weeks) but can occur acutely, and episodes typically last from weeks to months [20]. Overall, the disease course may be characterized as an isolated single clinical episode, relapsing–remitting MS, secondary progressive MS (following the relapsing–remitting phase), or primary progressive MS [290].

Psychosis is often said to be rare in MS [292, 294], but it can be the presenting feature [295]. More often, it follows the development of neurological symptoms [292]. One prospective study found hallucinations in 10% and delusions in 7% of patients with MS, in addition to depressive symptoms (79%), agitation (40%), anxiety (37%), irritability (35%), apathy (20%), euphoria (13%), and disinhibition (7%) [296]. Schizophrenia-like psychosis has been reported in up to 5% [94]. In a large Canadian population survey (n = 2.45 million), there was a significant association between the presence of psychotic disorders and MS, with odds ratios for the diagnosis of a psychotic disorder of 6.6 (in patients with MS aged 15–24 years), 2.2 (aged 25–44), 1.9 (aged 45–64), and 1.1 (aged ≥65) [297]. Psychosis in MS may be associated with temporal lobe lesions [292] or frontal and temporal periventricular lesions [94].

Mimics of MS reported to cause psychosis include X-linked adrenoleukodystrophy (Chapter 10.5.8 ▶), intravascular large-B-cell lymphoma (Chapter 7 ▶), diffuse sclerosis (Chapter 10.5.14 ▶), antiphospholipid syndrome (Chapter 13.1.2 ▶), and ADEM (Chapter 8.7.3 ▶). Multiple sclerosis may also sometimes be difficult to distinguish radiologically from intracranial tumours (Chapter 6.7 ▶, Chapter 7 ▶) including lymphoma.

6.9 Central pontine and extrapontine myelinolysis

Central pontine myelinolysis is a rare condition that is often precipitated following severe and prolonged hyponatraemia, particularly if corrected too fast. A typical history involves delirium secondary to prolonged hyponatraemia, rapid treatment and correction of the hyponatraemia with resolution of mental state, followed by neurological deterioration 48–72 hours later with confusion, horizontal gaze paralysis, and spastic quadriplegia, with MRI showing pontine demyelination [298]. The contribution of the rate of correction is debated [28]. In approximately 10% of patients, there is also extrapontine myelinolysis, and there is a case report of psychosis with delusions and hallucinations following central pontine and extrapontine myelinolysis that included the caudate [299].

6.10 Tuberous sclerosis

Tuberous sclerosis (**Bourneville disease**) is a disorder of cellular differentiation and proliferation causing the formation of multiple hamartomas, such as in the skin, brain, eye, kidney, and heart. It is named for the superficial resemblance of the lesions to a potato. It may occur spontaneously (60%) or have autosomal dominant inheritance. It has a birth incidence of 1:6000–1:15 000, and a prevalence variously estimated between 1:10 000–1:300 000 [28, 47, 300]. The severity is very variable. The most common symptoms are early-onset epilepsy (seizures are seen in 60–80% of patients), a degree of mental retardation (though a third have normal intelligence), and skin lesions, most typically hypopigmented macules (seen in 90% of patients), adenoma sebaceum (50%), a leathery "shagreen" fibromatous plaque over the lumbosacral or gluteal region, café au lait patches, fibromas (including subungual and periungual fibromas, seen in 20%, more commonly on the toes than the fingers), and angiomas [28, 47, 300].

The *primary features* are facial angiofibromas; multiple ungual fibromas; cortical tuber*; subependymal nodule or giant cell astrocytoma*; multiple calcified subependymal nodules protruding into the ventricle†, and multiple retinal astrocytomas. The *secondary features* are an affected first-degree relative; cardiac rhabdomyoma*†; other retinal hamartomas or achromic patch; cerebral tubers†; non-calcified subependymal nodules†; a shagreen patch; a forehead plaque; pulmonary lymphangiomyomatosis*; renal angiomyolipoma*†; and renal cysts*. The *tertiary features* are hypomelanotic macules; "confetti" skin lesions; renal cysts†; randomly distributed enamel pits in deciduous or permanent teeth; hamartomatous rectal polyps*; bone cysts†; pulmonary lymphangiomyomatosis†; cerebral white matter "migration tracts" or heterotopias†; gingival fibromas; hamartoma of other organs*; infantile spasms. (*Requires histological confirmation; †radiographic evidence; *†either.) The *diagnostic* *criteria* for definite tuberous sclerosis are one primary, two secondary, or one secondary plus two tertiary features; for probable tuberous sclerosis, one secondary plus one tertiary feature, or three tertiary features; for suspected tuberous sclerosis, one secondary or two tertiary features [28]. Magnetic resonance imaging shows the tubers, which often calcify. The EEG shows slowing and interictal epileptiform activity [20].

Early series described institutionalized patients with tuberous sclerosis frequently having psychosis, but only in the sense of bizarre behaviour in the context of mental retardation without access to the patients' mental state [25, 301]; catatonia was also common. Overt hallucinatory and delusional psychosis has also been described, sometimes resembling schizophrenia and without any mental retardation, and sometimes as the presentation leading to diagnosis [302–304]. Sometimes peri-ictal psychosis is suspected [305]. However, the overall prevalence of psychosis in patients with tuberous sclerosis appears low [306].

Chapter 7 Malignancy

Malignancy may cause psychosis via primary and metastatic intracranial mass lesions (Chapter 6.7 ▶), paraneoplastic limbic encephalitis/encephalopathy (Chapter 14.2 ▶), via delirium (Chapter 3 ▶), and via drugs used to treat cancer (Chapter 15.1 ▶). Thus, acute psychosis can sometimes herald undiagnosed tumours [307]. Overall, 5–10% of extracranial tumours cause some form of neurological or myopathic non-metastatic disease [29]. Psychotic presentations may be more common with tumours affecting anterior white matter; up to 20% of oligodendrogliomas, which commonly localize anteriorly, present with psychosis [94].

There is probably an increased risk of psychosis in survivors of childhood brain tumour [308]; the mechanisms are uncertain but plausible candidates include the effects of chemotherapy and radiotherapy.

Rarely, malignancy may produce psychosis via other mechanisms, as follows.

Phaeochromocytoma. Relapsing psychosis has been described as the presenting feature of phaeochromocytoma [309], a rare tumour (0.1–1% of hypertensives) causing catecholamine secretion. Its more typical symptoms are headache, sweating, and palpitations; there may be dizziness, paraesthesiae, tremor, palpitations, intense fear, and sometimes confusion and delirium. Hypertension is characteristic and may be paroxysmal; there may be episodic pallor, paroxysmal arrhythmias and heart failure. Initial screening is usually by measurement of urinary catecholamines and their metabolites (typically 24-hour urinary total catecholamines, vanillylmandelic acid, and metanephrines), or in patients at very high risk, the more sensitive but less specific test of plasma metanephrines [26, 310].

Carcinoid has also been described in association with psychosis [311]. This is a gastrointestinal (typically ileal) neuroendocrine tumour with an annual incidence of ~1 per 100 000 people. The tumours may produce many polypeptides and amines, including serotonin. Once liver metastases are present, serotonin is released into the systemic circulation, and causes carcinoid syndrome [312]. Common symptoms include diarrhoea, flushing, fatigue, wheeze and dyspnoea, palpitations, hypotension, and right-sided heart disease (typically tricuspid stenosis); mental state changes are less common. Diagnosis is by demonstration of elevated 24-hour urinary 5-hydroxyindoleacetic acid.

Lymphomatoid granulomatosis (neoplastic angioendotheliosis) is a form of B-cell lymphoma induced by EBV in the immunosuppressed that closely mimics Wegener's granulomatosis (Chapter 13.2.4 ▶), with pulmonary angiitis and granulomatosis. There is neurological involvement in ~25% [313], and this can include psychosis [314], though confusion, cranial neuropathies, ataxia, hemiparesis, and seizures are more common [25, 313]. Definitive diagnosis is histological [313], though MRI may show multiple high-intensity lesions on T2WI and angiography shows medium-sized vascular occlusions [47].

Intravascular large-B-cell lymphoma (intravascular lymphomatosis) is a rare form of lymphoma in which lymphoma cells proliferate in the lumina of small blood vessels (including capillaries and venules), without forming solid masses. It often presents in the CNS, and can mimic multiple sclerosis (Chapter 6.8 ▶) and CNS vasculitis (Chapter 13.2 ▶). Neurological symptoms and signs may be multifocal or non-specific (e.g. headache, confusion) and have included hallucinations. The mechanism of symptom production is likely ischaemia due to small-vessel occlusion. It may follow a relapsing–remitting or a relapsing–progressive course; it has a very high untreated mortality and is notoriously difficult to diagnose in life. While the skin, brain, and adrenals are often involved, lymph nodes are not. Magnetic resonance imaging typically shows multiple scattered abnormalities, with DWI being sensitive in the acute phase and FLAIR being most useful to establish disease extent. Definitive diagnosis is histological [315, 316].

Leptomeningeal carcinomatosis (carcinomatous meningitis), the infiltration of the leptomeninges by a carcinoma, has on occasion been reported to cause delirious psychosis [317]. Diagnosis is by CSF cytology [318, 319].

Chapter 8

Infectious and postinfectious syndromes

Many severe systemic infections can produce psychosis in the context of delirium (discussed above; Chapter 3 ▶). Other infections show particular neurotropism (as in infectious encephalitis), produce vasculitic phenomena affecting neural function, or cause postinfectious autoimmune neurological dysfunction. For some infectious agents, a role in psychosis has been postulated for chronic active infection, or developmental insult caused by maternal or childhood infection. For example, some studies have reported that maternal viral infections (including rubella, influenza, and HSV-2) increase the incidence of psychosis in the offspring [320]. This chapter will concentrate primarily on the role of acute infection and its sequelae.

Leptomeningitis (usually called simply **meningitis**) is inflammation of the leptomeninges (pia mater and arachnoid mater) and the subarachnoid CSF, which may be infective in origin. Its signs are headache, nausea, vomiting, irritability, photophobia, nuchal and back rigidity, and a positive Kernig's sign (resistance to passive extension of the knee while the hip is flexed) or Brudzinski's neck sign (flexion of the hip or knee in response to attempts at neck flexion). **"Meningism"** or "meningismus" refers to signs of meningeal irritation, particularly resistance to meningeal stretching (e.g. neck stiffness, Kernig's sign), photophobia, and headache. **Pachymeningitis** is isolated inflammation of the dura mater, and is usually due to infection entering via a skull defect, paranasal sinus infection, or cranial osteomyelitis [321]. **Encephalitis** is inflammation of the brain parenchyma; there is impairment of cerebral function, usually with an altered state of consciousness, and often with seizures and focal neurological signs [26]. It may be infective (usually viral) or non-infective (e.g. acute disseminated encephalomyelitis) [322]. In contrast, **encephalopathy** is non-inflammatory diffuse brain dysfunction (e.g. metabolic dysfunction, intoxication) [322]. **Cerebritis** is in one sense a synonym for encephalitis (Greek *enkephalos* = Latin *cerebrum* = brain) but the term cerebritis is usually used for focal bacterial infection preceding abscess formation [323]. **Subdural empyema** is pus within the subdural space, between the dura mater and arachnoid mater. **Ventriculitis** (ependymitis) implies extension of inflammation into the ventricular CSF, typically in meningitis [26, 47]. **Myelitis** denotes inflammation of the spinal cord.

Although it is wise to consider all CNS infections as potential causes of psychosis [22], some produce psychosis more commonly than others. We consider next specific intracranial infections in which psychosis has been described.

8.1 Bacterial infection

8.1.1 Pyogenic bacterial infection

Pyogenic bacterial meningitis may occur spontaneously (due to virulent organisms) or following neurosurgery or skull fracture (due to impaired host defences) [26]. The commonest cause worldwide is *Streptococcus pneumoniae*; other common causes of spontaneous meningitis include *Neisseria meningitidis, Streptococcus agalactiae, Haemophilus influenzae*, and *Listeria monocytogenes* [324]. The patient is typically extremely unwell, with fever and signs of meningitis; in the case of organisms such as *Neisseria meningitidis*, there may be systemic sepsis and septic shock as well as, or instead of, meningitis [26]. Though bacterial meningitis may cause delirium, and has an untreated mortality of 70–100% [26], it is unlikely to cause psychosis without significant meningeal and/or circulatory signs. Childhood meningitis, however, may increase the risk of adult psychosis including schizophrenia [325, 326].

Intracranial abscesses may be extradural (typically following skull osteomyelitis, mastoiditis, or sinusitis), subdural (subdural empyema, following sinus or middle-ear infection or secondary to haematogenous spread), or intracerebral (following middle-ear infection, sinusitis, and haematogenous spread). The oedema surrounding an abscess may contribute to substantial mass effect. Diagnosis is by CT or MR imaging [26]. Brain abscesses occasionally result in psychosis [327].

8.1.2 Neurosyphilis

Syphilis, archaically lues venerea, is caused by the spirochaete bacterium *Treponema pallidum* and is transmitted sexually or transplacentally. It is known as the "great imitator" because of the variety of symptoms and signs it can produce. The pathological mechanism is an infective arteritis.

Primary infection produces a painless but infectious chancre at the site of infection, 10–90 days after infection.

Secondary syphilis occurs 1–6 months later, and has a variety of forms, including a reddish-pink rash on the trunk and limbs (often non-pruritic and most marked on palms and soles), condylomata lata, fever, sore throat, malaise, weight loss, headache, and lymphadenopathy (and more rarely, meningitis, hepatitis, nephritis, gastritis, proctitis, colitis, arthritis, periostitis, iritis, and uveitis); patients are most infectious at this point, especially from wet mucocutaneous lesions. There is subsequently a latent period.

Tertiary syphilis usually occurs 1–10 years after initial infection, but sometimes up to 50 years later; it causes gumma formation (granulomas), neuropathic joint disease, cardiovascular syphilis (including aortitis, aortic aneurysm, and aortic regurgitation), and neurosyphilis. Neurosyphilis (neurolues) occurs in 25–35% of patients with untreated syphilis. Neurosyphilis typically causes meningovascular involvement early, and brain parenchymal involvement late. It may cause personality change, headache, weakness, vertigo, insomnia, focal peripheral sensorimotor neurological deficits, cranial nerve lesions, meningism, and ischaemic stroke. Argyll–Robertson pupils (bilaterally small pupils that are "accommodating but unresponsive" to light) may be seen. Tabes dorsalis is degeneration of spinal cord dorsal columns, with corresponding sensory deficits and hyporeflexia.

Treatment of primary and secondary syphilis does not exclude the subsequent development of neurosyphilis, as organisms may survive in the CSF [20, 28].

General paresis of the insane (dementia paralytica) is a severe form of neurosyphilis with progressive cognitive and memory decline, psychosis, and mood disorders. The presenting features are usually non-specific (headache, insomnia, lethargy, an insidious change in temperament), followed by episodic forgetfulness and deficits in concentration, heralding progressive cognitive decline. The psychiatric presentation can take virtually any form, including a schizophreniform psychosis. When first described, a grandiose presentation was the most common, but simple dementing and depressive forms are now more common. Syphilis is more rapidly progressive in those with HIV infection [22, 25, 328, 329].

In those infected congenitally, neurosyphilis may present after the normal latency period, such as in teenagers [20]. Patients with congenital syphilis may exhibit Hutchinson's triad of interstitial keratitis, sensorineural deafness, and Hutchinson's teeth (notched, widely spaced, and often tapering incisors). Other features include cataracts, frontal bossing, saddle nose and palatal destruction, arthropathy, and sabre tibia [330].

Despite a decline in prevalence, syphilis still presents as psychosis to modern-day psychiatrists, and if diagnosed is easily treatable [331–334]. A recent study found a serological prevalence of ~4% in a UK psychogeriatric inpatient population [335]. Tremor, dysarthria, and pupillary or tendon reflex abnormalities raise its likelihood [25]. Diagnosis is by serology using an appropriate method: CSF venereal disease research laboratory (VDRL) serology is more sensitive than serum VDRL alone [29] but sensitive blood assays are also available [336]. If confirmed, screening for other sexually transmitted diseases should be performed, typically via a genitourinary medicine service.

8.1.3 Lyme disease (borreliosis)

Lyme disease is caused by the spirochaete bacterium *Borrelia burgdorferi*, transmitted by *Ixodes* (black-legged or deer) ticks. Neuroborreliosis is the most common tick-borne neurological infection in Europe and North America. The exact strain of *Borrelia burgdorferi* varies with region, and the disease pattern varies with strain. In Europe, CNS disease is typically more severe, and *B. burgdorferi garinii* is the type most associated with neurological disease. The ticks have a three-stage life cycle (larva, nymph, adult); their preferred hosts are mice and deer. Humans are infected by nymph ticks 85% of the time, in spring to summer, and by adults 15% of the time, in autumn. Infection is rare unless the tick is attached to the human for 24–48 hours. However, the ticks are small and up to 64% of patients do not remember being bitten. In southern Sweden, the case rate is 69 per 100 000 per year. Following infection, there are three possibilities. First, the human may clear the infection asymptomatically, becoming seropositive; 5–10% of patients in endemic areas are seropositive without a history of symptoms. Secondly, the spirochaete may spread through the body and produce disease by direct invasion. For example, erythema migrans (described below) is probably due to an inflammatory response to *B. burgdorferi* in the skin. However, it is difficult to culture *B. burgdorferi*, and therefore difficult to confirm its presence in a specific organ. Thirdly, an immune response may produce symptoms with little evidence of bacterial invasion (e.g. Lyme arthritis). Lyme disease has peaks at age 5–9 and 50–70 years [26, 337–340].

Stage 1 Lyme disease is localized. *Erythema migrans* is an early feature, occurring 3–30 days after exposure. It is an erythematous lesion that increases in size over several days. It may be asymptomatic, itchy, or painful. It may persist for weeks (median duration 4 days in North America, 2–6 weeks in Europe). There may be multiple lesions (in 40% of patients) even following a single tick bite. Two-thirds of patients develop further symptoms. Typically, these begin with fever and myalgia (i.e. a 'flu-like illness). Systemic symptoms are less common in Europe [26, 337].

Stage 2 disease is disseminated. An *intermittent inflammatory arthritis* may occur, often a migratory polyarticular arthritis evolving over 1–2 days to a monoarticular arthritis (most commonly knee, ankle, and wrist). In ~66% of patients, the first episode of arthritis occurs within 6 months of erythema migrans. Each episode lasts about a week; many patients have recurrences approximately 2.5 months apart, which gradually become less severe and less frequent (and usually resolve within 10 years even untreated). Headaches are common. There may be *cranial nerve palsies*, the most common neurological feature. This is most common in children, and is often a facial palsy (in 5–10% of patients with neurological involvement), which may be bilateral and lasts less than 2 months. *Meningoradiculoneuritis* (Bannwarth syndrome) is neuritis characterized by severe radicular pain, especially at night; the meningitis may be mild. The radiculitis is more common in Europe. *Carditis* is manifested typically as atrioventricular node block, whose severity can vary (from asymptomatic ECG findings to syncope), and rarely lasts more than a week. *Malaise and fatigue* may be severe, and are common (80% of patients in the United States, though <35% in Europe) [22, 337].

Stage 3 disease is persistent. Approximately 10% develop a *chronic arthritis* (most commonly in the knee). There may be *chronic neuropathy and meningoencephalitis*, including abnormalities in mood, memory, and sleep, and in severe cases ataxia, spastic paresis, bladder dysfunction, seizures, and cognitive dysfunction. Brainstem arteritis may occur. Symptoms of *fibromyalgia and chronic fatigue* may develop, which do not appear to be due to active infection and whose origins are debated [22, 337, 338, 341].

Neuropsychiatric effects common early in the disease include depression, poor concentration, memory impairment, and sleep disturbance. Late effects include significant mood disorders, psychosis, panic attacks, severe dementia, catatonia, and mania [338]. However, there are several reports of Lyme disease presenting with schizophreniform or other psychosis [22, 342–344]. The overall prevalence of antibodies to *B. burgdorferi* may be higher in patients with psychiatric disease in an endemic area [345].

Culture is possible but requires specific techniques and yields are low. Inflammatory markers (white cell count, ESR, CRP) may be raised or normal; there are sometimes (~40%) abnormalities of liver function tests [346, 347]. Diagnosis is therefore clinical and by antibody testing. The false-positive rate is such that testing is not advised in patients who have not been in endemic areas. Erythema migrans may develop before antibodies. Extracutaneous involvement is almost invariably associated with antibody production, although in Europe neurological Lyme disease has been reported with seronegativity but with CSF antibody production. None of these tests can discriminate between exposure and current infection. In neuroborreliosis, the CSF findings typically show moderate lymphocytic or mononuclear pleocytosis, elevated protein, and normal or slightly low glucose [337, 339]. Cranial nerves may enhance on contrast MRI, and T2WI may show hyperintensities. Functional imaging abnormalities may be seen [338].

Similar presentations may be seen with **other tick-borne infections**, including *Bartonella* (Chapter 8.1.4 ▶), *Anaplasma*, *Babesia*, and *Ehrlichia*. There may be dual infection with one of these and *Borrelia*, or with each other. Encephalitis has been described with *Anaplasma* and *Ehrlichia* infection [348], though not psychosis.

The differential diagnosis includes Whipple's disease (Chapter 8.1.8 ▶) and cerebrotendinous xanthomatosis (Chapter 10.5.9 ▶) [20].

8.1.4 Bartonella infection

Bartonella species are facultative intracellular bacteria. They cause several well-recognized diseases, including trench fever (*Bartonella quintana*, transmitted by lice) and cat-scratch disease (*Bartonella henselae*, usually transmitted by cats). *Bartonella* infection can also be tick-borne [349]. *B. henselae* typically causes focal suppuration with regional lymphadenopathy (cat-scratch disease) but can cause a meningoencephalitis (~10% of cases) [350], and sometimes endocarditis [351]. Diagnosis is by serology. In immunocompromised patients, particularly in the setting of HIV infection, *B. henselae* and *quintana* can cause a multifocal angioproliferative syndrome called bacillary angiomatosis, most often visible in the skin as multiple subcutaneous nodules, but involving multiple organs [352]. Bacillary angiomatosis can present with psychosis [353].

8.1.5 Leptospirosis

Leptospirosis is the most common zoonosis worldwide. The spiral *Leptospira* bacteria enter humans via mucous membranes or abraded skin in contact with infected sources. The primary reservoirs are wild mammals of many species, of which rats are the most common. Urinary infection leads to transmission via contaminated water or food (sometimes with epidemics in the context of flooding). Occupational exposure accounts for 30–50% of human cases; at-risk occupations include those working with animals or animal products, in agriculture, in fishing, in sewage processing, and in the military [354].

After an incubation period of 2–20 days (typically 7–12 days), infection causes an acute febrile illness with renal and hepatic involvement. About 90% have a mild, anicteric form, and 10% have severe disease with jaundice (Weil's disease). There is an initial leptospiraemic phase of 4–7 days with 'flu-like symptoms, sometimes with sore throat, cough, chest pain, haemoptysis, rash, and meningoencephalitis. After a period of improvement of 1–3 days, a second ("immune" or leptospiruric) phase is seen, lasting 0–30 days. Aseptic meningitis is seen in 50% of patients, heralded by headache; cranial nerve palsies, encephalitis, and altered consciousness are less common. Renal involvement (50%), pulmonary involvement (20–70%), systemic symptoms, uveitis (2–10%), and muscle and joint pains are seen; there may be rashes, bleeding, and cardiac involvement [354].

A classic picture of Weil's disease is fever and confusion with jaundice and deranged LFTs, thrombocytopenia, leukocytosis, a raised ESR, and often a raised CK and renal involvement (renal failure or abnormal urinalysis). However, it can also present with mania and psychosis [355]. Definitive diagnosis is by culture and/or serology [354].

8.1.6 Tuberculosis

Worldwide, *Mycobacterium tuberculosis* infection is extremely common, with incidences up to 2% per annum in some regions of Africa and Asia. Tuberculous meningitis accounts for 5–9% of extrapulmonary tuberculosis [356]. It is associated with recent exposure to tuberculosis (particularly in children), tuberculosis infection elsewhere (particularly miliary tuberculosis), and with HIV infection. Tuberculous meningitis is notoriously difficult to diagnose early. It is a predominantly basal meningitis, preferentially affecting the sylvian fissures, basal cisterns, brainstem, and cerebellum. Most neurological consequences are due to an adhesive inflammatory exudate, granulomas coalescing to form tuberculomas (or sometimes abscesses), and an obliterative vasculitis [357].

The onset of tuberculous meningitis is often subacute. Symptoms include headache (50–80% of patients), fever (60–95%), vomiting (30–60%), photophobia (5–10%), and anorexia (60–80%). Signs include neck stiffness (40–80%), confusion (10–30%), coma (30–60%), cranial nerve palsy (30–50%, but particularly III [5–15%], IV, VI [30–40%], VII [10–20%]), hemiparesis (10–20%), paraparesis (5–10%), and seizures (children 50%, adults 5%). There may be signs of tuberculosis elsewhere (e.g. pulmonary, spinal), with systemic or other organ-specific symptoms (e.g. weight loss, night sweats, malaise, cough). Sometimes basal ganglia infarction occurs, with movement disorder (e.g. tremor, chorea, ballismus, myoclonus) [357]. Mental state change is more common in the elderly [356].

Evidence of active or past tuberculosis infection is seen on chest radiography in ~50%. There is hyponatraemia in 50%. Cerebrospinal fluid is normally (80–90%) clear, often with a raised opening pressure (>25 cmH_2O in 50%). There may be a neutrophil (10–70%) or lymphocyte (30–90%) CSF leukocytosis, typically with a raised protein (45–250 mg/dl); the CSF:plasma glucose ratio is <0.5 in 95% of cases. Contrast MRI may show basal meningeal enhancement, or sometimes tuberculomas or hydrocephalus. Diagnosis is by careful microscopy (with Ziehl–Neelsen staining for acid-fast bacilli) and specific culture of CSF, with PCR, particularly if antibiotics had been given prior to LP [357].

Rarely, tuberculous meningitis can present with paranoid psychosis [358], and auditory hallucinations have occurred in the context of intracranial tuberculoma [359]. Antituberculous therapy (e.g. isoniazid, ciprofloxacin, ethambutol; Chapter 15.1 ▶) can also cause psychosis.

8.1.7 Brucellosis

Brucellosis is a zoonosis caused by the bacterial genus *Brucella*, of which there are several species. Humans may catch it from ruminants (cows, goats, sheep, camels, buffalo, yaks), pigs, canines, and marine mammals. The most common route of human infection is consumption of unpasteurized goat's milk, but aerosolized body fluids may also cause occupational infection in vets and microbiologists. The incubation period is 1–8 weeks. *Brucella* invades and survives inside both phagocytic and non-phagocytic cells. It is rare in countries that screen and vaccinate domestic livestock, but common worldwide [360, 361]. It may present as an acute disease or a chronic infection.

Symptoms and signs are non-specific, but include fever (occurring in 98% of cases, but often intermittent), anorexia, weakness, fatigue, malaise, sweats, chills, joint paints, abdominal pain, constipation, diarrhoea, vomiting, headache, back pain, myalgia, cough, dyspnoea, weight loss, neuropsychiatric symptoms (including acute meningoencephalitis, myelitis and myelopathy, peripheral and cranial neuropathy, subarachnoid haemorrhage, anxiety, confusion, psychosis, depression, and insomnia), and testicular pain [360, 361]. Psychosis is not common, with one series exhibiting delusions and hallucinations in 1:750 cases, though it has been seen in acute and chronic brucellosis; delirium is more common [362–365]. However, psychiatric manifestations may be presenting features of CNS brucellosis [193]. Signs include hepatomegaly, splenomegaly, and relative bradycardia. There may be a variety of rashes (including ulcers, petechiae, purpura, and erythma nodosum) and inflammatory eye disease, and endocarditis also occurs. In chronic infection, low-grade fevers and neuropsychiatric symptoms predominate. Investigations may show non-specific findings such as leukopenia, relative lymphocytosis, pancytopenia, and slightly elevated liver enzymes. In neurobrucellosis, CSF often (88–98%) reveals a mild lymphocytic pleocytosis with elevated protein and normal glucose. Basal ganglia calcification occurs in about 14% of cases of CNS brucellosis [193]. Diagnosis is most commonly serological. Definitive diagnosis is by culture of blood or tissue (e.g. bone marrow, liver biopsy) with special culture techniques [360, 361].

8.1.8 Whipple's disease

Whipple's disease is a rare systemic infection caused by the *Tropheryma whipplei* (formerly *whippelii*) bacillus. Only of the order of 1000 cases have ever been reported. The most vulnerable group appear to be middle-aged white males but with an age range of 20–82. The mode of transmission is unknown but the organism has been described in the environment and faeco-oral transmission has been suggested. Microscopically, the jejunum is often involved, with a macrophage infiltration positive for the periodic acid–Schiff stain. However, there may be multi-organ infection. Untreated, it is fatal [366, 367].

Overall, the most common manifestations are diarrhoea, weight loss, abdominal pain, and arthralgia. There is a prodromal stage with a variety of non-specific symptoms, typically arthralgia and arthritis. The steady-state stage, on average 6 years later, is typified by weight loss and/or diarrhoea. Progression may be more rapid in the immunosuppressed. Classic Whipple's disease manifests with gastrointestinal symptoms as well as multi-organ involvement (e.g. joints, brain, heart, eyes), but pure neurological presentations can also occur, and culture-negative endocarditis may also be the initial feature [366].

Non-neurological features may include steatorrhoea and consequent malabsorption, abdominal masses, gastrointestinal bleeding, splenomegaly, and peritonitis; arthritis and arthralgia; myocarditis, pericarditis, and endocarditis; uveitis, other eye inflammation, and ophthalmoplegia; generalized hyperpigmentation sparing the buccal mucosa (occurring in 50%); generalized lymphadenopathy; pleuritis, pleural effusions, and pneumonitis [366].

Central nervous system involvement occurs in 10–50% of patients [366], and may be very varied. The commonest signs in CNS Whipple's disease [368] are cognitive changes (e.g. dementia) (71%), supranuclear gaze palsy (51%), altered consciousness (50%), and psychiatric signs (depression, euphoria, anxiety, psychosis, and/or personality change) (44%, though psychosis is not common [367]). Others include upper motor neuron signs (37%), hypothalamic dysfunction (polydipsia, hyperphagia, change in libido, amenorrhoea, changes in sleep–wake cycle, insomnia, hypersomnia) (31%), cranial nerve abnormalities (25%), myoclonus (25%), seizures (23%), ataxia (20%), and sensory deficits (12%). There may be hearing loss and vestibulo-ocular reflex impairment [366]. Extrapyramidal features are rare [369]. *Oculomasticatory myorhythmia* and *oculo-facial-skeletal myorhythmia* occur in only 20% [368] but are pathognomonic of Whipple's disease. Oculomasticatory myorhythmia is characterized by smooth, slow convergent–divergent pendular nystagmus with synchronous jaw contractions [366, 368]. Oculo-facial-skeletal myorhythmia is the same nystagmus associated with synchronous contraction of other body parts. These eye signs are always associated with supranuclear vertical gaze palsy. Sometimes there is chronic or recurrent meningitis [366].

The ESR is invariably raised and the malabsorption may cause iron or folate deficiency and hypoproteinaemia. Upper gastrointestinal endoscopy may reveal a range of changes including oesophagitis, gastritis, and duodenitis [366].

Diagnostic criteria for CNS Whipple's disease are as follows [368]. A diagnosis of *definite* CNS Whipple's disease requires any one of (1) oculomasticatory myorhythmia or oculo-facial-skeletal myorhythmia; (2) positive tissue histology; (3) positive tissue PCR. If the biopsy was not of CNS tissue, then for criteria 2 and 3 the patient must also display neurological signs. *Possible* disease requires (A) without another known cause, any one of (A1) fever of unknown origin; (A2) gastrointestinal symptoms (steatorrhoea, chronic diarrhoea, abdominal distension, or pain); (A3) chronic migratory arthritis or polyarthralgia; (A4) unexplained lymphadenopathy, night sweats, or malaise; *and* (B) without another known cause, any one of (B1) supranuclear vertical gaze palsy; (B2) rhythmic myoclonus; (B3) dementia with psychiatric symptoms (as defined above); (B4) hypothalamic manifestations (as defined above, excepting isolated somnolence). CSF PCR is a key initial diagnostic test for CNS Whipple's disease [370]. If the criteria for possible but not definite disease are met, multiple jejunal biopsies are indicated as the next step [368]. The differential diagnosis includes Lyme disease (Chapter 8.1.3 ▶) and cerebrotendinous xanthomatosis (Chapter 10.5.9 ▶) [20].

8.1.9 Other systemic bacterial infections with prominent neuropsychiatric effects

A large range of systemic bacterial infections can produce psychotic delirium (Chapter 3 ▶). Of these, some merit particular mention.

Typhus (Greek *tuphos* = smoke, vapour, stupor) [2] is caused by one of several *Rickettsia* infections. *Rickettsia* are bacteria that are obligate intracellular parasites. They are transmitted from arthropods (e.g. lice, ticks) and replicate in endothelium. The incubation period is about 2 weeks, varying with inoculation dose. Fever and headache are among the early symptoms, followed by a maculopapular or petechial rash at days 4–7. There may be generalized lymphadenopathy. Widespread endothelial damage may cause multi-organ involvement (e.g. increased vascular permeability, adult respiratory distress syndrome, myocarditis, rash, mild hepatosplenomegaly, encephalitis, renal impairment). There is a prominent inflammatory response, though the white cell count may be low early and then normal or mildly elevated. There may be hyponatraemia and mild elevation in hepatic transaminases. Diagnosis is clinical and by rash biopsy; serological diagnosis may provide later confirmation. Cutaneous eschars at the site of entry are not typical of typhus, though may occur with other rickettsial infections [26, 371]. Typhus caused neuropsychiatric disturbance in ~80% of one series frequently with psychosis [44].

Typhoid is due to infection with *Salmonella typhi*, transmitted faeco-orally. After an incubation period of 3–60 days (typically 7–14 days), high fever begins, often with constipation progressing to diarrhoea or dysentery and abdominal pain. There may be cough, sore throat, and epistaxis. There may be hepatosplenomegaly and a "rose spot" rash, which appears at the end of the first week. There is usually a normocytic anaemia, hyponatraemia, hypokalaemia, abnormal liver function tests, and deranged clotting [26]. Typhoid fever causes very frequent delirium (73%) with occasional acute psychosis (0.6%) [372], typically in the second to fourth week [26]. Diagnosis is by culture (of blood, urine, bone marrow, stool, CSF, bile, or rose spots) or serological/molecular techniques [26].

Rocky Mountain spotted fever is caused by *Rickettsia rickettsii*, transmitted by tick bites. It is restricted to the Americas, with most cases occurring in the USA, where it is the most common rickettsial infection with an annual incidence of 2.2 per million. The mean incubation period is 7 days (range 2–14). The classic triad is of fever, headache, and rash; this occurs in only 3% of patients within the first 3 days of illness, but in 60–70% of patients within the first 2 weeks following the tick bite. The disease typically begins with sudden-onset fever, malaise, and severe headache, usually with myalgia, anorexia, nausea, vomiting, abdominal pain, and photophobia. The rash occurs in 88–91% of patients and appears 2–5 days after the fever, beginning as 1–5 mm blanching erythematous macules on the wrists and ankles that spread to the palms and soles, and then to the limbs and trunk, evolving into a maculopapular rash with central petechiae. Other features may include pulmonary involvement (cough, pneumonia), hepatomegaly (clinically noticed in 12–25%), acute renal failure (in severe cases), ocular involvement (conjunctivitis [30%] and retinal vascular abnormalities including haemorrhage), muscular involvement (myositis), and neurological involvement (occurring in 40% of patients and including lethargy, photophobia, meningism, amnesia, bizarre behaviour, and transient deafness) [373]. Delusions or hallucinations were reported in 12% of one series, with mental state changes of some form in 60% [374]. Eschars are rare, as is myocarditis. Rocky Mountain spotted fever is virulent and may be fatal. There may be anaemia, thrombocytopenia, raised ALT and bilirubin, raised CK, and hyponatraemia. Antibodies are not detectable until 7–10 days after disease onset (and PCR of blood is not very sensitive, so antibody testing remains the gold standard for diagnosis) so treatment upon suspicion is vital [373].

Many of the "atypical pneumonias" may cause CNS involvement. ***Mycoplasma pneumoniae*** typically causes pneumonia with a dry cough, pharyngitis/otitis/conjunctivitis, and prominent systemic symptoms (malaise, headache), but neurological features occur in 6–7% [26, 375]. The most common neurological complication is meningitis or meningoencephalitis with alterations in mental status, and acute psychosis may be a feature [376]. ***Legionella pneumophila*** **(Legionnaire's disease)** is transmitted by droplet infection from contaminated water (e.g. air conditioning systems), with an incubation period of 7–10 days; this is followed by high fever, shivering, headache, and muscle pains. Dry cough progressing to dyspnoea is common. There are prominent extrapulmonary symptoms; diarrhoea and confusion are important clues to Legionnaire's disease [26], and there may be a relative bradycardia [375]. There is frequently leukocytosis with lymphopenia, hyponatraemia, and deranged liver function tests. Delirium and hallucinations are common, and encephalomyelitis may occur; cerebellar signs may also predominate [26, 376]. ***Coxiella burnetii*** **(Q fever)** is a zoonosis that may cause either a self-limiting febrile illness or a pneumonia typically associated with headache, dry cough, and sometimes pleuritic chest pain, nausea and vomiting, or diarrhoea. There are usually abnormalities of liver function tests, hyponatraemia, and thrombocytosis [26]. Q fever causes CNS manifestations in ~27% and can cause psychosis [377, 378]. Similarly, encephalitis and psychosis may feature in infection with ***Chlamydophila*** (formerly *Chlamydia*) ***pneumoniae*** [379], in which pharyngitis typically precedes pneumonia [26], and ***Chlamydophila psittaci*** **(psittacosis)**, which is transmitted from psittacine birds such as parrots and typified by headache, pneumonia with bloody sputum, and relative bradycardia [26, 375, 380]. Diagnosis of all of these is by CXR and serology, culture, or PCR to identify the organism (and, in the case of *Legionella*, urinary antigen detection).

8.2 Viral infection

Viral encephalitides will be considered here; the role of viral infection as a developmental insult predisposing to psychosis is discussed separately (Chapter 21.1 ▶).

Acute encephalitis should be suspected in any patient with fever, altered consciousness, and signs of diffuse cerebral dysfunction. Focal signs may also be present. A degree of leptomeningeal inflammation is invariably present, with corresponding signs and symptoms

[322]. Neuropsychiatric symptoms often predominate in encephalitis. In addition to aphasia, anosmia, agitation, and personality change [322, 1340], other psychiatric manifestations are common in acute viral encephalitis, with delusions (in 54% of patients in one series, preselected for psychiatric manifestations), hallucinations (auditory 44%, visual 13%, olfactory 3%, gustatory 1%), affective disorder (depression 21%, euphoria 6%), mutism (21%), catalepsy (16%), perseveration (9%), and perplexity, negativism, echolalia, and grimacing (1–4% each) [31, 33, 381]. Other forms of thought disorder and overexcitement may also feature [29]. In another series of patients with viral encephalitis not preselected for psychiatric disorder, but excluding HSV encephalitis and HIV, visual hallucinations were seen in 43% acutely, with auditory hallucinations in 28% and delusions in 27%; a year later, they were present in 10%, 8% and 7% respectively [1341].

In making the distinction between encephalitis and encephalopathy, the following may help to point towards encephalopathy: absence of fever, headache, and meningism; steady deterioration of mental status; absence of focal signs or focal seizures (except in hypoglycaemia); biochemical abnormalities consistent with a metabolic cause for encephalopathy; lack of a peripheral leukocytosis; normal CSF; diffuse slowing on EEG; normal MRI [322].

Establishing the cause of viral encephalitis requires a detailed history, usually from relatives. The geographical area and season are important clues. Recent foreign travel, insect bites, animal bites, and contact with individuals with infectious diseases must be sought [322]. Systemic examination may provide clues to viral or alternative diagnoses (e.g. rashes with VZV, rickettsial fever, Colorado tick fever, enteroviruses; mucous membrane lesions in herpes; upper respiratory tract infection with influenza and mycoplasmosis; parotitis in mumps; erythema nodosum in granulomatous infections such as tuberculosis and histoplasmosis). Neurological signs do not reliably differentiate the type of viral infection, but often include hemiparesis, aphasia, ataxia, pyramidal signs, cranial nerve deficits, myoclonus and tremors, and partial seizures; autonomic and hypothalamic dysfunction may also be seen (e.g. loss of temperature or vasomotor control, diabetes insipidus, SIADH). However, the constellation of frontotemporal signs with aphasia, personality change, and focal seizures is typical of HSV encephalitis, and multifocal lower motor neuron signs might suggest poliomyelitis [322]. Peripheral lymphocytosis is common in viral encephalitis. If acute encephalitis is suspected, emergency imaging (MRI if possible) should be performed, followed by CSF analysis unless there is a contraindication to LP, and EEG is strongly recommended; empirical aciclovir therapy for herpesvirus encephalitis is also usually used until CSF PCR results are available [322].

8.2.1 Herpesvirus encephalitis

All herpesviruses have the potential to establish latent infection, and are thus responsible for acute infections in the immunocompetent, and reactivation infections in the immunocompetent and the immunocompromised, depending on the virus [28]. Some cause significant primary infections and clinically obvious reactivation in the immunocompetent (e.g. HSV, VZV), while others cause very mild or no symptoms in primary infection and rarely reactivate symptomatically in the immunocompetent (e.g. CMV).

Herpes simplex virus (HSV) is the most common infectious cause of limbic encephalitis, and accounts for 11% of cases of acute encephalitis, with a case frequency of 1:250 000–1:500 000 per year. HSV-1 causes 90% of cases of herpes simplex encephalitis in adults and children, with an untreated mortality of 70%; HSV-2 is more common in neonates and the immunocompromised [28, 382]. The onset is acute or subacute (over <1 week). There is often (48%) a prodromal influenza-like illness [322]. Fever, headache, and mental state changes are common; the mental state changes include diminished consciousness, impaired memory and language, and personality change. Psychosis may be the presenting feature [383, 384]. Focal neurological deficits (e.g. hemiparesis) occur in ~50% of cases and seizures in ~66%. The CSF typically shows mild lymphocytic pleocytosis, increased protein, and normal glucose, with red cells in ~40%. MRI typically shows temporal lobe abnormalities on T2, FLAIR, and diffusion-weighted images; these may be unilateral or bilateral, and extratemporal abnormalities may also be seen. The insula, orbitofrontal region, and cingulate gyrus may also be affected. Occasionally the MRI is normal. The EEG is abnormal in ~85%, with focal slowing or lateralized epileptiform activity. Diagnosis is by MRI and then CSF PCR, which is >95% sensitive unless performed very early or late in the disease, and ~100% specific [47, 385, 1340].

Varicella zoster virus (VZV) accounts for 29% of CNS viral infections, making it the commonest cause of viral encephalitis [386]. Most typically, cerebral involvement with varicella presents as acute cerebellar ataxia, occurring in ~1:4000 children with varicella (primary VZV infection), within days to week of the varicella rash; this is probably a postinfectious syndrome (a benign variant of ADEM [Chapter 8.7.3 ▶]) [322]. In the immunosuppressed, VZV encephalitis may follow zoster (shingles; VZV reactivation) by days to months, or develop without a preceding rash. Symptoms may include fever, seizures, focal neurological deficit, and alteration in consciousness. Imaging in this context typically shows multifocal ischaemic and haemorrhagic infarctions, predominantly in white matter and at the grey–white matter junction [28], but the pattern can vary [387]. In the immunocompetent, a non-focal encephalitis is common, which may include psychosis [387]. Cerebrospinal fluid typically shows a lymphocytosis. Confirmation is by CSF serology or PCR [28].

Human herpesvirus 6 (HHV-6) is a ubiquitous neurotropic virus latent in most adults. It can lead to a limbic encephalitis, similar to that caused by HSV, typically following immunosuppression [388]. HHV-6 encephalitis has presented with psychosis in the immunocompetent, with normal MRI findings [389].

Cytomegalovirus (CMV) infection is extremely common, affecting 60–100% of adults depending on the country. Most primary infection is asymptomatic, though it may cause fever and lymphadenopathy. Occasionally it causes encephalitis, and has particular affinity for limbic structures [320]. In the immunodeficient, CMV encephalitis typically causes progressive cognitive impairment [28]. Confirmation is by CSF PCR [28]. CMV encephalitis has presented with schizophreniform psychosis [320]. Viruses related to CMV have been cultured from patients with psychosis and encephalopathy [390]. Studies of patients with schizophrenia have shown an association between negative symptoms and antibodies to CMV [391].

Epstein–Barr virus (EBV) infects 80–90% of children in developing countries by the age of 3, and has infected nearly 100% of adults by the third decade [28]. EBV infection causes infectious mononucleosis. Neurological involvement occurs in 1–5% and may include meningoencephalitis [22, 28, 392]. EBV infection may also cause psychosis without prominent systemic symptoms of infectious mononucleosis [393–396] and EBV antibody titres have been found to be significantly higher in patients with schizophrenia [397]. Infectious mononucleosis is diagnosed based on a positive heterophil antibody test, atypical lymphocytes appearing 1–4 weeks after disease onset, and/or changes in EBV-specific antibodies; CSF PCR does not distinguish latent from symptomatic EBV infection [28]. In AIDS, EBV can cause CNS lymphoma [28].

Casting the net broader, there are small studies suggesting an association of acute herpesvirus infection and psychosis without other manifestations of encephalitis. One study of patients admitted with first-onset psychosis found that 29% had a fourfold or greater elevation of serum and/or CSF antibodies over 2 weeks to one of a group of viruses including CMV, HSV-1, mumps, measles, VZV, and Japanese encephalitis virus [398]. Another found new-onset schizophrenia to be associated with higher levels of antibodies to CMV and *Toxoplasma gondii* (Chapter 8.3.2 ▶), and lower levels of antibodies to HHV-6 and VZV, but no differences in antibodies to HSV-1/2 or EBV [399].

The differential diagnosis of herpesvirus encephalitis includes other infectious encephalitides, PLE (Chapter 14.2 ▶) [400] and MELAS (Chapter 10.6 ▶) [401].

8.2.2 HIV encephalitis and AIDS dementia

Human immunodeficiency virus (HIV) is a lymphotropic and neurotropic virus that can cause psychosis directly, or by causing immunosuppression. The two forms, HIV-1 and HIV-2, are both originally zoonoses that are now transmitted sexually, vertically, and by blood contact [26]. The prevalence of HIV infection varies greatly, from 0.1% of adults in China to 26% in Swaziland [402]. Rates of infection are higher in patients with schizophrenia [34].

Acute infection produces a mild non-specific illness in 50–70% of patients, with fever, malaise, myalgia, lymphadenopathy, and pharyngitis. It typically occurs 2–6 weeks after exposure, and >50% of patients with seroconversion illness develop a rash (typically erythematous, maculopapular, and on the face and trunk). Acute encephalitis may occur during seroconversion [26], as may aseptic meningitis and myelopathy [33]. Symptomatically, fever and rash have the strongest association with primary HIV infection; fever and malaise have high sensitivity (80% and 68%, respectively); weight loss and oral ulceration have high specificity (86% and 85%) [403]. Diagnosis of HIV infection is by serology and/or PCR. Acute HIV infection is a time of viraemia but initial seronegativity. Seroconversion usually occurs within 3 months of infection, and very rarely after up to 6 months. Following acute infection, there is a latent period, lasting on average 10 years without therapy; this is a time of high viral turnover and load and high CD4-positive T-lymphocyte turnover but is asymptomatic, except that about a third of patients have persistent generalized lymphadenopathy. Overt immunosuppression characterizes AIDS. This is defined in Europe as HIV infection with at least one AIDS-defining infection or malignancy; the 1993 USA definition is broader, including also HIV infection with a CD4-positive T-cell count of <200/mm^3 [26, 404].

Central nervous system involvement is very common in HIV infection [405]. Psychosis may be the presenting manifestation of HIV infection or of AIDS [406, 407]. It may be a direct manifestation of HIV encephalopathy; the prevalence of new-onset psychosis in patients with HIV has ranged from 0.2–15%, and this included episodic and persistent psychosis [408].

However, established HIV infection greatly broadens the possible infectious differential diagnosis. The CD4-positive lymphocyte (T helper cell) count is a reliable indicator of HIV-related immunocompromise [26]; the normal CD4 count is >600/mm^3 and late HIV infection is associated with a CD4 count <200/mm^3. The most common neurological infections predisposed to by HIV are cerebral toxoplasmosis (Chapter 8.3.2 ▶), cryptococcal meningitis (Chapter 8.4 ▶), neurosyphilis (Chapter 8.1.2 ▶), and in late disease, progressive multifocal leukoencephalopathy (Chapter 8.2.4 ▶) and CMV encephalitis (Chapter 8.2.1 ▶) [26]. Failure to deal with viral infection also predisposes to CNS lymphoma. Ongoing HIV infection itself is not highly inflammatory [409].

Direct HIV neuronal infection causes HIV encephalopathy and AIDS dementia. Most patients dying of AIDS show neuronal loss, and up to 10% develop overt dementia. This begins with depression, poor concentration, and poor memory, but progressive intellectual and motor disability ensues (including slow movement, incoordination, weakness, and hyperreflexia), leading to a nearly vegetative state [26]. However, even in the early stages and in the absence of memory complaints, psychomotor speed impairment predicts progression to AIDS dementia. There is often early apathy, irritable mood, and anhedonia. Sleep disturbance, weight loss, restlessness, and anxiety are common. Psychosis develops in a significant number of patients (typically with paranoid delusions though hallucinations are also seen); in one series 15% of patients with HIV-associated dementia reported psychotic symptoms [33, 410]. In 5–8% of patients "AIDS mania" develops. Progression is rapid, with death typically within 2 years [22, 28]. Magnetic resonance imaging may show high-signal abnormalities on T2WI/FLAIR in the white matter and basal ganglia, possibly as a result of HIV neurotoxicity or HIV-induced vasculopathy, and cerebral atrophy [47]. Vitamin B_{12} deficiency (Chapter 11.4 ▶) occurs in up to 20% of patients with AIDS and can contribute to the neuropsychiatric syndrome, so should be checked for [411].

8.2.3 Other acute viral encephalitides

The range of viruses causing encephalitis is very wide. Many have been observed to cause psychosis, though as noted above, there is not often much to distinguish them in terms of neurological effects. Of the viral causes of acute encephalitis, herpesviruses and adenoviruses are DNA viruses; the rest are RNA viruses [28, 322].

Influenza A* virus accounts for 7% of viral encephalitis [386]. **Enteroviruses** (Coxsackie virus, echoviruses, other enteroviruses) account for 11% of viral encephalitis [386]. **Adenovirus** is a rare cause of acute encephalitis, though limbic encephalitis has been reported as a postinfectious syndrome following adenovirus infection [412]. A large range of **arboviruses** (arthropod-borne viruses, transmitted by mosquitos or ticks, of various genetic viral types including *Flaviviridae*, *Bunyaviridae*, and *Togaviridae*) can cause encephalitis. These include dengue, Colorado tick fever, Japanese B encephalitis*; the La Crosse strain of California virus; St Louis encephalitis virus*; West Nile encephalitis virus; Murray Valley encephalitis virus; lymphocytic choriomeningitis virus; Powassan virus; and Eastern*†, Western, and Venezuelan equine encephalitis viruses [28, 322]. **Other** causes of encephalitis include poliovirus (another enterovirus), measles*, mumps*, and rubella, each with a characteristic systemic syndrome, and Nipah virus* (a zoonosis characterized by encephalitis and respiratory disease). Diagnosis of all these specific viral encephalitides is typically by serum and/or CSF serology [28].

Of these, psychosis and catatonia have been reported in those marked * and †, respectively [31, 320, 413–421], but as discussed above, psychotic symptoms are a common manifestation of viral encephalitis in general. Encephalitis related to measles is rare but occurs as an early postinfectious autoimmune encephalitis, SSPE, or subacute measles encephalitis (Chapter 8.2.4 ▶).

Rabies is a specifically neurotropic virus, usually acquired from the bite of an infected mammal (e.g. dogs, foxes, skunks, raccoons, bats in endemic areas), or aerosolized secretions from a rabid animal. Human infection is rare. The virus enters peripheral nerves following inoculation, then spreads at 12–24 mm/day to the spinal ganglion, multiplies there (causing pain or paraesthesiae at the site of the inoculation in 50%; this is pathognomonic), spreads quickly (200–400 mm/day) to the CNS, causes a rapidly progressive encephalitis, and spreads to the periphery and salivary glands [422]. The incubation period depends on the size of the inoculum and its proximity to the CNS; it is usually 20–90 days, and is less than 1 year in >90% of cases, though the longest documented is 19 years. There is no immune response during the incubation period. If treatment is not initiated before the onset of symptoms, death is almost certain. The acute neurological phase (duration 2–7 days) is typically "furious" rabies, with agitation, hyperactivity, restlessness, thrashing, biting, confusion, or hallucinations. In 50%, hydrophobia and aerophobia occur; these are virtually pathognomonic. Attempts to drink, or having air blown in the face, trigger severe laryngeal and diaphragmatic spasms and a sensation of choking; even the suggestion of drinking may induce spasm. There may be autonomic instability, cranial nerve involvement, fasciculations, and seizures. After hours to days, the pattern becomes episodic, with brief furious episodes (spontaneous or triggered by visual, auditory, or tactile stimuli) lasting <5 minutes interspersed with calm and lucid periods. The furious phase may end in death, or paralysis. In 20% of patients, "dumb" rabies develops instead: in this, paralysis develops from the outset (commonly with fever and headache; paralysis is or rapidly becomes symmetric and may resemble Guillain–Barré syndrome). Coma follows within 10 days of onset of the acute neurological phase, and is followed by death. The most rapid test is based on nucleic acid sequence-based amplification (NASBA; essentially, a technique that is to RNA what PCR is to DNA) of saliva and CSF, but culture and skin biopsy may also be definitive [20, 422]. Rabies has presented with psychosis suspected of being schizophrenia, with persecutory delusions, and with mania [423, 424].

8.2.4 Other subacute viral encephalitides

Subacute sclerosing panencephalitis (SSPE) is a rare, slowly progressive encephalitis due to measles virus. There is degeneration of grey and white matter. Clinically, it begins several 7–12 years after measles infection in early childhood, and is characterized by neuropsychiatric abnormalities (which may include psychosis as the presenting feature, as well as forgetfulness, irritability, and mood changes) followed by intellectual deterioration, motor rigidity, and myoclonic jerks that progress to coma and death within 1–3 years, or rarely up to 10 years [22, 28, 425, 426]. The EEG typically shows generalized periodic complexes, often lasting up to 3 s, with 3–15 s between complexes [28]. MRI typically shows high-intensity lesions on T2WI/FLAIR in the periventricular regions, subcortical white matter, basal ganglia, cerebellum, and pons, later with diffuse cerebral atrophy [47]. In immunosuppressed patients, a **subacute measles encephalitis** can also occur, with features of encephalitis developing 1–9 months after exposure to, or overt, measles [28].

Progressive multifocal leukoencephalopathy (PML) is due to JC virus, a polyomavirus and papovavirus. This virus is ubiquitous (antibodies to it are present in 85% of people by the age of 9) and is latent in the kidneys. Impaired cell-mediated immunity (e.g. AIDS, chronic lymphocytic leukaemia, immunosuppressant drugs) allows viral reactivation and infection of oligodendrocytes, leading to demyelination. The clinical features are of focal neurological deficits, seizures, memory impairment, psychomotor retardation, and inattentiveness; catatonia has occurred [28, 427], as have hallucinations [428], though schizophrenia-like psychosis is rare [94]. There are multifocal demyelinating plaques involving subcortical white matter, which may be seen on MRI [47]. Diagnosis is by CSF PCR [429].

8.3 Protozoal infection

8.3.1 Malaria

Malaria is caused by infection with *Plasmodium falciparum*, *P. vivax*, *P. ovale*, or *P. malariae*, all transmitted by the female *Anopheles* mosquito but also exceptionally by blood-borne contact. Falciparum malaria is the most dangerous. The incubation period before symptoms is 6–14 days for falciparum malaria (rarely up to 4 months) or slightly longer for non-falciparum malaria. *P. vivax* and *P. ovale* can remain dormant in the liver; the longest reported incubation period for vivax malaria is 30 years. Symptoms occur when dividing parasites in the schizont stage rupture and erythrocytes are destroyed. Presentation can be gradual (resembling a viral illness) or fulminant. The majority of patients experience fever (>92% of cases), chills (79%), headaches (70%), and sweating (64%). Other common symptoms include dizziness, malaise, myalgia, abdominal pain, nausea, vomiting, mild diarrhoea, and dry cough. Physical signs include fever, tachycardia, jaundice, pallor, postural hypotension, hepatomegaly, and splenomegaly. Investigations typically show thrombocytopenia (60%), raised bilirubin (40%), anaemia (30%), and raised ALT (25%), usually with a neutrophilia, a normal or low lymphocyte count, and a raised CRP and ESR [430]. Severe malaria may cause severe haemolysis, haemoglobinuria ("blackwater fever"), acidosis, pulmonary oedema, cerebral oedema, hypoglycaemia, and renal failure. The combination of thrombocytopenia and raised bilirubin in hospitalized febrile returning travellers is strongly predictive of malaria [431].

Malaria can cause psychosis, sometimes as part of the presenting syndrome (in cerebral malaria), and sometimes after recovery from parasitaemia (postmalaria neurological syndrome) [430, 432–436]. The frequency of psychosis in cerebral malaria is approximately 5% [432]. Malaria must always be considered in the differential diagnosis of psychiatric disorders if the patient is in or has returned from an endemic area [29]. The key element in diagnosis is fever and a history of travel to an endemic area. All such patients require exclusion of malaria by examination of thick and thin blood films. PCR is more sensitive but is specific to a given species [430].

Note also that some antimalarials (chloroquine, hydroxychloroquine, mefloquine; Chapter 15.1 ▶) can cause psychosis [27, 437, 438].

8.3.2 Toxoplasmosis

Toxoplasma gondii is a protozoan that infects 20–60% of humans. Transmission is faeco-orally from cats (the definitive host), by consumption of undercooked meat containing tissue cysts, maternofetally, and rarely by transplantation [439, 440]. It has three forms: oocytes (produced in cats), tachyzoites (rapidly replicating parasites), and cysts. It has a high affinity for brain tissue as well as muscle, where tachyzoites may form tissue cysts and persist for the life of the host.

Symptomatic cerebral toxoplasmosis may manifest as seizures and/or focal neurological deficit, behavioural changes with psychosis and dementia, or chronic meningism with altered consciousness and/or seizures, reflecting a spectrum of focal encephalitis, multifocal encephalitis, and diffuse meningoencephalitis [440]. Acute *Toxoplasma* encephalitis can present with psychosis, with one study showing psychiatric symptoms in 21% of cases [441, 442]; such serious disease is more common in the immunodeficient (e.g. AIDS, malignancy, collagen-vascular diseases, drug-induced immunosuppression). Diagnosis of *Toxoplasma* infection is by serology, though PCR and biopsy is sometimes required. MRI is more sensitive than CT for the identification of overt cerebral toxoplasmosis [443, 444].

Toxoplasmosis also has more subtle behavioural effects. In rodents, *Toxoplasma* infection selectively alters the host's behaviour in a way that increases their exposure to predation by cats [445, 446]. Human behaviour is also different in those with latent *Toxoplasma* infection, as defined by the presence of antibodies [447]. Maternal *Toxoplasma* infection is a risk factor for schizophrenia in the offspring [448, 449]. In patients at ultra-high risk for developing psychosis, serum IgG levels against *T. gondii* are positively correlated with the severity of positive psychotic symptoms in *Toxoplasma*-positive individuals [450]. The prevalence of IgG antibodies against *T. gondii* is higher in patients with psychosis than controls, including in patients with first-episode schizophrenia [451–454]. Valproic acid and several antipsychotics, including haloperidol, are potent inhibitors of *T. gondii* replication [22, 446]. A meta-analysis has shown the odds ratio for schizophrenia risk associated with positive *T. gondii* serology to be 2.73 (95% CI 2.10–3.60) [320, 454].

8.3.3 Trypanosomiasis

African trypanosomiasis (sleeping sickness) is caused by *Trypanosoma brucei*, transmitted to humans by tsetse flies. The disease is confined to between latitudes 15° N and 20° S. East African trypanosomiasis (caused by *T. brucei rhodesiense*) has its onset rapidly, with symptoms beginning with 1 month, whereas West African trypanosomiasis (*T. brucei gambiense*) can have a latent period of months to a year; thus, it may present with psychiatric features in patients who have travelled to endemic areas [455].

Stage 1 disease is haemolymphatic. Occasionally a chancre develops at the site of the bite, 5–15 days after the bite. Subsequently, parasites replicate in the blood and lymphatics, causing intermittent fever, malaise, myalgia, and arthritis, usually 3 weeks after the bite. There may be generalized or local (posterior cervical, axillary, or inguinal) lymphadenopathy, splenomegaly, and weight loss. Transient urticarial, erythematous, or macular rashes may appear 6–8 weeks after onset. Sometimes there are oedematous, centrally pale, erythematous macules on the trunk. In a minority of patients the hypersensitivity reaction may include facial oedema. There may be haemolytic anaemia and pancarditis (which may lead to arrhythmia and death) [455].

Stage 2 disease involves CNS invasion; a meningoencephalitis causes behavioural and neurological changes. Typically, there are headaches, daytime somnolence and night-time insomnia, behavioural changes including irritability, mood swings, anorexia, and sometimes depression. There may be sensory disorders, speech disorders, extrapyramidal signs (including tremor and increased muscle tone), and sometimes ataxia and hemiparesis, but rarely meningism. There may be a delayed sensation of pain (Kerandel sign) [455]. Psychosis may be part of the presenting features [455–457], as may mania [455]. In children, there may be seizures. Stupor and coma may ensue. The two disease stages are less clearly separated in East African trypanosomiasis [455].

There is typically anaemia, hypergammaglobulinaemia (with particularly elevated IgM), a raised ESR, thrombocytopenia, and low albumin, but not eosinophilia or altered liver function. Cerebrospinal fluid shows a leukocytosis with elevated protein and IgM and raised intracranial pressure. Raised CSF IgM is very sensitive for CNS involvement. Definitive diagnosis is by demonstration of trypanosomes in blood, lymph nodes, CSF, chancre aspirates, or bone marrow [455].

In contrast, American trypanosomiasis (Chagas' disease) is caused by *Trypanosoma cruzi*. Catatonia (Chapter 19 ▶) has been described in Chagas' encephalitis [458], but not psychosis.

8.4 Fungal infection (mycosis)

Systemic fungal infections are rare except in the immunocompromised. They may be focal or disseminated. Neurological involvement may include brain abscess (e.g. *Aspergillus, Candida, Cryptococcus, Histoplasma capsulatum, Coccidioides*) [459], fungal vasculitis (e.g. *Histoplasma, Coccidioides*) (see Chapter 13.2.5 ▶) and meningitis/encephalitis (e.g. *Candida, Cryptococcus*). As for other causes of abscesses and encephalitis, psychosis can occur.

Of particular note, *Cryptococcus neoformans* infection (**cryptococcosis**) is the most common systemic fungal infection in patients with HIV, and occurs in other immunosuppressed groups; it is also the most common cause of chronic meningitis in Papua New Guinea. Its most common presentation is with a subacute meningitis or meningoencephalitis with fever, malaise, headache, and altered cognition, behaviour, and/or level of consciousness. Signs of meningism occur in only 25–33%. There may be cranial nerve palsies. The CSF usually has an elevated opening pressure, and shows a mildly elevated protein, normal or slightly low glucose, and a lymphocytic pleocytosis. Diagnosis is by India ink staining of the CSF to show the yeast, or cryptococcal antigen testing [26]. A significant finding on MRI is dilated Virchow–Robin spaces (the invaginations of the subarachnoid space into the brain associated with leptomeningeal vessels, seen in characteristic locations including the basal ganglia), as are miliary enhancing nodules [47]. The meningoencephalitis can present with psychosis [460].

8.5 Eosinophilic meningitis and meningoencephalitis, helminths, and macroparasites

Eosinophilic meningitis is defined as ≥10 eosinophils/μl of CSF, or eosinophilia of ≥10% of the total CSF leukocyte count. The most common cause is helminth infection. Psychosis has been reported in eosinophilic meningoencephalitis [461].

Parasitic causes of eosinophilic meningitis include *Angiostrongylus catonensis* (rat lungworm), the most common cause worldwide; gnathostomiasis (a worm hosted by dogs and cats); baylisascariasis (raccoon roundworm); other helminths; neurocysticercosis; cerebral paragonimiasis; neurotrichinosis; cerebral toxocariasis; and cerebral/spinal schistosomiasis.

Other infectious causes include *fungi* (*Coccidioides immitis*), *bacteria* (syphilis [Chapter 8.1.2 ▶], tuberculosis [Chapter 8.1.6 ▶]), *rickettsiae* (Rocky Mountain spotted fever [Chapter 8.1.9 ▶]), and *viruses* (coxsackie B4, chronic lymphocytic choriomeningitis virus) [462].

Non-infectious causes include *malignancy* (Hodgkin's disease, non-Hodgkin's lymphoma, eosinophilic leukaemia), *drugs* (ciprofloxacin, ibuprofen, intraventricular vancomycin, intraventricular gentamicin, intraventricular dye), *ventriculoperitoneal shunts, sarcoidosis* (Chapter 13.5 ▶), and *idiopathic hypereosinophilic syndrome* (Chapter 18.2 ▶) [462].

Neurocysticercosis, the most common parasitic disease of the nervous system, merits particular mention. It is due to infection with *Taenia solium*, the pork tapeworm. If humans ingest pig muscle infected with larval cysticerci, they develop an adult tapeworm (which excretes eggs), but if humans ingest eggs, the eggs release oncospheres that can develop into cysticerci in any organ, but particularly in muscle, brain, eyes, and subcutaneously. In the brain the cysticerci can cause epilepsy (in 70% of cases), headaches, intracranial hypertension, eosinophilic meningitis, and stroke [463]. It is a common cause of epilepsy worldwide. The presentation is frequently psychiatric, and it causes psychosis in 3–14% of cases, though depression (53%) and cognitive decline (16%) are more common [464]. Diagnosis is by imaging, CSF analysis, and serology.

8.6 Protein infection: Creutzfeldt–Jakob disease and other prion diseases

Creutzfeldt–Jakob disease (CJD) is a prion-induced spongiform encephalopathy. It may be sporadic, familial, or infectious. Infectious CJD may be variant CJD (vCJD) secondary to infection with bovine spongiform encephalopathy, or iatrogenic CJD secondary to cross-infection. Prion protein (PrP) can exist in two conformation states, PrP^{C} (the normal form) and PrP^{Sc} (the pathogenic form). PrP^{Sc} induces the conversion of PrP^{C} into PrP^{Sc}, initiating a vicious cycle of PrP^{Sc} formation, and PrP^{Sc} is deposited as amyloid. There is neuronal loss, gliosis, and spongiform change. CJD disease has an annual incidence of 1:1 000 000, except in Libyan-born Israelis and some populations in Slovakia, where the incidence is much higher. Most cases are sporadic; about 10% are familial [465]. Variant CJD has an incubation period that is estimated as 10–12 years [466]. The age of onset of vCJD is typically much earlier than sporadic CJD (29 years versus 65 years), and vCJD has slower progression [22].

Sporadic CJD typically presents with rapidly progressive cognitive impairment, cerebellar dysfunction, or both. Behavioural abnormalities, higher cortical dysfunction, cortical visual abnormalities, cerebellar dysfunction, and pyramidal and extrapyramidal signs all rapidly develop. Almost all patients with sporadic CJD develop myoclonic jerks involving a limb or the whole body (and 70% of those with vCJD develop myoclonus over the disease course, though myoclonus is rare at the onset of vCJD). Sensory symptoms (particularly limb pain) and psychiatric abnormalities are much commoner in the presentation of vCJD, including depression, poor memory and concentration, emotional lability, psychomotor retardation, paranoid delusions, and hallucinations [28, 465, 466]. Indeed, auditory or visual hallucinations, paranoid delusions, thought insertion, thought withdrawal, and inappropriate affect occur in up to 50% of patients with vCJD [22]. Psychiatric involvement of some sort occurs in 66% of patients at onset and 98% over the course of the disease [28]. However, even sporadic CJD commonly features depression, and an estimated 10% of cases are admitted under psychiatry [467].

During sporadic CJD, most patients develop characteristic EEG signs of periodic (~1 Hz) paroxysms of sharp waves or spikes on a slow background. These periodic complexes have a sensitivity of 67% and specificity of 87% on a single EEG; repeated EEGs demonstrate abnormalities in >90% of patients. In vCJD, the EEG is often normal. Magnetic resonance imaging is very useful and a combination of DWI and FLAIR imaging is sensitive and specific; the typical finding is of bilateral increased signal intensity in the globus pallidus, putamen, and caudate (CJD), or in the pulvinar and mediodorsal thalamus (vCJD). Cerebrospinal fluid typically contains 14-3-3 protein (sensitivity and specificity of ~96% in sporadic CJD but sensitivity 50% and specificity 91% in vCJD; it can also occur in MS, Chapter 6.8 ▶) [20] and/or tau protein (sensitivity 80% and specificity 94% in vCJD). Genetic testing of the PrP gene is available. Tonsil biopsy may be used to demonstrate PrP immunoreactivity, and brain biopsy is sometimes performed. Pathologically, vCJD is distinguished from CJD primarily by greater cerebellar involvement. Investigations must also be targeted at excluding other conditions, such as antithyroid antibody testing to exclude Hashimoto's encephalopathy (Chapter 14.1 ▶), and paraneoplastic antibodies with CT of the chest, abdomen, and pelvis to exclude a paraneoplastic syndrome (Chapter 14.2 ▶) [22, 28, 47, 465, 466]. See also NAIM (Chapter 14.3 ▶) and bismuth poisoning (Chapter 15.6.8 ▶), which can be mimics of CJD.

The other human prion diseases are **kuru**, **Gerstmann–Sträussler–Scheinker disease** (GSS), **fatal familial insomnia** (FFI), and **sporadic fatal insomnia**. All are rarer than CJD. Kuru was described in Papua New Guinea and is acquired via cannibalism (presumably initially from spontaneous CJD), while the others are due to mutations in the PrP gene; sporadic fatal insomnia can be due to spontaneous PrP gene mutation or spontaneous PrP protein conversion [465]. Of these, psychosis has been described in GSS [468] and as the presenting feature of FFI [469]. Gerstmann–Sträussler–Scheinker disease presents with a slowly progressive limb and truncal ataxia with dementia, and has autosomal dominant inheritance [465]. Fatal familial insomnia is an autosomal dominant disorder characterized by degeneration within a subset of thalamic nuclei (anterior, mediodorsal, dorsolateral, and pulvinar) (MIM 600072). It usually presents in patients aged 18–60 with severe insomnia, autonomic dysregulation (hyperthermia, hypertension, tachycardia, tachypnoea, hyperhidrosis), dementia, and motor paralysis [465]. It can produce psychosis and catatonia (MIM 600072); complex hallucinations representing disordered REM sleep may be one reason [33].

8.7 Autoimmune disease following infection

8.7.1 Sydenham's chorea and PANDAS

Sydenham's chorea (rheumatic chorea; St Vitus' dance) is chorea occurring in the setting of rheumatic fever. It is most common in children. In the USA, the annual incidence of rheumatic fever is low at 0.5–2 per 100 000, and chorea occurs in 10–20% of patients with rheumatic fever. Rheumatic fever is triggered by group A beta-haemolytic streptococcal infection (*Streptococcus pyogenes*), and antibodies cross-react with "self" tissues. Sydenham's chorea is associated with antineuronal antibodies that bind to the caudate and subthalamic nucleus. The neurological disease may lag behind the infection (and the arthritis and carditis) by some months, and children typically have diffuse chorea, motor impersistence (the inability to sustain simple voluntary acts), and variable degrees of weakness [28]. Psychiatric symptoms are prominent, and often precede the chorea; they typically include emotional lability, poor attention, and obsessive–compulsive symptoms [470–472]. Psychosis has been reported following acute Sydenham's chorea [473, 474], including in pregnancy, when the disease tends to be more severe (**chorea gravidarum**) [475]. A history of Sydenham's chorea has been reported to be more frequent in patients with psychosis than controls [476].

Diagnosis is clinical, supported by serological evidence of recent streptococcal infection (antistreptolysin O titre, anti-DNAse B) and anti-basal ganglia antibodies [474]. The Jones criteria for acute rheumatic fever [477] are as follows. *Major manifestations* are carditis (e.g. new murmur, heart failure, pericarditis), polyarthritis (almost always migratory), chorea, erythema marginatum, and subcutaneous nodules. *Minor manifestations* are arthralgia, fever, elevated acute phase reactants (ESR and/or CRP), and a prolonged PR interval on ECG. *Supporting evidence of preceding group A streptococcal infection* includes positive throat culture or streptococcal antigen test, or positive or rising antistreptococcal antibody titre (e.g. ASO). In the presence of such supporting evidence, two major manifestations, or one major and two minor manifestations, indicate a high probability of rheumatic fever.

Sydenham's chorea is part of a wider spectrum known as **paediatric autoimmune neuropsychiatric disorders associated with streptococcal infections (PANDAS)** of the group A beta-haemolytic type [478].

8.7.2 Encephalitis lethargica

Encephalitis lethargica (von Economo's disease) is a long-known disease, epidemic in 1916–1927, that presented with pharyngitis followed by sleep disorder (often hypersomnolence), basal ganglia signs (particularly parkinsonism, which often persisted as postencephalitic parkinsonism), cranial nerve palsies, and neuropsychiatric sequelae. Pathologically, it was an encephalitis of midbrain and basal ganglia. There is debate as to the cause, with influenza virus infection often suggested, but modern studies have cast doubt on this explanation and a recent similar series suggests that it may represent a postinfectious autoimmune disorder, with autoantibodies against the basal ganglia, thus resembling Sydenham's chorea [472]. Some patients in this series presented with psychiatric disturbance including mutism, paranoia, and hallucinations, and psychosis persisted in some [17, 25, 33, 472]. Postencephalitic parkinsonism was associated with a high frequency of delusions [36].

8.7.3 Postinfectious encephalomyelitis and acute disseminated encephalomyelitis

Postmeasles encephalomyelitis is an autoimmune syndrome occurring within 2 weeks of the onset of the measles rash, with a recurrence of fever associated with decreased consciousness, seizures, and multifocal neurological abnormalities; mortality is 20% [28]. Psychosis described soon after measles infection likely represents this entity [417].

Postinfectious encephalomyelitis is one form of acute disseminated encephalomyelitis (ADEM), a term that also encompasses post-vaccination encephalomyelitis. It is probably due to an autoimmune attack on myelin, and thus resembles MS in many ways. Acute disseminated encephalomyelitis is often very severe compared to acute events in MS, but is usually not relapsing nor progressive. It can occur in adults or children. It may follow a large number of immunological insults, including measles (1:1000), VZV (1:10 000) ("postvaricella encephalitis"), rubella (1:20 000), and the original Pasteur rabies vaccine (1:3000–1:35 000); there are many other recognized viral, bacterial, and vaccine triggers and it has even followed bee stings [28, 479].

An antecedent infection is identifiable in two-thirds of children but less than half of adults. Acute disseminated encephalomyelitis typically occurs 1–14 days after non-neural vaccines, and within a week of exanthematous illnesses. Neurological features are very variable, and may be focal or non-focal with an encephalopathy (which is almost invariable in measles-associated disease). Acute psychosis is an uncommon but recognized presentation of ADEM in adolescents and young adults [479, 480]. Cerebrospinal fluid shows a lymphocytic pleocytosis and elevated protein; CSF oligoclonal bands occur but less often than in MS. Magnetic resonance imaging may be normal until 5–14 days after symptom onset, and then typically shows demyelinating lesions [479].

Chapter 9 Endocrine disease

9.1 Hypothyroidism and hyperthyroidism

Hypothyroidism has long been known as a cause of psychosis ("myxoedema madness") in young and old, and psychosis can be the presenting feature [21, 481]. The prevalence of hypothyroidism is about 4.6% (0.3% overt, 4.3% subclinical), with a female:male ratio of about 2–8:1 [482] and psychosis occurs in perhaps ~2% of hypothyroid patients [25, 28, 483, 484]. Psychosis is common in hypothyroid elderly patients with concomitant cerebrovascular disease [485]. In older series, psychosis was reported in over 40% of patients [485], perhaps reflecting selection of more severe disease. Hypothyroidism may also cause mania, depression, cognitive impairment, memory impairment, and full-blown dementia. Systemically, it can cause fatigue, cold intolerance, dry skin, dry/thin hair, weight gain, constipation, nerve entrapment syndromes (e.g. carpal tunnel syndrome), deafness, ataxia, muscle weakness, muscle cramps, menstrual disturbance (menorrhagia and later oligomenorrhoea or amenorrhoea), infertility, bradycardia, diastolic hypertension, hoarseness, goitre, periorbital and peripheral oedema, galactorrhoea, yellow skin (due to carotenes), hyporeflexia, slow-relaxing tendon reflexes, and pleural/pericardial effusions. There may be hypercholesterolaemia, hyponatraemia (Chapter 12.5.1 ▶), hyperprolactinaemia, hyperhomocysteinaemia (Chapter 10.3.2 ▶), anaemia, CK elevation, and raised creatinine. Rarely, there may be myxoedema coma, with collapse, hypothermia, and cardiac failure [26, 482, 486, 487].

Worldwide, the most common cause of hypothyroidism is iodine deficiency. In iodine-replete areas, the most common cause is autoimmune (Hashimoto's) thyroiditis, which has a 7:1 female:male ratio, and is associated with other autoimmune disease. Other causes include congenital thyroid dysgenesis; thyroid injury (including by radiation and surgery); drugs that incidentally impair thyroid function (including lithium and amiodarone); antithyroid drugs (e.g. radioiodine, carbimazole); infiltrative diseases (e.g. haemochromatosis, amyloidosis, sarcoidosis); subacute (de Quervain's) thyroiditis and lymphocytic (postpartum) thyroiditis, both of which generally involve transient thyrotoxicosis followed by hypothyroidism; and hypothalamic or pituitary dysfunction [486]. Always consider inadequate thyroid hormone replacement in those known to be hypothyroid.

Hyperthyroidism is much less common than hypothyroidism (prevalence 0.05–1.3%) but psychosis is proportionally more common in hyperthyroidism at 10–20% [483, 485, 488], though some series put the estimate lower, at 1%, with most being depressive psychosis

[25, 33]. There is a slight female>male predominance. Hyperthyroidism can cause hyperactivity, irritability, heat intolerance, sweating, palpitations (sinus tachycardia or atrial fibrillation), insomnia, fatigue, weakness, weight loss with increased appetite (rarely weight gain), diarrhoea, steatorrhoea, polyuria, oligomenorrhoea, loss of libido, fine tremor, goitre, palmar erythema, onycholysis, pruritus, urticaria, alopecia, muscle wasting and proximal myopathy, hyperreflexia, eyelid retraction or lid lag, gynaecomastia, thyroid dermopathy (e.g. pretibial myxoedema), and thyroid acropachy. There may be hyperglycaemia, hypercalcaemia (Chapter 12.5.4 ▶), deranged LFTs, hypocortisolaemia (Chapter 9.3 ▶), leukocytosis, and (in thyrotoxic periodic paralysis) hypokalaemia (Chapter 12.5.5 ▶). In Graves' disease, 50–80% of patients have ophthalmopathy, including exophthalmos (proptosis). Rarely, hyperthyroidism causes chorea or impaired consciousness. In thyroid storm (thyrotoxic crisis), there is severe hypermetabolism with high fever, tachycardia, nausea and vomiting, tremor, agitation, and psychosis, progressing to coma with heart failure and hypotension; it is an emergency [26, 488].

Graves' disease, caused by TSH-receptor-stimulating antibodies, accounts for 60–80% of cases of hyperthyroidism. Most of the rest are accounted for by nodular thyroid disease (toxic multinodular goitre and toxic adenoma). Other causes include drugs (iodine excess, lithium, amiodarone), thyroid carcinoma, mutations of the TSH receptor or a stimulatory G-protein (these causes underlie many cases of toxic adenoma), ectopic thyroid tissue (the very rare struma ovarii), ingestion of excess thyroid hormone, a TSH-secreting pituitary tumour, tumours that secrete HCG, and gestational thyrotoxicosis. Rarely, hyperthyroidism occurs in the early phase of thyroid destruction, as stored thyroid hormone is liberated, such as in autoimmune thyroiditis ("hashitoxicosis"), subacute thyroiditis, and lymphocytic thyroiditis [26, 486, 489].

Psychosis in the early treatment of thyroid disease. Psychosis and mania have also occurred early in the initiation of levothyroxine hormone replacement treatment for hypothyroidism, sometimes while biochemical testing still indicated hypothyroidism [490–492], and sometimes early in the drug treatment of hyperthyroidism [25].

Diagnosis of thyroid abnormalities. Diagnosis is by clinical assessment of thyroid status, measurement of TSH, and if this is abnormal, free T4 ± free T3. Measurement of total T4 and T3 levels is unhelpful as the free (biologically active) hormone levels are related both to total hormone levels and to levels of binding protein, mostly thyroxine-binding globulin [26]. The basic principle underlying diagnosis is that hypothalamic TRH stimulates pituitary TSH release; pituitary TSH stimulates T4 production, with some T3 production and subsequent peripheral tissue conversion of T4 to T3; and thyroid hormones suppress TRH and TSH production via negative feedback.

Measurement of TSH is more sensitive than measurement of free thyroid hormone levels. A normal TSH is generally held to rule out clinically significant primary thyroid dysfunction [26], though see below. The most common patterns of abnormality in thyroid disease are a raised TSH with normal or low free thyroid hormone levels (subclinical or overt hypothyroidism, respectively) and a low TSH with normal or raised free thyroid hormone levels (subclinical or overt hyperthyroidism). Pituitary failure may cause hypothyroidism with a low TSH and consequent low free thyroid hormone levels, and a TSH-secreting pituitary adenoma may cause hyperthyroidism with a raised TSH and consequent raised free thyroid hormone levels. However, a number of other conditions may confuse the picture, as follows.

A raised TSH may be due to overt hypothyroidism (free thyroid hormone levels will be low), subclinical hypothyroidism (free thyroid hormone levels normal), sick euthyroid syndrome (low or normal), acute administration of dopamine antagonists (normal), a TSH-secreting pituitary adenoma (raised), thyroid hormone resistance syndrome (raised), or adrenal insufficiency (low or normal) [26]. A raised TSH with a normal or raised free T4 may also be due to non-compliance with thyroid replacement therapy until shortly before the blood test is due [493].

A low TSH may be due to overt thyrotoxicosis (free thyroid hormone levels will be raised), subclinical hyperthyroidism (free thyroid hormone levels normal), recently treated hyperthyroidism (normal), thyroid-associated ophthalmopathy without Graves' disease (normal), thyroxine over-replacement (normal or raised), sick euthyroid syndrome (low or normal), the first trimester of pregnancy (normal or raised), pituitary or hypothalamic disease (low or normal), anorexia nervosa (low or normal), acute administration of dopamine or somatostatin (normal), or glucocorticoids (normal) [26].

Abnormal TSH should prompt the measurement of free T4. Free T3 measurement is of no value in hypothyroidism, but is a sensitive test for hyperthyroidism, as it is usually raised more than T4 and sometimes is raised with a normal T4 ("T3 toxicosis") [493].

No biochemical test of thyroid function is wholly reliable in patients with non-thyroidal illness [493]. Any major illness can cause the "sick euthyroid" syndrome, in which T3 levels decrease and reverse T3 levels increase (due to peripheral conversion of T4 to inactive rT3 rather than active T3); T4 and TSH levels are usually normal, and there is no proven benefit to treatment. If there is no clear reason to suspect thyroid disease, the best approach is to repeat the tests when the patient is well [26].

Further investigation of hypothyroidism. Hypothyroidism should prompt measurement of antithyroid antibodies. Anti-thyroid peroxidase (a.k.a. anti-TPO, antimicrosomal) antibodies are positive in 95% of those with autoimmune thyroiditis [486]. Hypothyroidism must always prompt consideration of the possibility of adrenal or pituitary failure. Autoimmune adrenalitis and thyroiditis are associated with each other, treatment of hypothyroidism can worsen incipient adrenal failure (Chapter 9.3 ▶), and pituitary failure (Chapter 9.4 ▶) causes adrenal failure and hypothyroidism [493]. In postpartum psychosis (Chapter 9.6.2 ▶), consider Sheehan's syndrome (postpartum pituitary infarction) with pituitary failure in the differential. In the context of psychosis with a history of hypothyroidism due to autoimmune (Hashimoto's) thyroiditis, consider also Hashimoto's encephalopathy (Chapter 14.1 ▶).

Further investigation of hyperthyroidism. Graves' disease is caused by TSH-receptor-stimulating antibodies, but anti-thyroid peroxidase antibodies are present in ~75% of cases and are cheaper to measure [26]. Thyroid scintigraphy can differentiate Graves' disease (diffuse goitre with high radioiodine uptake), nodular thyroid disease (nodular uptake), and ectopic thyroid tissue, and will show virtually no uptake in destructive thyroiditis, or in factitious thyrotoxicosis (exogenous thyroid hormone overdose, in which thyroglobulin levels are uniquely low) [26]. Pituitary MRI is indicated if a pituitary tumour is suspected.

"Subclinical" disease. There are some controversies about subclinical hypothyroidism and hyperthyroidism, in which free thyroid hormone values are in the normal range for the population. In patients treated with levothyroxine, doses should normally be adjusted to normalize TSH [493, 494]; endogenous disease is considered next.

Some authors classify hypothyroidism as grade I (overt or clinical: thyroid hormone levels low, TSH raised), grade II (thyroid hormone levels in the population normal range, but TSH raised), and grade III (the mildest; thyroid hormone levels and TSH are normal but the TSH response to TRH stimulation is increased) [495]. By this classification, psychosis in grade I hypothyroidism is well known. Psychosis responding to levothyroxine has been described in grade II hypothyroidism [496, 497]. Note also that normal TSH levels are usually given as 0.4–4 mU/l. However, these are distributed logarithmically in the normal population with a geometric mean of 1.5 mU/l, and even TSH levels at the upper range of normal (e.g. >3 mU/l) may indicate mild thyroid dysfunction and the risk of progression to overt hypothyroidism, especially if thyroid autoantibodies are present [486]. Grade III hypothyroidism is associated with depression [498], and has been suggested to contribute to symptoms in bipolar affective disorder [499, 500], particularly if antithyroid antibodies are present [501]. Patients with subclinical hypothyroidism should have a careful search for symptoms (including psychiatric symptoms) and measurement of antithyroid antibodies, in addition to regular thyroid monitoring. Treatment of grade II subclinical hypothyroidism has been suggested to reduce cardiovascular risk, to prevent progression to overt disease, and to relieve mild symptoms, with some trials showing significant improvements, but there is no universal consensus [486, 502–504].

Subclinical hyperthyroidism is associated with increased risk of atrial fibrillation, other cardiac abnormalities, osteoporosis, and perhaps dementia and Alzheimer's disease. There is a weak association with affective disorders [501]. Pituitary dysfunction should be excluded, and regular thyroid monitoring performed. If the suppressed TSH persists for 3 months, radioisotope thyroid imaging should be considered. Subclinical hyperthyroidism due to nodular disease is more likely to progress to overt disease; this, and symptoms, may warrant antithyroid treatment, but when to treat is controversial and endocrinology advice should be sought [494, 503–505].

9.2 Glucocorticoid excess

Psychosis may be the presenting feature of Cushing's syndrome. **Cushing's syndrome** is glucocorticoid excess. **Cushing's disease** is pituitary-dependent glucocorticoid excess [26]. Having excluded exogenous steroid administration (Chapter 15.1 ▶), endogenous Cushing's syndrome may be divided into ACTH-dependent and ACTH-independent causes. *ACTH-dependent* glucocorticoid excess is usually (70%) caused by Cushing's disease, of which 90% of cases are due to an ACTH-secreting pituitary adenoma; rarely there is ectopic CRF production from a tumour elsewhere (e.g. thyroid, prostate). Other causes include ectopic ACTH production, usually paraneoplastic from a small-cell bronchial carcinoma. Some patients with Cushing's disease have nodular adrenal hyperplasia, which may be mistaken for adrenal tumours. *ACTH-independent* glucocorticoid excess may be due to adrenal adenomas and carcinomas (~10% each), mutations of proteins in control systems (Carney's syndrome, McCune–Albright syndrome, and aberrant responses to gut polypeptides), and alcohol-associated pseudo-Cushing's syndrome [26]. Endogenous Cushing's syndrome has an annual incidence of about 13 cases per million [506].

Psychiatric symptoms occur in 62% of patients with Cushing's syndrome [26], preceding the physical changes in 50% [485], and psychosis occurred in ~15% of one series [507]. It is often depressive psychosis [25, 33]. Cushing's syndrome causes weight gain, menstrual irregularity, hirsutism, psychiatric manifestations (depression, lethargy, poor concentration, emotional lability, paranoia, and overt psychosis), backache, muscle weakness, fractures, loss of scalp hair, obesity (truncal or generalized), plethora, moon face, hypertension, bruising, red/purple striae, muscle weakness, ankle oedema, pigmentation, steroid acne, diabetes (overt or impaired glucose tolerance), osteoporosis, renal calculi, susceptibility to infection, and gastric ulceration. Myopathy, bruising, and hypertension are common and discriminatory in the comparison to simple obesity. There may be a leukocytosis. In severe hypercortisolaemia, there may be hypokalaemic metabolic alkalosis [26, 506]. Occasionally, Cushing's syndrome is slowly cyclical [26].

To establish whether there is Cushing's syndrome, the first test should be the measurement of urinary 24-h free cortisol; if raised, this indicates hypercortisolaemia. However, it may be normal in 8–15% of patients with Cushing's syndrome. If suspicion is high, the usual next test is the low-dose dexamethasone suppression test, usually performed overnight. In Cushing's syndrome, exogenous dexamethasone fails to suppress plasma cortisol; the overnight version of the test has high sensitivity (false-negative rate <2%) and the 48-hour version has both high sensitivity and specificity. Patients with severe depression may show many of the biochemical features of Cushing's syndrome (including raised urinary free cortisol and failure of cortisol suppression with low-dose dexamethasone), and Cushing's syndrome can cause depression. The two states may usually be distinguished with the insulin tolerance test: insulin-induced hypoglycaemia causes a rise in ACTH and cortisol in normal people and patients with depression, and this does not usually occur in Cushing's syndrome [26].

If Cushing's syndrome is confirmed, further tests are needed to establish the cause; these will not be covered here.

9.3 Adrenal failure

Primary hypoadrenalism is glucocorticoid deficiency as a result of adrenal disease; it causes mineralocorticoid deficiency as well. Secondary hypoadrenalism is glucocorticoid deficiency secondary to ACTH deficiency, which does not cause mineralocorticoid deficiency [26]. *Primary hypoadrenalism* may be due to **congenital adrenal hyperplasia** (various inherited defects in adrenocortical hormone synthesis), or **Addison's disease**. The prevalence of Addison's disease is 40–60 cases per million [508]. Addison's disease is usually (70–89%) due to autoimmune adrenalitis in the West, and there are often (50%) other coexistent autoimmune diseases. Worldwide, tuberculosis is another common cause; rare causes include metastasis, lymphoma, infiltrative diseases including amyloid and haemochromatosis, haemorrhage following meningococcal sepsis (Waterhouse–Friedrichsen syndrome), other forms of adrenal infarction or infection, previous surgery, and adrenoleukodystrophies (~8% of primary hypoadrenalism) [26, 509]. *Secondary hypoadrenalism* is usually due to withdrawal of chronic exogenous steroids, but sometimes due to pituitary failure [26].

Mental state changes occur in 65–70% of patients with Addison's disease (usually apathy and mood symptoms), and psychosis in ~6%. Psychosis and delirium are probably associated with severe adrenal insufficiency, i.e. Addisonian crisis, which is an emergency and may be fatal, yet psychosis can be the presenting symptom [33, 510]. Primary adrenal insufficiency usually causes pigmentation of mucous membranes and sun-exposed areas, as MSH increases along with ACTH; secondary hypoadrenalism does not. In primary hypoadrenalism, mineralocorticoid deficiency may cause hypotension and circulatory failure (Addisonian crisis), which is usually triggered by infection or stress; anorexia, nausea, vomiting, diarrhoea, and sometimes abdominal pain precede the collapse. Chronic adrenal insufficiency usually presents with weakness, tiredness, weight loss, nausea, vomiting, abdominal pain, diarrhoea or constipation, malaise, muscle cramps, and symptoms of postural hypotension. There may be salt craving. There is almost invariably postural hypotension. There may be signs of associated autoimmune disease (e.g. vitiligo). In secondary hypoadrenalism, other signs of hypopituitarism (Chapter 9.4 ▶) may dominate (e.g. oligomenorrhoea and poor libido secondary to LH/FSH deficiency, weight gain and cold intolerance secondary to TSH deficiency, hypoglycaemia secondary to GH deficiency). In primary hypoadrenalism, there is usually hyponatraemia (90%) and hyperkalaemia (65%) with a raised urea. In secondary hypoadrenalism, there may be dilutional hyponatraemia with low or normal urea. Hypoglycaemia occurs in up to 50% of those with chronic adrenal insufficiency [26, 508]. Psychosis has also been reported in congenital adrenal hyperplasia [35].

Diagnosis is by a short synacthen (synthetic ACTH) test; plasma cortisol is measured in the morning, 250 μg of tetracosactrin (Synacthen®) is given i.m. or i.v., and the cortisol level is measured again at 30 min. A peak plasma cortisol of <550 nM is suggestive of adrenal insufficiency and warrants further urgent investigation as to the cause. In an emergency when the patient is critically ill and acute adrenal insufficiency is suspected, treatment should not be delayed; blood for ACTH and cortisol levels should ideally be taken before intravenous hydrocortisone, fluids ± glucose, and treatment for any precipitant are given urgently [26].

Aside from the likely electrolyte imbalances (Chapter 12.5 ▶), adrenal insufficiency and psychosis should raise the possibility of associated autoimmune encephalopathy (Chapter 13 ▶). In males particularly it should also raise the possibility of X-linked adrenoleukodystrophy (Chapter 10.5.8 ▶), which can also occur in a milder form in females (including psychosis; MIM 300100).

9.4 Hypopituitarism

Hypopituitarism (**Simmonds' disease**) may present with mental symptoms – commonly, confusion, disorientation, and drowsiness, often with lethargy and depression, and sometimes with psychosis and paranoia [485]. Hypopituitarism is diagnosed as a combination of multiple pituitary hormone deficiencies (see Chapter 9.1, Chapter 9.3 ▶), although there may be hypersecretion of one of them if the cause is a secretory pituitary adenoma. Hypopituitarism is rare (annual incidence 2–8 per 100 000) and most frequently caused by pituitary tumours, particularly adenomas but also craniopharyngiomas. Historically, necrosis secondary to postpartum haemorrhage (Sheehan's syndrome) was the commonest cause, and other causes include infarction and haemorrhage (termed pituitary apoplexy for its sudden onset), head trauma (as an immediate or delayed consequence), infiltration (e.g. sarcoidosis, Wegener's granulomatosis), and empty sella syndrome (herniation of the arachnoid through the sella turcica compressing the pituitary) [511]. The neurological features require both thyroid hormone and corticosteroid replacement [485].

9.5 Hypoparathyroidism and hyperparathyroidism

Hypoparathyroidism causes hypocalcaemia, and hyperparathyroidism causes hypercalcaemia. Psychiatric symptoms, including psychosis, are generally thought to be caused by the calcium abnormalities, but sometimes by associated hypomagnesaemia (either in hypoparathyroidism or hyperparathyroidism; in the latter there appears to be a magnesium-losing state and serum magnesium may drop when hyperparathyroidism is corrected surgically) [512–514]. In hypoparathyroidism, about 39% of patients have cognitive impairments, and 11% have psychosis [513, 515]. Psychosis can be the presenting symptom of primary hyperparathyroidism, sometimes even when calcium levels are only mildly elevated [514]; psychosis occurs in 5–20% of patients with hyperparathyroidism [485]. PTH itself may contribute to the neuropsychiatric consequences of renal failure (uraemic encephalopathy), in which secondary hyperparathyroidism is universal, possibly by facilitating calcium entry into neurons (see Chapter 12.4.1 ▶). See also Chapter 12.5.3, Chapter 12.5.4, Chapter 12.5.6 ▶.

The combination of hypocalcaemia with hypoparathyroidism and psychosis should also raise the possibility of velocardiofacial syndrome (Chapter 4.1 ▶). Basal ganglia calcification (Chapter 5.11 ▶) can be a sign of hypoparathyroidism. Hypoparathyroidism may also be caused by MELAS (Chapter 10.6 ▶).

9.6 Sex hormones and psychosis

9.6.1 Schizophrenia and sex hormones

Oestrogen may play a protective role against the onset of schizophrenic psychosis, perhaps by reducing dopamine D2 receptor sensitivity [516–521] or regulating COMT activity [522]. The onset of schizophrenia is later in women, schizophrenic symptoms are more prominent in low-oestrogen times of the menstrual cycle (perimenstrual and follicular phase), and onset is more likely at this time; an oestrogen effect may also explain why late-onset schizophrenia is more severe in women [523–526]. In one study, more antipsychotic drug treatment was needed for women in comparatively low-oestrogen states admitted with schizophrenia [527].

The relationship between psychosis and sex hormones in men has been studied less and is less clear. One study observed high DHEAS levels in males with early-onset psychosis [526]; these subjects were medicated but medication dose did not predict these particular hormonal abnormalities. Another study observed lower testosterone, oestradiol, and oestrone in men with first-onset psychosis or psychotic relapse, without a clear relationship to antipsychotic medication [528].

Of course, antipsychotics drugs themselves affect sex hormone status. Many antipsychotics cause hyperprolactinaemia by blocking pituitary dopamine receptors. Hyperprolactinaemia causes oligomenorrhoea, amenorrhoea, infertility, and galactorrhoea in women, and impotence, infertility, and gynaecomastia in men [493]. Sexual function is often impaired in patients with schizophrenia or schizoaffective disorder receiving antipsychotics, with some evidence of biochemical hypogonadism occurring in 92% of premenopausal women and 28% of men in one study, though subjective sexual functioning was not correlated with either prolactin or steroid hormone levels [529].

9.6.2 Puerperal (postpartum) psychosis and other oestrogen withdrawal states

Puerperal psychosis is a general term for psychosis occurring in the postpartum period or puerperium, the 6 weeks following delivery [530, 531]. It occurs in approximately 2.2 per 1000 deliveries [29]. Despite the traditional definition of the puerperium, the risk of psychosis extends to at least 90 days after childbirth, but is highest in the first 30 days [531]. The ICD-10 has a code for puerperal psychosis (F53.1), but no specific clinical or research diagnostic criteria [4, 10]. Additionally, bipolar affective disorder confers a very high risk of postpartum psychosis: in patients who cease lithium at the start of pregnancy, pregnancy itself does not alter the risk of relapse, but among those who remain well during pregnancy, 70% experience an affective relapse within the first 24 postpartum months [532], and postpartum psychosis occurs after 25–50% of deliveries in women with bipolar affective disorder [533].

Oestrogen and progesterone levels fall sharply from high levels after delivery. This may be an important trigger for puerperal psychosis via the induction of dopaminergic dysfunction. Such dopaminergic dysfunction predicts the recurrence of puerperal psychosis and mood disorders [534, 535]. Oestradiol has been used to treat refractory puerperal psychosis with low oestradiol levels [536], though its effectiveness is not well established and some studies have found no effect in preventing puerperal relapse [537, 538]. Psychosis has been reported in other conditions associated with oestrogen withdrawal, such as premenstrually, at menarche, cyclical psychosis occurring shortly before the onset of menses, on cessation of exogenous oestrogen (e.g. the combined oral contraceptive pill), and on administration of direct and indirect oestrogen antagonists [539].

In puerperal psychosis, consider also **Sheehan's syndrome** (postpartum pituitary infarction) with pituitary failure (Chapter 9.4 ▶) (which usually occurs in the setting of significant postpartum haemorrhage [533]), and hyper- or hypothyroidism (Chapter 9.1 ▶) due to postpartum thyroiditis, though the latter usually occurs 2–12 months postpartum.

Other causes of early postpartum psychosis include cerebral venous thrombosis (Chapter 6.1 ▶), paradoxical embolism (e.g. venous thromboembolism, amniotic fluid embolism, or venous air embolism, with a right-to-left intracardiac communication), subarachnoid haemorrhage, and subdural haematoma following epidural anaesthesia [540]. Postpartum cerebral venous thrombosis occurs after ~1:10 000 births, and typically presents with headache, vomiting, seizures, and focal signs; psychosis is uncommon. It usually occurs in the second postpartum week, but can occur in pregnancy or up to 4 weeks postpartum [540] (see also Chapter 6.1 ▶). Other rare causes include group B streptococcal meningitis (associated with delivery more than 6 hours after rupture of membranes) and meningioma [533].

9.6.3 Other relationships between sex hormones and psychosis

Administration of oestrogens has also been suggested to be associated with psychosis [539, 541] and with chorea triggered by oestrogenic contraceptives [542]. (Rarely, oral contraceptives can trigger chorea as a reactivation of Sydenham's chorea [Chapter 8.7.1 ▶], or possibly in association with other autoimmune disease with anti-basal ganglia antibodies [543].) However, the data supporting such an association are much weaker than for oestrogen withdrawal [539]. One large study (total $n > 16\,000$) found no association between oral contraceptive use and referral for psychiatric input, with a referral rate for psychotic illnesses of 0.46 per 1000 woman-years for users of an oral contraceptive, compared with 0.43 for diaphragm users and 0.53 for users of an intrauterine device [544]; thus, if any serious psychiatric complications of the oral contraceptive pill exist, they are very rare.

Anabolic steroids may also trigger psychosis (see Chapter 15.3 ▶).

Chapter 10 Inborn errors of metabolism

10.1 Hyperammonaemia and urea cycle disorders

Hyperammonaemia results from disruption of the hepatic urea cycle, which normally clears free ammonia by conversion to urea. Hyperammonaemia usually manifests as CNS toxicity.

Causes. Hyperammonaemia can result from several groups of disorders, as follows [545]. (1) Enzyme defects in the urea cycle. These include deficiencies of N-acetylglutamate synthetase, carbamoyl phosphate synthetase, ornithine transcarbamylase (OTC, or ornithine carbamoyltransferase), argininosuccinate synthetase (causing citrullinaemia), argininosuccinate lyase, and arginase. **OTC deficiency** is the most common; it is X-linked and occurs in 1:14 000 people. (2) Organic acidaemias. These usually cause ketosis and acidosis, but sometimes hyperammonaemia dominates. They include isovaleric acidaemia, propionic acidaemia, methylmalonic acidaemia, glutaric acidaemia type II, multiple carboxylase deficiency, and beta-ketothiolase deficiency. (3) Congenital lactic acidosis, including pyruvate dehydrogenase deficiency, pyruvate carboxylase deficiency, and mitochondrial disorders (Chapter 10.6 ▸). (4) Fatty acid oxidation defects, including acetyl-coenzyme-A dehydrogenase deficiency and carnitine deficiency. (5) Amino acid transport defects, including lysinuric protein intolerance and hyperammonaemia–hyperornithinaemia–homocitrullinuria. (6) Transiently in premature neonates, and in neonatal hypoxia. (7) In Reye's syndrome (Chapter 12.4.4 ▸) (cerebral and hepatic dysfunction usually occurring after a viral infection, and associated with aspirin use in children). (8) After drugs, particularly valproate, cytotoxic chemotherapy, and in salicylate poisoning. (9) In chronic liver disease and liver failure; ammonia is one of the neurotoxins that contributes to hepatic encephalopathy (Chapter 12.4.2 ▸) [546]. (10) In urinary tract infections with a urease-producing organism, more common after urinary tract surgery. (11) In parenteral nutrition with a high nitrogenous load.

Effects. Early-onset hyperammonaemia presents in neonates, and is unlikely to concern the psychiatrist except that treatment failure or nitrogenous loads can cause hyperammonaemic exacerbations in those known to have such a disorder. Excepting urinary infections and liver disease, late-onset hyperammonaemia is typically due to a urea cycle disorder. It may be due to a partial enzyme deficiency, such as in females with OTC deficiency, or OTC-deficient males with partial enzyme activity. Typically the hyperammonaemia is intermittent, and may be triggered by other medical conditions (e.g. postpartum, and following gastrointestinal bleeding, protein load, and surgery). The syndrome may present with intermittent ataxia or gait abnormalities, mild intellectual impairment, failure to thrive in children, mental state changes (including sleep disturbance, irritability, hyperactivity, mania, and psychosis), epilepsy, a recurrent picture of Reye's syndrome, and episodic headaches with vomiting. There may be stroke-like episodes (e.g. diplopia, hemiparesis, pyramidal signs). There may be a history of protein avoidance (such as vegetarianism or anorexia). Severe hyperammonaemia produces depression of consciousness and coma. Ammonia increases extracellular glutamate and NMDA receptor activation, though it has many other neurometabolic effects [115, 545]. Urea levels can be low in those with urea cycle disorders [547].

Primary psychiatric presentation has been documented for a number of urea cycle disorders; the presentation may be acute, and obviously can be recurrent. In general, there are attacks of confusion, bizarre behaviour, and delusions triggered by high protein intake or situations of protein catabolism [115]. Hyperammonaemia can cause psychiatric features before frank encephalopathy is evident [548]. Citrullinaemia may present in childhood or in adulthood, with episodic bizarre behaviour, mania, and psychosis all being features (MIM 603471). Hyperammonaemia secondary to mild argininosuccinate synthetase deficiency has presented for the first time as postpartum psychosis [549] and hyperammonaemia secondary to N-acetylglutamate synthetase deficiency has presented as mental state change in an adolescent [550]. Partial N-acetylglutamate synthase deficiency has presented with vomiting, psychosis, and confusion in puberty (MIM 237310). Ornithine transcarbamylase deficiency has also presented as mental state change postpartum [551]. Valproate can induce hyperammonaemia, and has precipitated mania, aggression, psychosis, lethargy, confusion, seizures, and coma in patients with pre-existing mental disorders [552]. Portosystemic shunting has been associated with hyperammonaemia and disorientation and hallucinations in a child [553].

Diagnosis is by serum ammonia levels, followed by investigation as to the cause [545]. The next step is to measure urine organic acids; a decision tree proceeds to the diagnosis [see 28]. Magnetic resonance imaging may be normal, or show cerebral oedema or high cortical signal intensity on T2WI [115].

10.2 Porphyria

The porphyrias are a group of disorders of haem biosynthesis. They are over-represented in psychiatric hospitals, with an inpatient prevalence that may be as high as 1:500 [554]. They may be divided clinically into acute and non-acute porphyrias. Acute porphyrias include **acute intermittent porphyria** (porphobilinogen deaminase deficiency), **variegate porphyria** (protoporphyrinogen oxidase deficiency), **hereditary coproporphyria** (coproporphyrinogen oxidase deficiency), and **Doss porphyria** (aminolaevulinate dehydratase deficiency). They cause neurovisceral symptoms and are typically precipitated by environmental factors, though spontaneous attacks may occur. All are autosomal dominant except Doss porphyria, which is autosomal recessive. Non-acute porphyrias (congenital erythropoietic porphyria, protoporphyria, porphyria cutanea tarda, and hepatoerythropoietic porphyria) are characterized by photosensitivity [26, 555], and will not be considered further. The overall frequency of heterozygosity for acute porphyria is generally given as approximately 1:10 000, of whom 10–20% will develop an acute attack [26], though one study of blood donors found inherited porphobilinogen (PBG) deaminase deficiency in 1:500 [33, 556]. Latent porphyria is equally common in males and females, but symptomatic acute porphyria is commoner in females (female:male ratio 2:1) [26]. Lead poisoning (Chapter 15.6.4 ▶) and hereditary tyrosinaemia (Chapter 10.3.1 ▶) can mimic porphyria by inhibiting aminolaevulinate dehydratase. There is a single case report of psychosis with erythropoietic protoporphyria [557], a type not usually associated with neurovisceral attacks, and it is unclear if this was causal.

Porphyria was known historically as the "little imitator" for its many features. The classic triad of acute porphyria is of "neurovisceral" attacks, with intermittent abdominal pain (often non-localized), polyneuropathy, and psychiatric symptoms (which have been estimated to occur in 25–75% of patients). However, psychiatric symptoms may be the only feature of porphyric attacks, and may include psychosis, apathy, delirium, anxiety, agitation, and depression [26, 33, 554, 555]. Psychosis may be acute and brief or persist for weeks to months [558]. Neuropathies may be sensory and/or motor. Visceral signs may also include vomiting, constipation, ileus, diarrhoea, dysuria, urinary retention or incontinence, tachycardia, and hypertension. Seizures and limb or trunk pain may occur [559]. A wide variety of drugs, including steroids and many psychotropics, may precipitate or worsen a porphyric attack [27], as may fasting, alcohol, infections, menstruation, and pregnancy [115, 554]. If related to menstruation, symptoms are usually worse 1–2 days before menstruation begins [26]. Since psychiatric manifestations can occur alone, the diagnosis should be considered in any of the following situations: (a) unexplained leukocytosis, (b) unexplained neuropathy, (c) aetiologically obscure neurosis or psychosis, (d) "idiopathic" seizure disorder, (e) unexplained abdominal pain, including a history of laparotomy, or severe constipation, (f) dissociative (conversion) disorders, and (g) susceptibility to stress [25, 560].

Hyponatraemia occurs during attacks in 40% of patients, due to SIADH [265, 555, 559]. A variety of brain MRI changes are sometimes seen but are non-specific [115, 559]. The EEG may show diffuse slowing or be normal [33]. Occasionally severe attacks cause PRES (Chapter 6.4 ▶).

Demonstration of elevated urinary porphyrins (5-aminol[a]evulinate [ALA] and/or PBG) in a 24-h urine collection during a symptomatic period is indicative of porphyria, and a negative result makes acute porphyria unlikely as the cause of acute symptoms, but does not exclude latent porphyria or some rare forms. Urinary porphyrins may be normal between attacks. False negatives are possible if there is a delay between sample collection and testing, or improper sample transport, as porphyrins are photosensitive. If urinary porphyrins are elevated, the urine may turn purple or amber in sunlight, or appear pink or red [26, 555]. Faecal porphyrin measurement is used to distinguish between types of acute porphyria, or to detect some types of porphyria between acute attacks. Faecal porphyrins are always low in acute intermittent porphyria and Doss porphyria, but usually increased (between and during attacks) in variegate porphyria and hereditary coproporphyria [555]. Another test is to measure red cell monopyrrole porphobilinogen deaminase [560]; in ~95% of patients with acute intermittent porphyria (the commonest acute porphyria), porphobilinogen deaminase activity is reduced to 50% of normal levels, and this test can be performed at any time [554].

Thus, a diagnostic strategy is as follows. If acute porphyria is suspected, urinary porphyrins (PBG and ALA) should be analysed using a quantitative method, paying careful attention to specimen packaging and transport methods. A positive result (which typically is of very substantial elevation of porphyrins) confirms acute porphyria, and subsequent testing is directed at identifying the type of porphyria. A negative result makes an acute attack unlikely. In remission, if the clinical suspicion of porphyria is high, consider porphobilinogen deaminase assay (as above), faecal porphyrins (as above), and fluorescence emission spectroscopy of plasma (the most sensitive test for variegate porphyria in remission) [265].

In addition to the mimics of porphyria discussed above, the differential diagnosis also includes arsenic and thallium poisoning (Chapter 15.6.2, Chapter 15.6.3 ▶) [20].

10.3 Disorders of amino acid metabolism

10.3.1 Hereditary tyrosinaemia

Hereditary tyrosinaemia has not been reported to cause psychosis in isolation, but is mentioned because of the similarity of its neurovisceral crises to porphyria. It comes in a number of forms. Hereditary tyrosinaemia type I causes acute and chronic liver failure, renal Fanconi's syndrome, and hepatocellular carcinoma. Untreated, death occurs in the first few years of life. However, it also causes aminolaevulinate dehydratase (ALA-D) inhibition, and neurovisceral crises that resemble acute intermittent porphyria (Chapter 10.2 ▶). These crises can include mental state changes including self-mutilation, peripheral neuropathy, vomiting or ileus, muscle weakness and paralysis. Tyrosinaemia type II is primarily ocular but can involve mental retardation and self-mutilation; type III is exceptionally rare but also can cause seizures, ataxia, and mental retardation. Diagnosis of any tyrosinaemia is usually in infancy by elevated blood tyrosine [26, 561–563].

10.3.2 Hyperhomocysteinaemia and homocystinuria

Homocysteine is metabolized by two pathways. The first, remethylation to methionine, requires folate (vitamin B_9) and cobalamin (vitamin B_{12}) and its failure leads to neuropsychiatric disease. This pathway involves the enzyme *methylenetetrahydrofolate reductase* (MTHFR) to make methyltetrahydrofolate (MTHF), ultimately from folate. *Methionine synthase* then converts MTHF plus homocysteine to tetrahydrofolate and methionine. In mammals, methionine synthase requires cobalamin as a cofactor. The other pathway is through the irreversible synthesis of cystathionine, by *cystathionine synthase.*

If metabolism fails, homocysteine builds up, causing hyperhomocysteinaemia (hyperhomocysteinaemia) and homocystinuria (homocysteinuria). Several clinical variants are recognized.

Severe hyperhomocysteinaemia is caused by deficiencies of key enzymes. **Deficiency of cystathionine synthase** causes classic homocystinuria, with increased methionine levels, and a clinical picture similar to Marfan's syndrome (e.g. abnormal body habitus, lens dislocation), sometimes with thromboembolism. **Deficiency of MTHFR** causes a syndrome of neuropsychiatric dysfunction and thromboembolism, discussed further below, with normal methionine levels [115, 564–566]. **Other cobalamin metabolism defects (Cbls)** can have similar psychiatric presentations [115] (see also Chapter 11.4 ▶).

Milder hyperhomocysteinaemia may be caused by folate deficiency, cobalamin deficiency, or a thermolabile form of MTHFR [566]. As will be apparent from the sequence outlined above, the reaction catalysed by MTHFR may also be impaired by **folate deficiency** (Chapter 11.5 ▶). As methionine synthase requires cobalamin, **cobalamin (vitamin B_{12}) deficiency** (Chapter 11.4 ▶) also produces hyperhomocysteinaemia. In addition, homocystinuria caused by vitamin B_{12} deficiency is associated with methylmalonic acidaemia and methylmalonic aciduria [565], as cobalamin is also required for methylmalonyl-coenzyme A metabolism (MIM 277400). Hypothyroidism (Chapter 9.1 ▶) may also elevate homocysteine levels.

Hyperhomocysteinaemia triggered by a dietary methionine load, as distinct from fasting hyperhomocysteinaemia, may be caused by **pyridoxine (vitamin B_6) deficiency**

(Chapter 11.3 ▶), which also disrupts homocysteine metabolism, or by a heterozygous cystathionine synthase defect [566].

The clinical phenotype of MTHFR deficiency is varied, and it has presented with delusions, hallucinations, and catatonia. Depression, memory disorders, mild mental retardation, confusion, movement disorders, weakness, ataxia, peripheral neuropathy (e.g. paraesthesiae), subacute degeneration of the spinal cord, strokes, and thromboembolism have all been reported (MIM 236250) [115]. There is also MTHFR polymorphism in the general population. A homozygous C677T mutation reduces overall enzyme activity to <30% of normal, and the homozygous prevalence is >5%; it is the most common genetic cause of hyperhomocysteinaemia [567]. Recent meta-analyses have confirmed that both raised plasma homocysteine and the C677T mutation are associated with schizophrenia, and the C677T polymorphism is also associated with unipolar and bipolar depression [568–570]. There is debate about the sex specificity of the effect, and there are other MTHFR polymorphisms that have been associated with bipolar disorder and schizophrenia [571]. Individuals with folate- or vitamin B_{12}-responsive schizophrenia-like symptoms have been documented as a result of MTHFR deficiency [572, 573]. Within patients with schizophrenia, the C677T genotype is associated with some executive function deficits [574], and interacts with COMT mutations [575]. Independent of the C677T MTHFR mutation, low folate levels have also been suggested to represent a risk factor for schizophrenia [576]. Administration of methionine can worsen psychosis in schizophrenia [577].

Homocysteine remethylation defects can present with acute, subacute, or chronic psychiatric symptoms [115]. Homocystinuria due to cystathionine synthase deficiency usually produces a chronic picture [115]. Psychosis is seen in MTHFR deficiency [115], cobalamin C disorder (cblC; MIM 277400), and cblD [376].

Initial diagnosis of homocysteine metabolism disorders is by measurement of plasma (and/or urinary) homocysteine. Magnetic resonance imaging may be normal or show leukoencephalopathy or spinal cord changes of subacute degeneration [115].

10.3.3 Hartnup's disease

Hartnup's disease is one of the most common amino acid disorders, with an incidence of about 1:14 000 births. It causes defective transport of neutral amino acids in the small intestine and kidneys. Tryptophan transport is affected, and consequently niacin synthesis is reduced. Clinical features of pellagra (Chapter 11.2 ▶) are seen. Non-psychiatric symptoms include pellagra-like rashes and cerebellar ataxia. Psychiatric symptoms include anxiety, emotional instability, mood changes, and rarely psychosis and delirium. It usually presents in childhood but occasionally in adults. There is gross aminoaciduria [173, 578, 579].

10.3.4 Maple syrup urine disease

Maple syrup urine disease is an autosomal recessive aminoacidopathy in which there is failure to catabolize leucine, isoleucine, and valine. The overall frequency is approximately 1:180 000 births, though it is much higher in some inbred populations. It leads to encephalopathy and progressive neurodegeneration in infants. In classic maple syrup urine disease, the disease develops very early in life, with infants being ketotic and having urine smelling of maple syrup. Less common is intermittent maple syrup urine disease, in which patients develop with normal intelligence and growth, but develop neurological features during catabolic stress (e.g. infections). These features include ataxia, lethargy, seizures, and coma [580]. There is a single case report in which these intermittent episodes were associated with hallucinations [581]. Diagnosis is by plasma (and/or urinary) amino acid measurement: the presence of alloisoleucine is diagnostic [580].

10.4 Wilson's disease

Wilson's disease (WD; hepatolenticular degeneration) is an autosomal recessive disease that causes reduced biliary copper excretion, and failure to transfer copper onto apocaeruloplasmin to form caeruloplasmin. Failure to excrete copper into bile leads to copper accumulation and toxicity in hepatocytes and, with increasing liver dysfunction, copper spills into the blood and accumulates, causing toxicity, in the CNS (particularly the basal ganglia and within them the putamen), cornea, kidneys, and other organs. WD has a carrier frequency of about 1:90 and a disease frequency of about 1:5000 to 1:30 000. It presents with psychiatric manifestations in 10–20% of cases, and 60% of patients with neurological disease have psychiatric symptoms. Overall, 51% of patients have psychiatric symptoms [26, 153, 159, 582, 1342]. Untreated, it is lethal. A similar, secondary (acquired) form of chronic copper toxicity may also occur secondary to chronic cholestasis (such as biliary atresia or primary biliary cirrhosis) [26].

Hepatic presentation tends to occur in younger patients (8–12 years); neuropsychiatric presentations usually occur in those aged 14–40. Most typical are movement disorders including dystonia. Dysarthria, decreasing physical performance in sports, and clumsiness are common early features, progressing to tremor and abnormal movements. Psychiatric presenting features include a deterioration in intellectual ability, depression, anxiety, phobias, OCD-like features, aggressive/antisocial behaviour, psychosis, and memory loss [20, 26, 153, 582–586]. In one series psychosis occurred in ~2% of patients, so a true association with psychosis has been questioned, though other studies have given frequencies of up to 11%. Personality change, disinhibited behaviour, cognitive impairment, and depression are more common [17, 33, 159, 587]. In another series, the main neurological features were parkinsonism in 62%, dystonia in 35%, cerebellar signs in 28%, pyramidal signs in 16%, chorea in 9%, athetosis in 2%, myoclonus in 3%, and behavioural abnormalities in 16% [588]. There may be early osteoarthritis and other joint abnormalities; rarely, there may be a grey hyperpigmentation of the skin with a bluish discolouration of the nail lunulae [26]. Occasionally seizures develop [33].

Kayser–Fleischer rings are present in most patients with neurological WD, and about 50% of patients with hepatic WD. They are almost pathognomonic [26, 589, 1342], though not quite, occurring also in primary biliary cirrhosis and autoimmune hepatitis [33]. They are due to copper deposition in the limbus of the cornea and appear as a brown ring surrounding a grey-blue iris, or a grey ring surrounding a brown iris. They are best seen on slit-lamp examination but can be seen with the ophthalmoscope or naked eye when more pronounced [26]. Their presence correlates with copper deposition in the brain [1342]. Sometimes there are sunflower cataracts [33]. There may be signs of chronic liver disease, sometimes with portal hypertension.

There may be features of acute or chronic haemolytic anaemia, features of liver dysfunction (such as deranged LFTs, raised PT, and hypoalbuminaemia), renal tubular acidosis, and osteomalacia (due to renal loss of phosphate) or hypoparathyroidism.

Serum caeruloplasmin is reduced or absent in 95% of patients with Wilson's disease, though it can also be low in low-protein states including liver synthetic failure, protein-losing enteropathy, and nephrotic syndrome, and as caeruloplasmin is an acute-phase reactant, low levels can be raised to normal in the context of inflammation. Total serum copper is usually low, through "free" copper (that not bound to caeruloplasmin) is high. Urinary copper excretion is usually raised, and the combination of a low caeruloplasmin and increased urinary copper indicates Wilson's disease. Hepatic copper is raised. Obviously, these findings may be modified in treated patients [26, 153]. MRI is reasonably sensitive, with 75% of patients exhibiting generalized cerebral atrophy on T1WI, 66% showing basal ganglia hypointensities on T1WI, and 33% showing hyperintensities in the basal ganglia, white matter, thalamus, or brainstem on T2WI. Occasionally the midbrain "face of the giant panda" or pontine "face of the miniature panda" signs are seen on T2WI [1342]. Genetic testing may be helpful, but there are many possible mutations in the ATP7B gene that can cause WD [1342]. A thorough workup is needed to exclude other liver disorders [26]. Treatment is by chelation therapy ± liver transplant.

10.5 Storage diseases

The storage diseases are characterized by pathological intracellular accumulation of abnormal material in the nervous system; they include neuronal ceroid lipofuscinoses, cerebral lipidoses (gangliosidoses, sphingomyelinoses, cerebrosidoses, mucopolysaccharidoses, and so forth), and leukodystrophies [28].

10.5.1 Neuronal ceroid lipofuscinosis

The neuronal ceroid lipofuscinoses (NCL, CLN) are a heterogeneous group of neurodegenerative disorders characterized by intracellular accumulation of lipopigment. The clinical course includes progressive dementia, seizures, and progressive visual failure. Classification was originally by age of onset: CLN1 (Santavuori–Haltia disease) has infantile onset, CLN2 (Janský–Bielschowsky disease) has late infantile onset, CLN3 (Batten's disease or Spielmeyer–Vogt–Sjögren–Batten disease) has juvenile onset, and CLN4 (**Kufs' disease**) has adult onset. However, classification is now according to the underlying gene defect (CLN1–10), and it is clear that CLN1 as well as CLN4 can begin in adulthood. The CLNs may be the most common group of neurodegenerative diseases in children (MIM 256730), with a frequency of 2–4 per 100 000 live births, but adult-onset forms are rare, representing only 1.3% of all cases [590].

In adult-onset CLN, visual loss is less common than in childhood-onset forms, and either seizures and myoclonus or dementia with extrapyramidal and cerebellar dysfunction predominate [590]. Other psychiatric disturbances such as alterations in personality have been reported in several types of CLN. Visual hallucinations have been reported in adult-onset CLN1 (MIM 256730) and hallucinations (not specified) in CLN9 (MIM 609055). Episodic psychosis has been reported in adult-onset CLN4, which is usually autosomal recessive but sometimes autosomal dominant (MIM 204300) [590]; the rate of psychosis has been reported as being up to 20% [17].

Diagnosis may be aided by biopsy showing lipofuscin accumulation (e.g. in muscle or skin) on electron microscopy, but the sensitivity of extracerebral biopsy is not known and ultimate diagnosis is by examination of brain tissue. Urinary sediment dolichol levels may be elevated [590]. Although it is typically an infantile-onset form, assay for palmitoyl-protein thioesterase deficiency allows diagnosis of CLN1 (MIM 256730).

10.5.2 Niemann–Pick disease, type C

Niemann–Pick disease is a lipid storage disorder in which sphingomyelin is accumulated in reticuloendothelial cells and neurons. Type A is an infantile form leading to death within the first few years of life, while type B involves the viscera but not the brain. Type C may concern the psychiatrist as it may begin in childhood or with insidious onset and slow progression in adolescence or adulthood. It is an autosomal recessive disorder with a highly variable phenotype. The term "type C" encompasses other variants sometimes called type D (MIM 257220). The prevalence of type C is approximately 1:211 000 [591].

In adult-onset Niemann–Pick type C disease, psychiatric disease is the presenting feature in 36% of patients, usually with psychosis, though mood disorders and obsessive–compulsive disorder have been seen. Most patients presenting with psychosis are neurologically normal. The psychiatric course can be progressive or acute, with spontaneous fluctuation. Vertical oculomotor apraxia (vertical supranuclear ophthalmoplegia; vertical supranuclear gaze palsy) is characteristic but while it usually appears early, it can be very subtle initially, or appear later, and does not appear at all in 20% of patients [115]. The rate of schizophrenia-like psychosis has been reported as 25–40% [17, 94]. Sometimes there is dementia. Other neurological features include ataxia and dysarthria (often early features) and dystonia and seizures (often later) (MIM 257220). There may have been a preceding episode of hepatitic jaundice in infanthood or childhood, but this typically resolves [26].

Splenomegaly and/or hepatomegaly are usually seen on ultrasound (>90% of patients). Foamy Niemann–Pick cells and "sea-blue" histiocytes may be seen in the bone marrow. Liver biopsy may show cirrhosis. Plasma chitotriosidase activity may be increased. There are characteristic histological features on skin biopsy, and fibroblast culture (from skin biopsy) may demonstrate free cholesterol accumulation, reduced sphingomyelinase activity, and a reduced ability to esterify exogenous cholesterol. Molecular genetic testing may be confirmatory (MIM 257220) [115].

10.5.3 Hexosaminidase deficiency (GM_2 gangliosidosis)

The GM_2 gangliosidoses are lysosomal storage disorders in which GM_2 gangliosides accumulate. They include **Tay–Sachs disease** (type 1 GM_2 gangliosidosis, prevalence ~1:201 000 in Australia but significantly more common in Ashkenazi Jews) and **Sandhoff disease** (type 2 GM_2 gangliosidosis, prevalence ~1:384 000). Both are due to mutations affecting subunits of hexosaminidase and they are clinically indistinguishable (MIM 606869, 272800, 268800) [591]. Classic Tay–Sachs disease presents in infancy with developmental retardation followed by paralysis, dementia, and blindness, with very early death. However, there are many forms of late-onset GM_2 gangliosidosis having onset in older childhood or adulthood.

Late-onset GM_2 gangliosidosis usually presents with lower motor neuron disease, cerebellar ataxia, or dystonia. Cherry-red macular spots are a feature. Psychiatric features occur in 20–40% of patients, and may predate motor signs by years or appear later. Acute psychotic episodes are characteristic, and often involve persecutory delusions, thought disorder, agitation, and hallucinations, with variable persistence between attacks. Mania and depression are less common [17, 115]. Intermittent confusion, emotional lability, and upper motor neuron signs may also be seen, along with progressive dementia over years; there may also be cardiac involvement (MIM 268800). Tricyclic antidepressants and phenothiazines may aggravate the condition [115]. Initial diagnosis is by blood hexosaminidase assay [115]; rectal, muscle, and nerve biopsy are also sometimes used.

10.5.4 Mucopolysaccharidosis

Mucopolysaccharidosis type 1H/S (**Hurler–Scheie syndrome**) is due to alpha-L-iduronidase deficiency, leading to accumulation of partially degraded mucopolysaccharides (glycosaminoglycans). It is a condition intermediate between Hurler syndrome (a severe mucopolysaccharidosis with onset in childhood and death at a mean age of 6 years) and Scheie syndrome (mild with late onset, primarily with stiff joints, corneal clouding, little or no intellectual impairment, and aortic regurgitation). The prevalence of Hurler–Scheie syndrome is approximately 1:88 000. It causes short stature, depression of the nasal bridge, micrognathia, corneal clouding, stiff joints, umbilical hernia, dysostosis multiplex, hepatosplenomegaly, variable mild cardiac abnormalities, and frequent respiratory infections (sometimes with abnormal airways), typically with little or no intellectual dysfunction. Psychosis has been described, and it has presented as acute paranoia in a young adult. It may be diagnosed by fibroblast enzyme assay (MIM 607015) [591]. Head MRI may show thickened meninges and ligaments, atrophy, atlantoaxial subluxation, cribriform or cystic areas within the white matter and/or basal ganglia, delayed myelination, and hydrocephalus [47].

10.5.5 Fabry's disease

Fabry's disease (Anderson–Fabry disease) is an X-linked lysosomal storage disorder resulting from α-galactosidase A deficiency. Glycosphingolipids accumulate in the plasma and in lysosomes throughout the body. Female heterozygotes are not free of disease (MIM 301500). Its prevalence is approximately 1:117 000 [591].

The most characteristic symptom is lancinating pain in the extremities, which worsens with exercise and with extremes of temperature, with background burning pain; this usually begins in early childhood. Affected males have small, red, raised vascular lesions (angiokeratomas), particularly around the buttocks and genitalia. They are seen in smaller numbers in affected heterozygote females (e.g. in restricted dermatomes), due to X-chromosome inactivation mosaicism. Cataracts are common (whorl-like corneal opacifications). Diarrhoea shortly after eating, and abdominal pain associated with febrile attacks, are also seen. Most males have a loss of peripheral sweating, and impotence is common. Many of these features result from autonomic neuropathy, which may also reduce saliva and tear formation. Subsequently, impaired capillary circulation and progressive renal disease (glomerular, interstitial, and tubular) lead to proteinuria and renal failure. Cardiac involvement may include left ventricular hypertrophy and conduction defects. Vascular involvement also leads to stroke [26, 28].

Fabry's disease also affects the CNS, and schizophrenia-like psychosis may occur [22, 592], though it is undoubtedly rare.

Diagnosis is by demonstrating abnormal glycolipid in urine or plasma, and by α-galactosidase A assay from tears, plasma, white cells, or other tissue [26].

Diffuse angiokeratomas are also seen in some other rare lysosomal enzyme disorders, including aspartylglucosaminuria (Chapter 10.5.6 ▶).

10.5.6 Aspartylglucosaminuria

Aspartylglucosaminuria (aspartylglycosaminuria) is a lyosomal glycoprotein storage disorder caused by N-aspartyl-β-glucosaminidase (glycoasparaginase) deficiency (MIM 208400). Its prevalence is generally very low, at 1:2 111 000 in Australia [591], but it is much commoner in Finland at 1:26 000, with one study in eastern Finland showing a prevalence of 1:3600, making it the third most common genetic cause of mental retardation in Finland (MIM 208400).

The typical presentation is with severe mental retardation, thick sagging skin of the cheeks, broad nose and face, short neck, cranial asymmetry, scoliosis, periodic hyperactivity, recurrent infections, and vacuolated lymphocytes (MIM 208400). Psychosis is not typical but has been reported [593].

Diagnosis is by demonstrating increased urinary oligosaccharides, then by aspartylglucosaminidase (glycoasparaginase) assay.

10.5.7 Metachromatic leukodystrophy

Leukodystrophies are characterized by non-inflammatory demyelination [26]. Metachromatic leukodystrophy (MLD) is an autosomal recessive disease in which the lysosomal enzyme arylsulfatase A is deficient, leading to accumulation of "metachromatic material" (cerebroside sulfate) in oligodendrocytes, microglia, and Schwann cells, and consequently demyelination. Accumulation also occurs in non-neural tissue including the kidneys and gallbladder. The incidence is estimated at 1:40 000 births. There are late infantile, juvenile, and adult-onset forms. Schizophrenia-like psychosis is prominent in the later-developing forms, with a prevalence of psychosis of ~53% in forms with onset in adolescence and young adulthood. A related condition, arylsulfatase A pseudodeficiency, is common (16% of the general population), and thought to be due to heterozygotic deficiency. It is usually asymptomatic, though heterozygotes have been observed to have increased rates of cognitive abnormalities and psychopathy [17, 594–597].

Late infantile MLD presents with weakness and hypotonia and is usually fatal by age 5. Juvenile and adult-onset MLD (arbitrarily divided from each other at age 16) are more slowly progressive; they typically present either with motor or neuropsychiatric abnormalities [594]. The neuropsychiatric features include conduct disorder, non-verbal learning disability, drug abuse, depression, and schizophrenia-like psychosis, often with prominent negative symptoms. The cognitive profile resembles that of a subcortical dementia, with impaired verbal fluency, poor memory retrieval, executive dysfunction, disinhibition, anosognosia, complex delusions, bizarre behaviour, and auditory hallucinations. Occasionally, extrapyramidal signs, seizures, and peripheral neuropathy occur, but motor signs can be absent for decades after the psychiatric presentation [594]; thus, adult-onset MLD is often diagnosed as schizophrenia (MIM 250100). The rate of schizophrenia-like psychosis is 25–40% [94].

White matter abnormalities on MRI are characteristic (typically periventricular leukoencephalopathy), and usually relatively symmetrical and confluent. Diagnosis is by demonstrating low arylsulfatase A levels in leukocytes or cultured fibroblasts, or by genetic testing. Metachromatic leukodystrophy may be distinguished from arylsulfatase A pseudodeficiency by urine sulfatide levels, functional cell assay, or genetic testing [115, 594, 597].

10.5.8 X-linked adrenoleukodystrophy

X-linked adrenoleukodystrophy (ALD) is a peroxisomal disorder in which very long chain fatty acids (VLCFA), meaning fatty acids with more than 22 carbon atoms, accumulate in peroxisomes due to a defect in fatty acid beta-oxidation [598, 599]. Its frequency has been estimated as 1:20 000 [598]. The molecular deficit is a lack of functional ALD protein, a transporter that allows the enzyme that degrades VLCFA to enter the peroxisome. VLCFA accumulate in all cells, but preferentially affect the adrenal cortex, the Leydig cells of the testes, and myelin-producing cells of the peripheral and central nervous system [598]. If the disease involves the brain clinically, it is called cerebral adrenoleukodystrophy. There are subtypes of X-linked adrenoleukodystrophy, including **adrenomyeloneuropathy**, the most common adult form (dominated by a progressive spastic paraparesis).

Childhood-onset X-linked adrenoleukodystrophy, the classic form, typically begins at 3–8 years with symptoms of attention-deficit disorder followed by progressive neurological deterioration followed by death within a few years. Adolescent-onset X-linked adrenoleukodystrophy is less severe, and may present with adrenal failure, neurological dysfunction, or psychiatric symptoms. Death usually occurs within 1–2 years of cerebral involvement [598]. There are also adult-onset forms, which may present with adrenal insufficiency, gonadal dysfunction (including impotence), neurological involvement (typically gait abnormalities and upper motor neuron lesions preferentially affecting the lower extremities, but also peripheral sensory deficits, visual defects, seizures, dysarthria, and cerebellar signs), or psychiatric symptoms (including mania, psychosis, personality change, cognitive impairment, disinhibition, and depression) [115, 598]. Schizophrenia-like psychosis is rare, and affective psychosis more common [94], with one estimate that psychosis occurs in 30% of patients [17]. The age of onset varies considerably, as does the phenotype within a family. Although the X-chromosome linkage means that males are typically affected, 20–50% of female heterozygotes also have neurological dysfunction (following random inactivation of the "good" X chromosome via lyonization). Affected females typically have disease onset in their 30s, milder symptoms, and a slower disease course; their symptoms often resemble multiple sclerosis (Chapter 6.8 ▶), and only 3% have cognitive decline and <1% have adrenal dysfunction [598].

Investigations may reveal features of adrenal insufficiency (Chapter 9.3 ▶) and testicular failure (with a low testosterone:LH ratio). Most patients with neuropsychiatric disease have evidence of demyelination on brain MRI, typically with hyperintensities on T2WI. Definitive diagnosis is by measurement of serum VLCFA, which are elevated in X-linked adrenoleukodystrophy [598].

10.5.9 Cerebrotendinous xanthomatosis

Cerebrotendinous xanthomatosis is a rare autosomal recessive lipid storage disease in which large deposits of cholesterol and cholestanol are found in virtually every tissue. The brain is an organ particularly affected. The disease is characterized by progressive neurological dysfunction, premature atherosclerosis, and early-onset cataracts. Tendon xanthomas are common and chronic diarrhoea may feature. Neurological disease is typically characterized by cerebellar ataxia beginning after puberty, spinal cord involvement, and a phase of pseudobulbar palsy leading to death. There may be peripheral neuropathy, spastic paraparesis, parkinsonism, and dementia (MIM 213700) [115]. Psychosis occurs but is not common, occurring in 9% of one small series, though other estimates put the incidence rate of schizophrenia-like psychosis at 10–30%. Catatonia has also occurred [17, 94, 600]. Plasma cholesterol is low-normal. Magnetic resonance imaging may show leukoencephalopathy, or abnormal signal in the deep grey matter (especially the dentate nucleus and globus pallidus), and CT may show dentate nucleus microcalcification [47]. Diagnosis is by demonstrating elevated cholestanol in serum or tendon tissue [115]. Specific treatment is available [600]. The differential diagnosis includes Whipple's disease (Chapter 8.1.8 ▶) and Lyme disease (Chapter 8.1.3 ▶) [20].

10.5.10 Alpha-mannosidosis

Alpha-mannosidosis is an autosomal recessive lysosomal storage disease caused by lysosomal α-mannosidase deficiency. There is a broad phenotype, from a severe infantile form (Type I), fatal in childhood, to a less severe juvenile- or adult-onset form (Type II) (MIM 248500).

The late-onset form is characterized by mild mental retardation, progressive sensorineural hearing loss, immunodeficiency (recurrent respiratory and gastrointestinal infections), dysmorphism (e.g. coarse features, macroglossia, flat nose, large ears, widely spaced teeth, large head/hands/feet, tall stature, bowed femurs, and radiographic skeletal abnormalities such as spondylolisthesis), sometimes hepatosplenomegaly, and progressive neurological dysfunction including visual impairment, cerebellar ataxia, and pyramidal signs. From puberty or adolescence, there may be recurrent episodes of confusion, psychosis (including delusions and auditory and visual hallucinations), and/or depression; these episodes typically last 3–12 weeks and are followed by a period of tiredness and somnolence (MIM 248500) [115, 601]. Occasionally α-mannosidosis has been considered to be schizophrenia for many years [602]. Diagnosis is by urine oligosaccharide analysis and blood α-mannosidase assay [115].

10.5.11 Krabbe's disease (globoid cell leukodystrophy)

Krabbe's disease (globoid cell leukodystrophy, Krabbe leukodystrophy) is an autosomal recessive PNS and CNS white matter storage disorder caused by deficiency of galactosylceramidase beta-galactosidase (galactocerebrosidase) leading to accumulation of galactosylceramide and psychosine. Histologically, microglia (of monocyte-macrophage lineage) accumulate the abnormal material and appear as "globoid" cells. The clinical form is variable, with infantile and late-onset (including adult-onset) forms (MIM 245200). The frequency is approximately 1:100 000 births in the USA and Europe, with a few isolated communities in Israel having much higher disease rates [603]. The adult forms typically present with signs including pes cavus, optic disc pallor, progressive spastic tetraparesis, a sensorimotor demyelinating neuropathy, and brain demyelination on MRI (typically hypodense lesions in the parieto-occipital periventricular white matter) [604]. Nerve conduction studies and EEG may be abnormal but often are not in the late-onset disorder (MIM 245200). Psychosis is very uncommon in Krabbe's disease [94], though a "dementia–psychosis" variant at onset has been described [605, 606]. Diagnosis is by leukocyte enzyme assay.

10.5.12 Gaucher's disease

Gaucher's disease is an autosomal recessive lysosomal storage disorder caused by deficiency of glucosylceramidase, an acid β-glucosidase, and consequent accumulation of glycolipids in macrophages (termed Gaucher cells) and brain [607]. The disease frequency is approximately 1:57 000–1:86 000, though founder effects led to higher rates in some specific populations (Ashkenazi Jewish, Spanish, Portuguese, Swedish, Jenin Arab, Greek, and Albanian). The spectrum is broad and includes various combinations of primary CNS involvement (bulbar signs, pyramidal signs, cognitive impairment, oculomotor apraxia, ataxia, seizures, progressive myoclonic epilepsy), bone disease (osteopenia, lytic/sclerotic lesions, osteonecrosis, pathological fractures, joint collapse, febrile episodes of bone pain), visceral disease (splenomegaly, hepatomegaly, pulmonary disease, mitral/aortic valve calcification) and other (cytopenia, skin changes) [607, 608].

Gaucher's disease is categorized as non-neuronopathic type I, acute neuronopathic type II, and subacute neuronopathic type III, of which types II and III have CNS involvement, and type III is associated with survival beyond infancy, though usually with juvenile onset. These represent the typical phenotypic continuum of mutations in the same underlying gene (MIM 230800, 230900, 231000). Type III can exhibit neurological, bone, and visceral manifestations [608].

Adult-onset neuronopathic Gaucher's disease is rare, but psychosis is not infrequent within it, and psychosis is also seen in the juvenile-onset form [609, 610].

Diagnosis is by leukocyte enzyme assay.

10.5.13 Vanishing white matter leukoencephalopathy

In vanishing white matter leukoencephalopathy (leukodystrophy) (VWM), the white matter of the cerebral hemispheres undergoes diffuse cystic degeneration. It is an autosomal recessive disease (MIM 603896). It usually begins in childhood, but adolescent- and adult-onset forms are also well described. It has presented in late life with dementia and psychosis [611], and at the age of 25–30 with psychosis and contemporaneous mild motor disturbance or subsequent overt ataxia [612].

Suggested diagnostic criteria (MIM 603896) are as follows. (1) Initial motor and mental development is normal or mildly delayed. (2) Neurologic deterioration has a chronic progressive and episodic course; episodes of deterioration may follow minor infection and minor head trauma and may lead to lethargy or coma. (3) Neurologic signs consist mainly of cerebellar ataxia and spasticity (though there may also be optic atrophy, epilepsy, and cognitive impairment). (4) MRI may indicate symmetric involvement of the cerebral hemispheric white matter; part or all of the white matter has a signal intensity close to or the same as CSF on proton-density, T2WI, T1WI, and FLAIR images; and cerebellar atrophy varies from mild to severe and primarily involves the vermis. Magnetic resonance spectroscopy may also be supportive: white matter spectra show a very substantial decrease in all normal signals and the presence of some lactate and glucose.

10.5.14 Diffuse sclerosis

Diffuse myelinoclastic sclerosis presents as pseudotumoural demyelinating lesions (clastic from Greek *klastos*, broken in pieces). It is more common in children than adults. Similar diseases must be excluded, including SSPE (Chapter 8.2.4 ▶), leukodystrophy (e.g. adrenoleukodystrophy [Chapter 10.5.8 ▶], metachromatic leukodystrophy [Chapter 10.5.7 ▶]), encephalitis (Chapter 8 ▶), acute disseminated encephalomyelitis (Chapter 8.7.3 ▶), acute MS (Chapter 6.8 ▶), mitochondrial cytopathies (Chapter 10.6 ▶), and Krabbe's disease (Chapter 10.5.11 ▶). Having excluded these, diffuse sclerosis is exceedingly rare and there is debate as to whether it is a distinct entity [613]. It is sometimes termed **Schilder's disease**, though this eponym is best avoided as it was originally applied to a series that turned out to represent several unrelated disorders, and its use subsequently broadened further [614].

Cognitive impairment (confusion, aphasia, memory disturbance, disorientation, mental dullness), mental state changes (including psychosis, personality change, and behavioural disturbance), and deafness are common. Other brainstem and cerebellar signs may be seen, as may cortical blindness, hemiparesis, and cortical somatosensory deficits. Seizures and extrapyramidal manifestations are uncommon [33, 613].

Diagnostic criteria are (1) one or two roughly symmetrical large plaques, >2 cm in at least two dimensions, chiefly in the centrum semiovale, and if there is more than one, one should be in each hemisphere; (2) no other lesions; (3) no abnormalities of the peripheral nervous system; (4) normal adrenal function; (5) normal serum VLCFA; (6) biopsy or autopsy confirming acute or chronic myelinoclastic diffuse sclerosis (histologically indistinguishable from multiple sclerosis) [613].

10.6 Mitochondrial encephalopathies

Mitochondria generate ATP by oxidative phosphorylation, and host other processes including beta oxidation and the Krebs cycle. They contain multiple copies of mitochondrial DNA, and can contain a mix of different DNAs, sometimes normal and abnormal, known as heteroplasmy. Some nuclear mutations may also cause mitochondrial disease. Mitochondrial disease is clinically and genetically heterogeneous, and is not rare, with a prevalence of ~1:10 000. Its common features are: eye manifestations of *ptosis, ophthalmoplegia*, and *retinopathy*; somatic manifestations of *diabetes, deafness, short stature, cardiac involvement, renal involvement*, and *sideroblastic anaemia*; and CNS manifestations of *dementia, ataxia, myoclonus, seizures, and stroke-like episodes*. *Myopathy* and *peripheral neuropathy* may also occur. Combinations of any of these features should raise the suspicion of mitochondrial disease. Mitochondrial encephalopathies can present at any age, though presentations in childhood are more commonly associated with multisystem disease. They may conform to the acronyms MERRF (myoclonic epilepsy with ragged red fibres [on muscle biopsy]) or **MELAS (mitochondrial encephalopathy with lactic acidosis and stroke-like episodes)** but more often do not [615, 616]. MELAS is classically associated with stroke-like episodes before the age of 40, seizures and/or dementia, and ragged red fibres and/or lactic acidosis; and sometimes with diabetes mellitus, cardiomyopathy (hypertrophic leading to dilated), bilateral deafness, pigmentary retinopathy (retinitis pigmentosa), and cerebellar ataxia. Migraine (Chapter 6.3 ▶), hypoparathyroidism (Chapter 9.5 ▶), basal ganglia calcification (Chapter 5.11 ▶), and CVAs (Chapter 6.1 ▶) may occur [26]. Psychiatric manifestations are rare in isolation but may include auditory and visual hallucinations, delusions, cognitive impairment, and behavioural disorganization [17, 617–620]. In one series with psychosis (mostly in the context of MELAS), the mean age of onset of psychosis was 24.7 years, with a similar age of onset of physical symptoms but, on average, considerable diagnostic delay [17].

Suspected mitochondrial disease requires a hunt for other evidence of respiratory chain disease, including cardiac assessment (ECG and echocardiography), endocrine assessment (oral glucose tolerance test, thyroid function tests, alkaline phosphatase, fasting calcium, and parathyroid hormone levels), and urinary organic and amino acids (which may be abnormal even in the absence of overt tubular disease). Measuring blood and CSF lactate levels may be helpful (but less so in adults than children); the differential of blood and CSF lactic acidosis is quite wide and includes fever, sepsis, dehydration, seizures, and stroke. Cerebrospinal fluid protein may be elevated. Serum CK may be raised but is often normal. Neurophysiology may identify a myopathy or neuropathy. The EEG may show diffuse slow-wave activity consistent with a subacute encephalopathy, or evidence of seizure activity. Magnetic resonance imaging may show lesions of the basal ganglia (including calcification), white matter hyperintensity, or generalized cerebral atrophy [26, 33].

Specific diagnosis of a mitochondrial disease is often by genetic testing, but is sometimes guided by skeletal muscle biopsy [26]. An important differential diagnosis is CADASIL (Chapter 6.1 ▶) [20]. See also DIDMOAD (Chapter 4.8 ▶). For a review of the relationship between mitochondrial dysfunction and schizophreniform psychosis, see also [17].

10.7 Glucose-6-phosphate dehydrogenase deficiency

G6PD deficiency is a common X-linked disorder, with highest prevalence (gene frequency 5–25%) in the Mediterranean, Middle East, tropical Africa, parts of Asia, and Papua New Guinea. G6PD protects cells against oxidative stress, which in G6PD deficiency provokes acute haemolysis (typically triggered by infections, oxidative drugs, or fava [broad] beans) [621] (MIM 305900). There is some, albeit weak, evidence for an association between G6PD deficiency and psychosis [35, 622].

Chapter 11 Nutritional deficiency

11.1 Thiamine (vitamin B_1) deficiency

Thiamine is a water-soluble vitamin that is required as a cofactor by several enzymes involved in carbohydrate metabolism. It is present in all vegetables and the outer layers of grains. Body stores are small, normally lasting a total of approximately one month, and healthy individuals usually develop symptoms of thiamine deficiency within a week of no thiamine intake, with a resting tachycardia, weakness, decreased deep tendon reflexes, and sometimes a peripheral neuropathy. Thiamine deficiency is usually caused by inadequate dietary intake. In the developed world, this is most common in alcoholism, which is associated with low thiamine intake but also impaired uptake and storage, increased destruction, and additional neurotoxic effects of alcohol. Dietary deficiency can also occur in starvation and on fad diets, including diets rich in thiaminases (milled rice, raw freshwater fish or shellfish, ferns), anti-thiamine factor (tea, coffee, betel), and processed foods rich in sulphites (which destroy thiamine). Absorption may be impaired by chronic intestinal disease and malabsorptive states, alcoholism, malnutrition, gastric bypass surgery, and in folate deficiency (be it dietary or induced by chemotherapy such as methotrexate; Chapter 11.5 ▶), since folate is required for thiamine use by cells. Thiamine may be lost by diarrhoea, vomiting (especially hyperemesis gravidarum), diuretics, peritoneal dialysis, and haemodialysis. Severe liver disease impairs its use. It is consumed more rapidly in high metabolic states including hyperthyroidism, pregnancy, lactation, fever, and physical exercise; in diets high in carbohydrate or saturated fats; and if intravenous fluids with a high glucose content are given [26, 623].

Thiamine deficiency (**beriberi**) causes neurological and cardiac manifestations – sometimes termed dry and wet beriberi, respectively, though these terms have been used in different ways [624]. The typical neurological effects include symmetrical peripheral neuropathy (sensory and motor) secondary to demyelination (often with paraesthesiae and neuropathic burning pain as well as decreased vibration sense, absent distal reflexes, muscle atrophy, and eventually foot drop), fatigue, poor memory, irritability, sleep disturbance, and muscle cramps [26, 623]. **Wernicke's encephalopathy** is the neuropsychiatric consequence of acute and severe thiamine depletion [33]. The three classic features of Wernicke's encephalopathy are (1) mental state change, with lethargy and inattentiveness, confusion, memory impairment, and progressive cognitive impairment; (2) eye signs, with ophthalmoplegias and diplopia (most commonly nystagmus on lateral or vertical gaze, sixth nerve palsy, or defects of conjugate gaze); and (3) ataxia [26, 623]. However, these three features are *not* always present [625]. A prodrome of anorexia, nausea, and vomiting may occur, and hallucinations and delusions may be present in the acute phase [33]. There may also be hypothermia, and it may progress to stupor, coma, and death. Wernicke's encephalopathy is seen in up to 3% of admissions for alcohol complications, and the untreated mortality is 20% [623]. If the patient survives, the chronic features of **Korsakoff's syndrome**, or Korsakoff's "psychosis", may emerge. Despite the name, delusions and hallucinations are not typical features [626]. There is often severe anterograde amnesia secondary to mammillary body damage in the diencephalon. The patient is alert but disoriented in time and place, and remote memory is intact. Gaps in memory are often covered by confabulation. Wernicke's and Korsakoff's syndromes are the acute and chronic phases of the same process, collectively termed **Wernicke–Korsakoff encephalopathy**. Pathologically, there are hyperaemic areas of dilated capillaries with perivascular haemorrhage in the upper brainstem, hypothalamus, thalamus, and mammillary bodies, often with associated alcohol-induced cortical, cerebellar, and peripheral nerve damage [26]. Magnetic resonance imaging may show high or abnormal signals in the mammillary bodies, and sometimes in the mammillothalamic tract, paraventricular and mediodorsal thalamus, periaqueductal grey, and surrounding the third ventricle [47]. The EEG may show diffuse slowing or be normal [33]. Autopsy evidence of Wernicke–Korsakoff syndrome is seen in up to 12.5% of alcoholics, most not diagnosed during life; the prevalence of thiamine deficiency in alcoholics is 30–80% [624, 627].

Wet beriberi may present chronically (with periperal vasodilatation and a high-output cardiac state, followed by sodium retention and peripheral oedema, and then cardiac failure) or acutely (acute fulminant cardiovascular beriberi, or Shoshin beriberi, in which cardiac muscle dysfunction occurs early). Clinically, there may be tachycardia, chest pain, and left and/or right ventricular failure, sometimes with vasodilatation. There may be anorexia, abdominal discomfort, and constipation [623].

Diagnosis and treatment. There are a number of tests possible for thiamine deficiency; however, thiamine is non-toxic and the usual method of diagnosis is clinical and by assessing the effects of thiamine replacement. Wernicke–Korsakoff syndrome must be suspected in any patient with unexplained confusion, stupor, or coma, particularly in the presence of eye signs, peripheral neuropathy, or a history of alcoholism or excessive vomiting. All such patients should be given thiamine, parenterally and at adequate doses until the deficit has been replaced, at which point oral maintenance treatment can be given. Oral absorption is low and variable and must not be relied upon in this acute situation. Thiamine must always be given if intravenous glucose is to be administered to alcoholic or chronically malnourished patients, or to patients with stupor or coma of unknown cause, to avoid precipitating Wernicke's encephalopathy. Giving glucose without thiamine to those with Wernicke–Korsakoff syndrome can cause deterioration and death; give thiamine first or simultaneously [26, 628]. Beriberi short of Korsakoff's syndrome responds extremely quickly to thiamine replacement, though only half of patients with frank Korsakoff's syndrome respond significantly; therefore, treatment before this stage is a priority. Treatment is until all symptoms have gone [623], and supplementation will probably be needed for longer. Supplements that also provide niacin (typically as nicotinamide) will treat any coexistent pellagra encephalopathy (Chapter 11.2 ▶), and any hypomagnesaemia should also be corrected to improve the response to treatment [25, 33].

11.2 Niacin (vitamin B_3, nicotinic acid) deficiency

Niacin is a B-group vitamin found in food as nicotinic acid, as NAD or NADP, and as nicotinamide. It is in meat, poultry, fish, wholemeal cereals, pulses, and coffee. It also occurs in maize as niacytin, though this is only absorbed if it is hydrolysed externally; humans eating diets based on maize are prone to niacin deficiency. Nicotinic acid can be synthesized in the liver from tryptophan (60 mg of tryptophan makes ~1 mg of nicotinic acid), though this requires vitamin B_6 (pyridoxine) and riboflavin (vitamin B_2); deficiency of either can exacerbate niacin deficiency. Maize is also poor in tryptophan. There are no substantial body stores of niacin, and 1–2 months' dietary deficiency leads to **pellagra**. In addition to dietary deficiency, other risk factors for niacin deficiency include malabsorption, pyridoxine deficiency (Chapter 11.3 ▶) (e.g. caused by isoniazid therapy; Chapter 15.1 ▶), Hartnup's disease (an inborn error of tryptophan metabolism; Chapter 10.3.3 ▶), hepatic cirrhosis, diabetes mellitus, prolonged fever, prolonged diarrhoea, and HIV infection [26, 629]. Alcoholics are predisposed to niacin deficiency, known in its neuropsychiatric form as **alcoholic pellagra encephalopathy** or **acute nicotinic acid deficiency encephalopathy** [25, 33, 625], though this is much less common than Wernicke–Korsakoff syndrome.

Niacin deficiency, or pellagra, classically causes the triad of dementia, diarrhoea, and dermatitis. Neurological involvement is the most constant feature, and encephalopathy may be the only feature of niacin deficiency in industrialized countries, particularly in alcoholics. Diarrhoea occurs in 50% and dermatitis in 30%. The neurological features may include dementia and confusion, increased limb tone, and grasping/sucking reflexes. Early neurological changes include anxiety and irritability with poor concentration. There may be paraesthesiae and a burning sensation with loss of proprioception and vibration sense. The encephalopathy can progress to mania, depression, delusions and hallucinations ("pellagra psychosis"), and stupor (followed by coma and death).

The chronic form of the disease has seasonal periodicity. There are often sebaceous follicles of the nose early in the condition, but later there is a dermatosis in sun-exposed areas, also exacerbated by heat, friction, and pressure. There may be itching and burning of the lesions; they may blister early on but become hyperpigmented (or relatively depigmented in dark skins) and have sharp margins. The skin looks sunburnt in chronic pellagra. There is weight loss and poor stamina, with a predisposition to bacterial and parasitic infections. In severe cases, there are gastrointestinal disturbances with poor appetite, nausea, epigastric discomfort, abdominal pain, increased salivation, diarrhoea, glossitis, angular stomatitis, cheilosis, and oral infections [26, 28, 629].

Sometimes, the onset of nicotinic acid deficiency encephalopathy is acute, usually in patients with malnutrition and/or alcoholism, or in response to increased metabolic demand (e.g. severe physical illness, surgery, and rarely carcinoid syndrome). The neuropsychiatric manifestations can occur alone, typically with delirium and hallucinations or delusions, though glossitis/stomatitis or other features of pellagra and extrapyramidal signs may give an indication as to the cause [25, 33].

Diagnosis is clinical and by therapeutic response to niacin, though serum and urinary measurements of niacin and metabolites can be used to confirm the diagnosis [629].

See also Hartnup's disease (Chapter 10.3.3 ▶) and pyridoxine deficiency (Chapter 11.3 ▶).

11.3 Pyridoxine (vitamin B_6) deficiency

Isolated pyridoxine deficiency is very rare as pyridoxine is widespread in foods, though malnutrition or a diet restricted to unenriched grains increases the risk. Acquired deficiency is usually associated with one or more of: inflammatory disorders and catabolic states, malnutrition, coeliac disease, hepatitis and biliary obstruction, chronic renal failure, dialysis, alcoholism, and a number of drugs including cycloserine, hydralazine, penicillamine, pyrazinamide and isoniazid (Chapter 15.1 ▶) [630].

Pyridoxine phosphate is a cofactor in many synthetic pathways. Deficiency of pyridoxine can exacerbate niacin deficiency and can on its own cause a syndrome identical to pellagra. Pyridoxine deficiency can also impair homocysteine metabolism, causing homocystinaemia and homocystinuria. The syndrome of pyridoxine deficiency can therefore encompass the signs of pellagra (Chapter 11.2 ▶) (dermatological, neurological, gastrointestinal; q.v.), homocystinaemia (Chapter 10.3.2 ▶) (e.g. increased risk of thromboembolism, neurological dysfunction; q.v.), and sometimes sideroblastic anaemia. Pyridoxine-responsive seizures may occur in people with a version of CNS glutamic acid decarboxylase that has a low affinity for pyridoxine. Pyridoxine deficiency may also play a part in isoniazid-induced psychosis (Chapter 15.1 ▶) [631] and psychosis in homocystinuria (Chapter 10.3.2 ▶) [632], and the use of pyridoxine has been suggested in certain other psychotic states, though it appears more useful for tardive dyskinesia than schizophrenia itself [633–635]. Unusually for a vitamin, pyridoxine excess can also cause neuropathy [630].

Whole-body pyridoxine levels may be assayed by serum pyridoxal 5′-phosphate (PLP) [630].

11.4 Cobalamin (vitamin B_{12}) deficiency, and methylmalonic aciduria

Vitamin B_{12} is an umbrella term for a group of vitamers (different molecules with the same vitamin activity) required as a cofactor for the use of folate in DNA synthesis, and in other processes less well understood. They contain cobalt and corrin ring structures, and include cyanocobalamin (a synthetic form) and natural cobalamin molecules, which are made only by certain forms of bacteria. Many animals harbour B_{12}-synthesizing bacteria in their gut and have behavioural mechanisms (e.g. rumination, coprophagia) for absorbing the B_{12} thus produced. Humans obtain B_{12} from foods of animal origin, including meat and milk. Vegans are thus vulnerable to B_{12} deficiency. Absorption by humans requires secretion of intrinsic factor from gastric parietal cells. The intrinsic factor binds B_{12} and the complex is absorbed in the terminal ileum; 1% of free cobalamin is also absorbed. Body stores are 2–5 mg, mostly in liver and bone marrow, and there is recycling via the enterohepatic circulation, keeping the daily requirement down to about 2 μg/day (more in pregnancy and lactation). Deficiency after malabsorption therefore occurs in 2–5 years, and deficiency in vegetarians usually after 10–20 years [636], assuming normal initial stores.

Causes. The prevalence of deficiency is not known precisely because of variation in assays (radioassay and chemiluminescence) and cut-offs, but deficiency below blood levels of 200 ng/l by radioassay has a prevalence of 3–16% in the USA and 1.6–10% in Europe [636]. B_{12} intake may be deficient in strict vegetarianism, though this is rare. It is usually claimed that 75% of cases of B_{12} deficiency are due to pernicious anaemia, an autoimmune attack on gastric parietal cells or intrinsic factor [636]. Gastrectomy and *Helicobacter pylori* gastritis can also cause intrinsic factor deficiency. Defects of gut pH regulation (including atrophic gastritis, pancreatic insufficiency, and PPI use) may hinder absorption, as may terminal ileal disorders (e.g. tropical sprue, coeliac disease, Whipple's disease [Chapter 8.1.8 ▶], resection). In fact, recent studies suggest that malabsorption due to failure to release B_{12} from food or intestinal transport proteins ("food–B_{12} malabsorption"), particularly in the presence of hypochlorhydria, accounts for 60–70% of cases of B_{12} deficiency in the elderly, usually due to atrophic gastritis [637]. Metformin also hinders absorption [638]. B_{12} requirements are increased in hyperthyroidism (Chapter 9.1 ▶) and α-thalassaemia. Late-stage HIV infection (Chapter 8.2.2 ▶) is associated with B_{12} deficiency via several mechanisms [636]. Rarely, inherited disorders of cobalamin metabolism lead to methylmalonic aciduria and homocystinuria (Chapter 10.3.2 ▶) in infancy, and features of B_{12} deficiency. Nitrous oxide (N_2O) (Chapter 15.1 ▶) can precipitate vitamin B_{12} deficiency, and recreational inhalation of N_2O has been suggested to precipitate cobalamin-responsive psychosis with only slightly low B_{12} levels [639].

Effects. B_{12} deficiency causes damage to peripheral and optic nerves, the posterior and lateral columns of the spinal cord (subacute combined degeneration of the cord; myelopathy), and the brain, and disrupts haematopoiesis. Sometimes haematological and neurological features dissociate. The onset is usually gradual (subacute), though exposure to nitrous oxide can make it faster. The classic symptoms are weakness, a sore tongue, and paraesthesiae, but the onset is often with cold, numbness, or tightness in the tips of the toes and then the fingertips; isolated paraesthesiae occur in 33% of patients. This may be followed by ascending paraesthesiae, sometimes a sensation of truncal constriction, and later limb weakness and ataxia (with gait abnormalities in 12% of patients). There is often poor joint position sense and vibration sense distally, and absent ankle reflexes. Neuropsychiatric symptoms occur in 8% of patients (recent memory loss, poor attention, depression, paranoid psychosis with auditory or visual hallucinations, violent behaviour, personality change, blunted affect, and/or emotional lability). Psychosis in this context is sometimes called "megaloblastic madness". More rarely (0.5%), visual acuity decreases, usually secondary to optic neuropathy. There may be lightheadedness, and impaired taste and smell. Autonomic neuropathy can occur. Non-neurological symptoms and signs include anorexia and weight loss (50%), low-grade fever (33%), a yellow waxy pallor, mild jaundice, fatigue, malaise, syncope, dyspnoea, biventricular failure, orthopnoea, tachycardia, palpitations, angina, heartburn, flatulence, constipation, diarrhoea, a sore tongue (glossitis), and early satiety [636, 640]. There is some debate as to the prevalence of neuropsychiatric disorders without other (e.g. haematological) features of B_{12} deficiency [641, 642].

There is often macrocytic anaemia; the probability of B_{12} deficiency with a normal MCV is <25%, while B_{12} deficiency is almost certain if the MCV is >130 fl [636]. Neutrophil hypersegmentation is typical, and thrombocytopenia is common. There may be an element of haemolysis, with an elevated unconjugated bilirubin and LDH. However, 25% of patients have no anaemia or macrocytosis [28]. B_{12} deficiency is associated with hyperhomocysteinaemia (Chapter 10.3.2 ▶), a cardiovascular risk factor.

Low serum cobalamin levels indicate B_{12} deficiency. Deficiency should prompt testing for antiparietal cell antibodies (positive in 90% of pernicious anaemia cases) and anti-intrinsic factor antibodies (positive in 70%); if either is positive, pernicious anaemia is confirmed (and requires specialist input for long-term cancer surveillance, in addition to B_{12} treatment). If they are negative, the specialist Schilling test can be used to determine the aetiological class of the deficiency [636].

Sometimes there is doubt as to whether a low serum B_{12} result truly indicates deficiency, or whether deficiency is present despite a normal serum B_{12} result, as current commercial assays are imperfect. The usual next step is to measure methylmalonic acid and homocysteine, which are usually both elevated in B_{12} deficiency (see hyperhomocysteinaemia, Chapter 10.3.2 ▶), but the clinical picture is also important [28, 636, 643, 644].

Methylmalonic aciduria. Finally, there are also inherited disorders of B_{12} usage that can present with psychosis, such as **cobalamin C disease** (cblC; MIM 277400). This causes methylmalonic aciduria with homocystinuria. It usually presents in infancy but can present in adults with a clinical picture resembling B_{12} deficiency and including psychosis; B_{12} cannot be used by the body, and the enzyme blockades that result cause elevated levels of methylmalonic acid and homocysteine (Chapter 10.3.2 ▶) in the blood and urine [645].

11.5 Folate (vitamin B_9) deficiency

Folic acid can refer to pteroylglutamic acid, but the term folic acid or folate is more often applied to a group of substances with similar nutritional activity. They underpin key one-carbon metabolic pathways required for a variety of processes including DNA synthesis. Folates are synthesized by plants and microorganisms and there are a variety of dietary sources for humans, amongst which the most significant are green vegetables, citrus fruits, and animal products. Folates are destroyed by prolonged exposure to heat. In the healthy state, body stores are 5–20 mg and the daily requirement is 50–100 μg, so deficiency can manifest after a few months. A serum folate <3 ng/ml (<6.8 nM) and a red cell folate <140 ng/ml (<317 nM) indicate a high risk of deficiency [644, 646, 647]. High homocysteine levels are also a marker of folate deficiency (see Chapter 10.3.2 ▶, Chapter 11.4 ▶). The prevalence of folate deficiency varies according to geographical region and whether folate supplementation or fortification (e.g. of flour) is in use. Before fortification, the prevalence of deficiency was 16% in the USA [647]. Aside from inadequate intake, deficiency may arise from malabsorption (e.g. widespread jejunal disease, intestinal bacterial overgrowth, zinc deficiency), increased demands (pregnancy, infancy, diseases associated with rapid cellular proliferation), or be drug-induced. Methotrexate directly blocks folate metabolism, but other drugs causing folate deficiency include anticonvulsants (phenytoin, primidone, phenobarbital), oral contraceptives, sulfasalazine, triamterene, trimethoprim, and alcohol [644, 647, 648].

Substantial failure of the metabolism of folate can cause psychosis, as in MTHFR deficiency (see Chapter 10.3.2 ▶). Folate is required for normal metabolism of homocysteine (see Chapter 10.3.2 ▶, Chapter 11.4 ▶) and normal use of thiamine (Chapter 11.1 ▶). However, although simple folate deficiency may play a role in depression and cognitive impairment, and is linked (likely via hyperhomocysteinaemia) to atherosclerosis and cardiovascular risk (Chapter 6.1 ▶) [28, 33, 649], its role in psychosis is not clear: it may be an exacerbating factor, but there is no good evidence that it is causal on its own. In randomized controlled trials, methylfolate improved clinical outcome scores in schizophrenia [650] and a combination of folic acid, vitamin B_{12}, and pyridoxine improved symptoms of schizophrenia in patients who also had hyperhomocysteinaemia [651].

Symptoms of folate deficiency include glossitis and angular stomatitis, other gastrointestinal symptoms (anorexia, nausea, vomiting, abdominal pain, diarrhoea), fever, hyperpigmentation of mucous membranes and skin (particularly on the dorsal aspects of fingers, the toes, and on the creases of palms and soles). Cognitive impairment may be present, with irritability and sleep disruption. There may be macrocytic anaemia with neutrophil hypersegmentation, as for B_{12} deficiency [647].

Diagnosis of folate deficiency is by red cell or serum folate measurement. Red cell folate reflects long term stores and is generally considered the better measure of deficiency, though in practice serum folate measurement usually gives similar results [644, 647, 652]. Note that folate should never be given alone if there is coexistent vitamin B_{12} deficiency, as it may precipitate subacute degeneration of the spinal cord [653].

One other mechanism of neurological folate deficiency is the **cerebral folate deficiency syndrome**. This is a term applied to any neuropsychiatric condition where there are low levels in the CSF of 5-MTHF, the active CSF folate metabolite, with normal folate metabolism outside the central nervous system (indicated by normal haematological values, normal serum homocysteine levels, and normal serum and red cell folate). This condition is often associated with autoantibodies blocking transfer of folate from plasma to brain tissue and CSF, though there are other mechanisms, and it can be treated with folinic acid. Usually it presents in infancy (typically with irritability, sleep disturbance, reduced head growth, developmental delay, psychomotor retardation, movement disorders, seizures, and visual or hearing loss) [654, 655] but it has recently been suggested, in a single case study, that it can present with catatonic schizophrenia [656]. Diagnosis is clinical and by LP, measuring 5-MTHF [655].

11.6 Zinc deficiency

One uncontrolled study depleted zinc acutely, using histidine in patients with systemic sclerosis, producing anorexia, disruption of taste and smell, dizziness, cerebellar dysfunction, depression and tearfulness, memory impairment, lethargy, auditory and visual hallucinations, and paranoid ideation. These symptoms were related to zinc levels and reversed by zinc administration even in the continued presence of histidine [657]. Aside from one other case study (see [25, 33]) there appear to be no studies suggesting zinc deficiency to be a cause of psychosis encountered in clinical practice.

11.7 Omega-3 fatty acids

Essential fatty acid levels have been found to be reduced in lipid membranes of patients with schizophrenia, though this may not derive from dietary deficiency [658]. Omega-3 fatty acid (ethyl-eicosapentaenoic acid) supplementation has been shown to be of some benefit in first-episode psychosis and schizophrenia, though not all studies have found an effect [659–661]. Methods for assessing essential fatty acid levels are not available in routine clinical practice.

11.8 Starvation

Visual hallucinations of food have been reported during prolonged starvation [662]. Similarly, olfactory hallucinations, typically pleasant food-related ones, were reported by 29% of inpatients with severe eating disorders (anorexia nervosa, bulimia nervosa, or both) in one study [17, 663]. There is clearly scope in this situation for overlap with other nutritional deficiencies (Chapter 11 ▶) and metabolic disturbances (Chapter 12 ▶). Starvation has preceded recurrent psychosis in such patients, and transient psychosis (with delusions, hallucinations, and/or thought disorder) has been observed in patients with severe anorexia nervosa [664, 665]. See also Chapter 21.13 ▶.

Chapter 12 Other acquired metabolic disorders

12.1 Global cerebral hypoxia

Acute hypoxia (**hypoxic encephalopathy**) is a cause of psychosis (see delirium, Chapter 3 ▶), with hallucinations being frequent when cerebral hypoxia or hypoperfusion is induced in healthy individuals [666, 667]. **Post-anoxic encephalopathy** (post-hypoxic encephalopathy, post-ischaemic encephalopathy, ischaemic–hypoxic encephalopathy) may occur following recovery from anoxia or global cerebral ischaemia causing coma; there may be amnesia or a delirium, sometimes with delusions and hallucinations [20]. See also carbon monoxide poisoning (Chapter 15.7.1 ▶).

12.2 Disturbances of pH and hypercapnic encephalopathy

Respiratory alkalosis is caused by hyperventilation lowing $PaCO_2$. The alkalosis causes neuronal hyperexcitability: H^+ ions and Ca^{2+} ions compete for plasma protein binding, so alkalosis can lead to ionic hypocalcaemia (Chapter 12.5.3 ▶) and thus neuronal hyperexcitability. Respiratory alkalosis can cause anxiety and panic, perceptual disturbances (including paraesthesiae), feelings of unreality and impending doom, and dyspnoea, but psychosis is not typical [668] (though see psychosis occurring during panic attacks; Chapter 21.11 ▶). The causes are spontaneous and psychogenic hyperventilation; reflex hyperventilation (e.g. pulmonary disease, pulmonary embolism); mechanical overventilation; and other stimulation of the respiratory centre: chemical (tissue hypoxia), toxins (e.g. salicylates, liver failure), after recovery from metabolic acidosis with respiratory compensation, and local lesions of the respiratory centre [669].

Metabolic alkalosis can precipitate psychosis with auditory and visual hallucinations and delusions [668]. The causes are alkali excess (milk–alkali syndrome, therapeutic alkali); inappropriate loss of acid renally or intestinally (pyloric stenosis, other persistent vomiting, potassium depletion other than in renal tubular acidosis, chloride depletion, hyperaldosteronism); "contraction alkalosis" (rapid diuresis); and perhaps failure of urea generation (fulminant hepatic failure) [669].

Respiratory acidosis is caused by excess CO_2, due to structural and mechanical pulmonary disease (chronic obstructive pulmonary disease, large airway obstruction, and, uncommonly, severe asthma); neuromuscular and mechanical chest wall problems (of which the many causes include e.g. poliomyelitis, myasthenia gravis, drug-induced neuromuscular blockade, motor neuron disease, acute chest injury, and severe kyphoscoliosis); and respiratory centre failure (e.g. direct CNS disease, drugs depressing respiratory function). The CNS effects of respiratory acidosis obviously overlap with **hypercapnic encephalopathy (CO_2 narcosis)** , with the two only uncoupled by metabolic compensation for chronic respiratory acidosis (at which point CO_2 remains high but pH moves towards normal). CO_2 intoxication causes confusion and headache, sometimes hallucinations, then narcosis [33]. There may be coexistent **hypoxic encephalopathy** (Chapter 12.1 ▶).

Metabolic acidosis has a range of causes, and while psychosis can be a feature of a number of them, it is not clear that "isolated" metabolic acidosis has been described as a cause of psychotic symptoms. The causes of metabolic acidosis are an inability to excrete normally produced acid (renal failure, hypoaldosteronism [see Chapter 9.3 ▶], type 1 or distal renal tubular acidosis); renal bicarbonate loss (type 2 or proximal renal tubular acidosis, acetazolamide); gastrointestinal bicarbonate loss (e.g. diarrhoea, fistulae, cholestyramine); and increased acid load. Increased acid load may be due to lactic acidosis (overproduction of lactate, due to tissue underperfusion or underoxygenation, or failure of lactate metabolism, due to organ failure, inborn errors of metabolism, or toxins); ketoacidosis (diabetes, starvation, alcoholism); or exogenous acid poisoning (e.g. salicylates, methanol, ethylene glycol). An important clinical feature of metabolic acidosis is deep and rapid (Kussmaul) breathing [670, 671]. Metabolic acidosis and psychosis should prompt a careful search for the cause in the normal way but also raise the possibility of mitochondrial disease with lactic acidosis (Chapter 10.6 ▶), renal failure (Chapter 12.4.1 ▶), and poisoning (Chapter 15 ▶).

12.3 Hypoglycaemia

Hypoglycaemia may produce a wide variety of mental state derangements via neuroglycopenia, and this includes psychosis and focal neurological deficit, as well as the typical features of acute neuroglycopenia (anxiety, agitation including violence, sweating, tremor, tachycardia, hunger, paraesthesia, confusion, fatigue, speech and visual disturbances) and subacute neuroglycopenia (decreased activity, somnolence, poor concentration, personality change, amnesia), both of which can progress to coma and death [26, 33, 672, 673]. Sympathetic overactivity is usually present as a compensatory mechanism, but may be attenuated by drugs that block adrenergic or cholinergic function, or by disease. Those with a history of frequent hypoglycaemia may lose awareness of the early symptoms and develop subacute neuroglycopenia. The cause of hypoglycaemia is usually exogenous insulin or oral hypoglycaemic drugs taken in excess of food (acutely or sometimes chronically), reactive hypoglycaemia (hypoglycaemia secondary to insulin release following a dietary carbohydrate load, though this is rarely severe enough to cause severe neuroglycopenic symptoms), or poisoning (e.g. alcohol, typically 2–16 hours after heavy consumption), and less commonly endogenous insulin excess (e.g. insulinoma), a deficiency in glucose synthesis or mobilization (e.g. adrenal insufficiency, hypothyroidism, liver failure), serious infections (e.g. malaria), prolonged starvation, and a wide range of other causes [26, 29, 674, 675]. Initial diagnosis of hypoglycaemia should be obvious if fingerprick glucose testing is undertaken along with clinical history and examination; hypoglycaemia is usually defined as a glucose level below 3 mM [26]. Emergency treatment with oral or intravenous glucose (according to level of consciousness) is required, with oxygen if necessary [49]. Hypoglycaemia requires explanation: if the cause is not obvious, it should be hunted for thoroughly.

12.4 Organ failure

12.4.1. Renal failure

Renal failure causes the syndrome of **uraemia** primarily through the accumulation of waste products normally cleared by the kidneys [676]. Normal GFR in young adults is 100–120 ml/min/1.73 m^2 body surface area. Neurological manifestations including **uraemic encephalopathy** occur in severe renal failure, acute or chronic, and symptoms can include psychosis. Early neuropsychiatric deficits include impairments in attention and memory performance and "higher" cognitive function, detectable at a GFR of 30–60 ml/min/1.73 m^2. Overt uraemic encephalopathy typically begins when GFR falls to ~10% of normal [677]; to give a very rough approximation, this would equate to a creatinine of the order of ~500 μM in a young man of average size. Its features include drowsiness, confusion, impaired sleep (fragmented, sometimes with brief apnoea), headache, visual abnormalities, tremor, muscle twitching/myoclonus and restless leg syndrome, psychosis, chorea, seizures, and ultimately catatonia and coma [676, 678, 679]. Meningism may also develop [33]. Many of these manifestations are helped by dialysis. Secondary hyperparathyroidism (Chapter 9.5 ▶) is universal in chronic renal failure, and PTH itself may contribute to uraemic encephalopathy [677, 680–683].

Chronic renal failure can also lead to many other conditions that can worsen neurological function. Encephalopathy in renal failure may also be due to Wernicke's encephalopathy (thiamine deficiency [Chapter 11.1 ▶]), "dialysis dementia" (aluminium toxicity [Chapter 15.6.7 ▶]), transplant rejection encephalopathy (headache, confusion, or convulsions with systemic signs of organ rejection, secondary to cytokine production during rejection), hypertensive encephalopathy (Chapter 6.4 ▶), "dialysis disequilibrium" syndrome (headache, nausea, muscle cramps/twitching, delirium, and seizures; it is a self-limiting condition of uncertain aetiology, possibly due to an osmotic plasma–brain gradient developing during rapid dialysis, and preventable by adjusting the dialysis parameters), electrolyte disturbances (hypercalcaemia, hypermagnesaemia, hypernatraemia, hyperosmolality, hyponatraemia, hypoosmolality), and drug toxicity by immunosuppressives or by drugs excreted by the kidney [33, 678]. Renal failure also causes or predisposes to atherosclerosis, ischaemic and haemorrhagic stroke, subdural haematoma, osmotic myelinolysis, infections, and intracranial hypertension (pseudotumor cerebri secondary to dialysis or steroids) [678].

Diagnosis is by demonstration of a raised urea and creatinine. Causes must be sought, and are most usefully classified as prerenal (impaired renal perfusion, the most common, usually due to hypovolaemia and hypotension), renal (intrinsic kidney disease), and postrenal (urinary outflow obstruction). Always consider renal ultrasound to exclude obstruction and urine dipstick ± microscopy to exclude haematuria, proteinuria, cells, or casts secondary to an intrinsic renal cause, in addition to ensuring adequate vascular filling. Renal failure of a degree sufficient to cause psychosis, and acute renal failure whatever the degree, is an emergency. Hyperkalaemia must be sought (including by ECG) and treated immediately. Indications for emergency dialysis are pulmonary oedema, severe acidosis, or refractory hyperkalaemia. The patient with acute or acute-on-chronic renal failure should be managed in a hospital with full medical facilities. In uraemic encephalopathy, EEG typically shows diffuse slowing [678]; the CSF may have a slightly raised opening pressure and protein, and sometimes features of aseptic meningitis with lymphocytes and neutrophils [33].

12.4.2 Hepatic encephalopathy

Hepatic encephalopathy is a neuropsychiatric syndrome caused by acute or chronic liver failure. Acute liver failure leads to hyperammonaemia (see also Chapter 10.1 ▶), cerebral oedema, disrupted cerebral blood flow autoregulation, and often multi-organ failure with reduced systemic vascular resistance and hypoperfusion. In addition there is a coagulopathy (secondary to failure of liver synthetic function), and hypoglycaemia and sepsis may also ensue. In this context, hepatic encephalopathy indicates severe disease and fulminant hepatic failure. Hepatic encephalopathy may also develop in chronic cirrhosis with liver failure, and may be caused and is exacerbated by portosystemic shunts (spontaneous, or surgical to reduce portal pressure), which bypass hepatic metabolism [684, 685]. Encephalopathy in this chronic context is often termed **portosystemic encephalopathy**. Neurotoxins that contribute to hepatic encephalopathy include ammonia (see Chapter 10.1 ▶) and manganese (Chapter 15.6.5 ▶), though 10% of patients with significant encephalopathy have normal ammonia levels. Constipation, gut protein loads, gastrointestinal bleeding, infection, renal failure, hypokalaemia, and alkalosis may exacerbate hyperammonaemia and thus hepatic encephalopathy; hypoxia, hypoglycaemia, hypokalaemia, and sedative drugs may also trigger it [28, 685, 686].

Acute liver failure is most often caused by drugs (most commonly paracetamol and idiosyncratic drug reactions but also herbal remedies) and viral hepatitis (A, B, D, E, and less typically CMV, HSV, and EBV herpesviruses [Chapter 8.2.1 ▶], paramyxoviruses, and haemorrhagic fevers). Other causes are legion [684] but include other toxins (e.g. the death cap mushroom *Amanita phalloides*, cyanobacteria, and carbon tetrachloride), acute fatty liver of pregnancy, hepatic vein thrombosis (Budd–Chiari syndrome) and hepatic veno-occlusive disease, portal vein thrombosis, ischaemic hepatitis, autoimmune hepatitis, Reye's syndrome (Chapter 12.4.4 ▶), and Wilson's disease (Chapter 10.4 ▶).

Chronic liver failure secondary to cirrhosis is most often caused by hepatitis C, alcoholic liver disease, and hepatitis B; other causes include non-alcoholic steatohepatitis, autoimmune hepatitis, primary biliary cirrhosis, primary sclerosing cholangitis, haemochromatosis, Wilson's disease, α-1-antitrypsin deficiency, granulomatous diseases, glycogen storage diseases, drug-induced liver disease, hepatic vein obstruction, and cryptogenic cirrhosis [687].

Hepatic encephalopathy is graded as shown in Table 12.1, with the usual EEG changes also indicated [22, 28, 684, 685]. Psychosis may be part of the encephalopathy [25, 29, 688]. Occasionally there may be seizures and focal neurological signs [20]. Liver failure also increases the chance of drug-induced psychosis (e.g. flumazenil [Chapter 15.1 ▶] [689]) and other mental state changes, through changes in brain vulnerability and drug clearance.

Diagnosis of hepatic encephalopathy is by establishing liver failure, be it acute (with jaundice, elevated liver enzymes, and prolonged PT) or chronic (e.g. with peripheral stigmata of chronic liver disease such as spider naevi, palmar erythema, Dupuytren's contractures, gynaecomastia, and loss of body hair; portal hypertension with ascites, splenomegaly, and caput medusa; coagulopathy; ± jaundice) [26], with encephalopathy as above, and by excluding non-hepatic causes of altered mental state, excluding other contributing factors related to hepatic failure (e.g. hypoglycaemia, hyponatraemia, renal impairment), and identifying causes and precipitants. Serum ammonia levels and EEG may be helpful where there is doubt [22, 685].

Table 12.1 Grades of hepatic encephalopathy

Grade 0	Subclinical. Abnormalities only on psychometric testing; minimal changes in memory, concentration, intellectual function, and coordination. Asterixis is absent. Normal EEG.
Grade 1	Day/night sleep reversal or insomnia/hypersomnia, restlessness, forgetfulness, mild confusion, agitation, irritability/depression/euphoria, tremor/asterixis, apraxia, incoordination, impaired handwriting. Triphasic 1.5–3 Hz waves on EEG.
Grade 2	Lethargy or apathy, slowed responses, intermittent disorientation to time, disinhibition, inappropriate behaviour, obvious asterixis, dysarthria, ataxia, hypoactive reflexes. Triphasic 1.5–3 Hz waves on EEG.
Grade 3	Somnolence, confusion, disorientation to place, intermittent aggressive behaviour, asterixis, muscular rigidity, upgoing plantar reflexes, hyperreflexia. Triphasic 1.5–3 Hz waves on EEG.
Grade 4	Coma with or without response to painful stimulation, decerebration. Generalized delta frequency slowing on EEG.

12.4.3 Pancreatic encephalopathy

Pancreatic encephalopathy is a rare complication of severe acute pancreatitis. It occurs in the first 2 weeks of the pancreatitis and is characterized by fluctuating neurological signs that may include seizures and focal neurological deficit, and/or behavioural change, delirium, and hallucinations. The serum amylase is markedly elevated. Diagnosis depends on the exclusion of other causes of delirium; the exact aetiology is not known [690, 691].

12.4.4 Reye's syndrome

Reye's syndrome is an acute non-inflammatory encephalopathy with hepatic failure. Its aetiology is unknown but it typically follows a viral illness (e.g. upper respiratory tract infections including influenza, varicella, or gastroenteritis), usually within the preceding 3 weeks, and is associated with the use of aspirin during the illness. The peak ages are 5–14 years (median 6) and it is rare in those over 18. Since the warning in 1986 to avoid aspirin in children, the incidence in the UK has fallen from 0.63 to 0.11 cases per 100 000 per year. A number of other drugs and toxins are associated with Reye's or a Reye-like syndrome [692].

The pathogenesis appears to involve mitochondrial dysfunction (see also Chapter 10.6 ▶). Hyperammonaemia (see Chapter 10.1 ▶) is characteristic, and many patients have retrospectively been identified as having an inborn error of metabolism. The differential diagnosis includes fatty-acid oxidation defects, urea cycle abnormalities, amino and organic acidopathies, primary carnitine deficiency, and disorders of carbohydrate metabolism. Inborn errors of metabolism are suggested if symptoms recur with precipitants (e.g. fasting, dietary change, metabolic stress) or if there is a family history [692].

The clinical course is characterized by abrupt onset of vomiting (12 hours to 3 weeks after a viral insult), followed within 24–48 hours by neurological symptoms (typically lethargy with progressive neurological decline, which may include irritability, restlessness, delirium, seizures, and coma). There is hyperammonaemia with evidence of hepatic dysfunction (raised ALT, bilirubin, and PT, ± hypoglycaemia) and its consequences. There may be renal impairment. The EEG may show slowing or flattening [692]. Psychosis may be part of the encephalopathy [693].

The diagnostic criteria are: (1) acute non-inflammatory encephalopathy with altered consciousness; (2) hepatic dysfunction, with a liver biopsy showing fatty metamorphosis or a >3-fold increase in ALT, AST, and/or ammonia levels; (3) no other explanation for cerebral oedema or hepatic abnormality; (4) CSF with WBCs (which are usually lymphocytes) $\leq 8/mm^3$; (5) brain biopsy showing cerebral oedema without inflammation [692].

12.5 Electrolyte disturbances

12.5.1 Hyponatraemia

Severe hyponatraemia can cause psychosis, though rarely, and is associated with some other causes of psychosis.

Hyponatraemia has a wide range of causes and is common, with an in-hospital prevalence of ~2.5% and an in-hospital daily incidence of ~1% for sodium <130 mM [694].

(1) *Hypertonic* hyponatraemia is due to an osmotically active molecule in serum (e.g. glucose, mannitol) causing a water shift from the intracellular to the extracellular compartment.

(2) *Normotonic* hyponatraemia (pseudohyponatraemia) is an artifact that may occur if there are substantial excesses of fat and/or protein in plasma and if the sodium level is measured with respect to the entire plasma rather than the plasma water.

(3) *Hypotonic* hyponatraemia is the most common, and is due to the inability of the kidneys to excrete free water to match water intake. It may be further divided as follows.

   (a) *Hypovolaemic*: due to volume depletion (with salt and water loss) with the defence of intravascular volume taking priority over the defence of osmolality, via ADH release (primary sodium loss with secondary water retention). The cause is fluid loss with replacement by inappropriately hypotonic fluids or very severe sodium depletion (e.g. vomiting, diuresis, salt-wasting nephropathies, adrenal failure causing hypoaldosteronism).

   (b) *Hypervolaemic*: there is increased total body water and sodium (primary sodium gain with excessive water gain), with oedema or ascites, but a water-conserving response nonetheless, secondary to a decrease in effective circulating volume (renal hypoperfusion) or a failure of renal water excretion. Causes include heart failure, hepatic cirrhosis, nephrotic syndrome, severe hypoproteinaemia, and renal failure.

   (c) *Euvolaemic*: there is excessive water intake or failure to excrete it (primary water gain). It may be due to polydipsia that overwhelms the kidney's ability to excrete free water (e.g. psychogenic polydipsia, beer potomania), or much more commonly ADH excess in the absence of the normal physiological triggers to ADH secretion of hyperosmolality or severe hypovolaemia [493, 695–698]. Note that non-osmotic secretion of ADH is a very common cause of euvolaemic hyponatraemia [694], but ADH is raised in most patients with hyponatraemia, regardless of the cause [493] and the diagnosis of SIADH requires exclusion of hypovolaemia, hypotension, oedema-forming states, and abnormal renal or adrenal function [26, 493, 699]. Hyponatraemia should produce a maximally dilute urine (50–80 mOsm/kg), so urine more concentrated than this in the presence of hyponatraemia suggests SIADH [700]. SIADH has many causes, including paraneoplastic secretion (e.g. bronchial carcinoma), lung diseases (e.g. pneumonia, mechanical ventilation), cerebral disease (e.g. head injury, encephalitis, intracranial tumours), pain, physical/

emotional stress, hypoxia, hypercapnia, hypothyroidism, porphyria, SLE, a large number of drugs, and idiopathic SIADH.

Mild hyponatraemia is often asymptomatic. Severe hyponatraemia (≤120 mM) causes clouding of consciousness (in 76% of one series) including coma, pyramidal motor signs (6%), seizures (3.3%), tremor (1%), mild cognitive impairment with normal conscious level (0.5%), hallucinations (0.5%), other acute psychosis (0.5%), and death (4.3%) [701]. Coma is usually associated with sodium levels <110 mM [26].

There also appears to be an association of psychosis, intermittent hyponatraemia, and polydipsia (PIP syndrome) [702]. In this state, there appears to be excess ADH secretion at any given plasma osmolality, in addition to other osmoregulatory defects [703]. Within-subject measurements have shown that cognitive performance is impaired during hyponatraemia in these patients [704], and experimental induction of psychosis in schizophrenics can trigger ADH release [705].

Diagnosis of hyponatraemia is by routine biochemistry, followed by clinical assessment of volume status and further investigations as indicated. Severe hyponatraemia must not be corrected too rapidly, as this carries a risk of central pontine myelinolysis (Chapter 6.9 ▶) and other neurological sequelae [701].

In the context of hyponatraemia with psychosis, consider also hypothyroidism (Chapter 9.1 ▶), adrenal insufficiency (Chapter 9.3 ▶), porphyria (Chapter 10.2 ▶), SLE (Chapter 13.1.1 ▶), and anti-voltage-gated potassium channel encephalopathy (Chapter 14.2.1 ▶).

12.5.2 Hypernatraemia

Hypernatraemia is due to water deficiency (dehydration), salt excess, or both [706, 707]. It is much less common than hyponatraemia. Hypovolaemic hypernatraemia indicates water deficiency in excess of sodium deficiency (e.g. diarrhoea, vomiting, burns, diuretics, renal disease, decreased thirst, central or nephrogenic diabetes insipidus). Apparently euvolaemic hypernatraemia involves water deficiency but mostly from intracellular and interstitial spaces (the causes are as for hypovolaemic hypernatraemia). Hypervolaemic hypernatraemia indicates salt intake in excess of water intake (e.g. iatrogenic, salt ingestion, mineralocorticoid excess). Severe hypernatraemia (typically >160 mM), especially if acute, has neurological effects via reduced intracellular fluid volume and cell shrinkage. Effects can include severe thirst, confusion, agitation, irritability, weakness, hyperreflexia, focal neurological deficits, coma, and seizures [26, 706, 708]. Psychosis has also been reported [709], though rarely. The relationship with psychiatric symptoms can be bidirectional: psychosis can cause a lack of fluid intake [e.g. 710]. Diagnosis is by routine biochemistry. Severe hypernatraemia is an emergency, with high mortality. It must not be corrected too rapidly, to avoid cerebral oedema [706].

12.5.3 Hypocalcaemia

Calcium binds to fixed negative charges on the surface of neurons, increasing the local electrical potential on the outside surface of the cell membrane, thus increasing the resting transmembrane voltage gradient and reducing neuronal excitability [711]. Hypocalcaemia causes neuronal excitability. When severe, this can cause hallucinations and delusions [513, 712, 713]. Other manifestations include bronchospasm or stridor (due to smooth muscle contraction), bradycardia or ventricular tachyarrhythmias, dysphagia, biliary or intestinal colic, bladder dysfunction, muscle spasm and tetany, paraesthesiae and numbness, Chvostek's and Trousseau's signs, irritability, confusion, extrapyramidal movement disorders, and seizures. Calcium concentrations should always be measured in a form related to the free ionic concentration (e.g. corrected for serum albumin). Causes of a low corrected calcium include PTH deficiency or resistance, vitamin D deficiency or resistance, hypomagnesaemia (magnesium is required for PTH release and action), hyperphosphataemia, acute pancreatitis, rhabdomyolysis, sepsis, malignancy, drugs (e.g. bisphosphonates, calcitonin, citrate), and poisoning (e.g. fluoride, ethylene glycol [Chapter 15.7.2 ▶]) [26, 712]. Diagnosis is by routine biochemistry; if the cause is not obvious, the next step in diagnosis is to measure PTH levels.

Hypocalcaemia and psychosis should also raise the possibility of velocardiofacial syndrome (Chapter 4.1 ▶).

12.5.4 Hypercalcaemia

Hypercalcaemia is a clear cause of psychosis, sometimes as the presenting symptom, and psychosis, like other psychiatric manifestations, can occur even with relatively mild hypercalcaemia [513, 514], though mental state changes become common with serum calcium levels >3.2 mM [33]. Serum calcium is maintained by the action of PTH. Hypercalcaemia may be caused by PTH excess in primary hyperparathyroidism and in "tertiary" hyperparathyroidism (in which parathyroid secretion gains autonomy after a long period of exposure to hypocalcaemia). Other causes include malignancy (Chapter 7 ▶, through lytic bone lesions or paraneoplastic production of PTHrP); granulomatous diseases such as tuberculosis (Chapter 8.1.6 ▶) and sarcoidosis (Chapter 13.5 ▶, associated with elevated vitamin D synthesis); endocrine diseases including hyperthyroidism (Chapter 9.1 ▶), Addison's disease (Chapter 9.3 ▶), phaeochromocytoma (Chapter 7 ▶), and other rare disorders; drugs (including substances containing vitamins D and A, thiazide diuretics, and lithium – the last two can cause an elevation of PTH); and calcium-rich alkaline foods [26].

Hypercalcaemia can cause depression, anxiety, lethargy, mild cognitive disturbance (e.g. poor memory and concentration), paranoid psychosis, delirium, stupor, weakness, nausea and vomiting, indigestion, abdominal pain (including that due to gastric ulceration), flank pain (renal stones), constipation, weakness, joint and muscle aches, polyuria, and headaches. Traditionally, this is summarized as "moans, groans, stones, and bones – with psychic overtones". There may be hypertension, bradycardia, drowsiness, dehydration, proximal muscle weakness, and hyperreflexia [513, 514, 714]. Clinical examination should be focused on finding occult malignancy, which is a common cause of hypercalcaemia.

Diagnosis is by routine biochemistry. Calcium concentrations should always be measured in a form related to the free ionic concentration (e.g. corrected for serum albumin). Persistent, even mild, hypercalcaemia always requires investigation. The next step after finding hypercalcaemia is to measure PTH levels. As indicated above, hypercalcaemia is associated with other causes of psychosis including hyperthyroidism (Chapter 9.1 ▶) and granulomatous diseases such as sarcoid (Chapter 13.5 ▶).

12.5.5 Hypokalaemia

Hypokalaemia has been described as a cause of psychosis [715, 716], although there have been few clear documented demonstrations. Hypokalaemia can be caused by renal losses (e.g. renal tubular acidosis, hyperaldosteronism, magnesium deficiency), leukaemia), gastrointestinal loss (e.g. vomiting, diarrhoea), drugs (e.g. diuretics, beta-adrenergic agonists, steroids, aminoglycosides), a shift into cells (e.g. insulin, alkalosis, thyrotoxic periodic paralysis [Chapter 9.1 ▶]), leukaemia (multifunctional) and malnutrition [716, 1343]. Hypokalaemia is correlated with, and likely caused by, agitation and muscular activity in psychosis [717].

Hypokalaemia can cause palpitations, weakness, muscle cramps, paralysis, paraesthesiae, constipation, nausea, vomiting, abdominal pain, polyuria and polydipsia, delirium, hallucinations, and depression [716]. Symptoms are uncommon until the potassium level is <3 mM [33]. Hypokalaemia is dangerous primarily because it causes a variety of cardiac arrhythmias. Diagnosis is by routine biochemical testing; obviously, a cause should be sought carefully.

12.5.6 Hypomagnesaemia

Hypomagnesaemia causes neuronal hyperexcitability, and is a cause of psychosis [513, 718]. Psychosis has been observed with hypomagnesaemia and normal calcium levels in the context of both hypoparathyroidism and hyperparathyroidism (Chapter 9.5 ▶) [512, 719]. Magnesium deficiency (with or without hypomagnesaemia) is common in alcoholism; its relationship to delirium tremens and alcoholic encephalopathy is unclear, but it may worsen Wernicke–Korsakoff encephalopathy (Chapter 11.1 ▶) [720–722]. Intriguingly, competition between Li^+ and Mg^{2+} ions has also been suggested to be important in the mechanism of action of lithium in bipolar affective disorder [723, 724]. Causes of hypomagnesaemia are legion, and include GI loss and malabsorption, malnutrition, decreased renal tubular reabsorption, drugs (especially diuretics and alcohol), pregnancy and lactation, and endocrine disorders (e.g. hyperaldosteronism, hypoparathyroidism [Chapter 9.5 ▶], and, hyperthyroidism [Chapter 9.1 ▶].

Neuromuscular excitability in hypomagnesaemia can cause weakness, tremor, seizures, paraesthesiae, tetany, Chvostek's and Trousseau's signs, and nystagmus. The ECG may show non-specific T wave changes, U waves, QT interval prolongation, ectopics, and tachyarrhythmias including VT [718, 725]. Hypokalaemia and hypocalcaemia may occur (Chapter 12.5.5, 12.5.3 ▶).

Diagnosis of hypomagnesaemia is by blood magnesium levels, though assessment of the consequences of magnesium deficiency is complicated by the fact that blood magnesium levels may bear little relationship to tissue magnesium [720]. Magnesium abnormalities commonly co-occur with abnormalities of potassium, calcium, and phosphate; these should be measured and a cause sought for the magnesium abnormality.

12.5.7 Hypophosphataemia

Severe hypophosphataemia (defined as less than 1 mg/dl or 0.32 mM; normal range 2.5–4.5 mg/dl or 0.8–1.46 mM) [726] has been suggested to cause psychosis in one case with sudden-onset severe hypophosphataemia (0.4 mg/dl or 0.13 mM) [727]. The psychosis reversed on correction of the hypophosphataemia.

Hypophosphataemia may be caused by a *shift in phosphate from extracellular to intracellular fluid* (respiratory alkalosis due to hyperventilation; refeeding syndrome in which carbohydrate triggers insulin release; insulin administration in diabetic ketoacidosis; catecholamines; beta-adrenoceptor agonists; intracellular consumption in anabolic states and in rapidly growing malignancies such as leukaemias and lymphomas; thyrotoxic periodic paralysis), *increased urinary excretion* (hyperparathyroidism; acute volume expansion triggering PTH release; diuretics; metabolic acidosis including diabetic ketoacidosis; insulin deficiency leading to a phosphate shift from intracellular to extracellular fluid; malnutrition; certain primary renal disorders), *decreased intestinal absorption* (e.g. chronic diarrhoea or vomiting; malabsorption; phosphate-binding drugs), or *decreased dietary intake* (e.g. anorexia nervosa; alcoholism). Rates are especially high in those with HIV and falciparum malaria [726].

The primary manifestations are muscle weakness (skeletal, smooth, or cardiac muscle, involving any muscle group; thus clinical features include proximal myopathy, ophthalmoplegia, ileus, dysphagia, respiratory insufficiency, and myocardial depression), rhabdomyolysis, neurological dysfunction (confusion, seizures, coma, peripheral neuropathy, extrapontine myelinolysis), and haematological impairments (haemolytic anaemia, impaired oxygen delivery, impaired leukocyte function). Diagnosis of hypophosphataemia is by serum phosphate levels, but these do not directly reflect intracellular stores [726].

Chapter 13 Autoimmune rheumatic disorders and vasculitides

This group includes subsets of the connective tissue disorders, the primary inflammatory vasculitides, and some other autoimmune conditions. Likewise, many vasculitides can cause psychosis. Conditions that overlap considerably with these major groups of diseases are also included here.

13.1 Connective tissue disorders

Amongst the connective tissue disorders, CNS involvement is extremely rare in rheumatoid arthritis, though rheumatoid nodules, rheumatoid meningitis, and rheumatoid vasculitis can affect the CNS [25, 728, 729]. Many of the others, however, have been associated with CNS manifestations including psychosis.

13.1.1 Systemic lupus erythematosus

Systemic lupus erythematosus is an autoimmune condition that can present with symptoms virtually anywhere. Its underlying aetiology is unknown, but autoantibody production is a prominent feature. It is a chronic disease with flares of activity, which can give rise to episodic neuropsychiatric and systemic manifestations. In the UK, the annual incidence of SLE is approximately 4:100 000, with a female:male ratio of 10–20:1 [26]. The prevalence also varies with race, in the order Chinese > Afro-Caribbean > Indo-Asian > Caucasian [730]. About 57% of patients with SLE have manifestations of neuropsychiatric SLE (NPSLE) at some point in the course of their illness [731], although primary neuropsychiatric presentation is relatively rare [732]. Psychosis occurs in about 16% [29, 733, 734], this figure having probably declined over the years due to earlier recognition and treatment of SLE [33]. Systemic lupus erythematosus has an extremely wide range of presenting signs and symptoms. The following are well-described systemic features [26].

- *Musculoskeletal.* Arthralgia and arthritis, tenosynovitis, myalgia, myositis.
- *Cardiopulmonary.* Dyspnoea, pleurisy, pleural effusion, pneumonitis, interstitial fibrosis, pulmonary function test abnormalities, cardiomegaly, pericarditis, cardiomyopathy, myocardial infarction.
- *Gastrointestinal.* Anorexia, nausea, vomiting, diarrhoea, ascites, abdominal pain, hepatomegaly, splenomegaly.
- *Renal.* Haematuria, proteinuria, urinary casts, hypoalbuminaemia, impaired renal function (raised serum creatinine, reduced creatinine clearance).

- *Haematological.* Anaemia (iron deficiency, anaemia of chronic disease, autoimmune haemolytic anaemia), leucopenia, lymphopenia, thrombocytopenia (see also TTP, Chapter 13.7 ▶), circulating "anticoagulants" (see below).
- *Dermatological.* Butterfly rash, erythematous maculopapular eruption, discoid lupus, relapsing nodular non-suppurative panniculitis, vasculitic skin lesions, livedo reticularis, purpuric lesions, alopecia.

The following are recognized neuropsychiatric manifestations of SLE [735].

- *Central nervous system.* Aseptic meningitis, cerebrovascular disease, demyelinating syndrome, headache (including migraine and benign intracranial hypertension), movement disorder (chorea), myelopathy, seizure disorders, acute confusional state, anxiety disorder, cognitive dysfunction, mood disorder, psychosis. Catatonia can occur [736, 737].
- *Peripheral nervous system.* Acute inflammatory demyelinating polyradiculopathy (Guillain–Barré syndrome), autonomic disorder, mononeuropathy (single/multiplex), myasthenia gravis, cranial neuropathy, plexopathy, polyneuropathy.

Systemic lupus erythematosus is a one of a few conditions that often causes a raised ESR with a normal CRP, though the ESR can also be normal in SLE; in one series of patients with CNS lupus, the ESR was elevated in 50% and the CRP in 9% [732]. Leucopenia and/or lymphopenia are also a feature. Renal impairment, anaemia, and hypoalbuminaemia may be present. Complement is typically low [26]. SIADH can occur [738].

Antinuclear antibody testing is the initial screening test. One estimate is that it has 99% sensitivity and 49% specificity for SLE [739]; this gives a negative predictive value of >99.9% in any patient group with a prevalence less than 4.6% [23], making SLE very unlikely with a negative ANA. Others estimate the sensitivity of ANA as being lower, at 93% [740], highlighting a small number of patients with SLE but without ANA [741]. In part this discrepancy is because the prevalence of ANA across the course of the disease is very high, but only 76% of patients have ANA at disease onset [742].

If the ANA test is positive, the immunology laboratory will further categorize the ANA. Anti-dsDNA and anti-Sm antibodies are strongly suggestive of SLE. Other antinuclear antibodies associated with SLE are anti-Ro, anti-La, and anti-RNP [743]. Systemic lupus erythematosus can also exist in the absence of ANA, though this is harder to diagnose; most commonly, ANA-negative SLE patients are positive for anti-Ro [744], if specifically tested for. Neuropsychiatric SLE with psychosis has been associated in particular with anti-Sm and anti-Ro ANAs [745], anti-RNP [746, 747], and anti-NR2 NMDA receptor autoantibodies [748, 749]. Mechanisms of antibody neurotoxicity have been described, and depend on compromise of the blood–brain barrier [750, 751] (though see also [752]). The role of antiphospholipid antibodies in SLE is discussed further below (see Chapter 13.1.2 ▶).

The American College of Rheumatology research criteria for classification of SLE [739, 753] are 4 of the following 11 features, not necessarily at a single time (shown here in the order of the convenient mnemonic "SOAP BRAIN MD"):

1. serositis: pleuritis (convincing history of pleuritic pain, or a pleural rub or effusion) or pericarditis (demonstrated on ECG, or a pericardial rub or effusion);
2. oral or nasopharyngeal ulceration (usually painless);

3. arthritis (non-erosive arthritis involving ≥2 peripheral joints, with tenderness, swelling, or effusion);
4. photosensitivity (rash in reaction to sunlight);
5. blood (haematological) disorder: haemolytic anaemia (with reticulocytosis), or leucopenia ($<4.0 \times 10^9$/l) on ≥2 occasions, or lymphopenia ($<1.5 \times 10^9$/l on ≥2 occasions), or thrombocytopenia ($<100 \times 10^9$/l) in the absence of drug causes;
6. renal disorder: persistent proteinuria (>0.5 g/24 h or 3+ on dipstick), or cellular casts;
7. antinuclear antibody in raised titre (in the absence of drugs known to be associated with drug-induced lupus);
8. immunological disorder: raised anti-dsDNA antibody, or anti-Sm antibody, or positive antiphospholipid antibodies;
9. neurological disorder: seizures or psychosis (in the absence of drug precipitants or known metabolic derangements);
10. malar rash (fixed erythema, flat or raised, over the malar eminences, tending to spare the nasolabial folds);
11. discoid rash (erythematous raised patches with adherent keratotic scaling and follicular plugging; atrophic scarring may occur in older lesions).

These criteria have 96% sensitivity and 96% specificity for SLE [739].

Additional clues (the "St Thomas's alternative criteria" based on clinical experience) are (1) teenage growing pains, (2) teenage migraine, (3) teenage prolonged "glandular fever", (4) severe reactions to insect bites, (5) recurrent miscarriages, (6) allergy to sulphonamides including co-trimoxazole, (7) agoraphobia, (8) finger flexor tenosynovitis, (9) premenstrual exacerbations, (10) family history of autoimmune disease, (11) a dry Shirmer's test of lacrimation, (12) a borderline-low complement C4, (13) a normal CRP with a raised ESR, and (14) lymphopenia [754].

A characteristic imaging sign of NPSLE, best seen on a FLAIR sequence, is high-signal-intensity lesions in the periventricular white matter, suggestive of a vasculitis. However, structural MRI has low sensitivity for NPSLE and images can be entirely normal in the presence of NPSLE [755]. This is likely because NPSLE is often due to an antibody-mediated encephalopathy, mediated through direct injury to neurons, or due to a vasculopathy, rather than being a true vasculitis [756]. Other imaging techniques such as DWI and MRS are at a research stage [757]. LP is not necessarily required, but can show an elevation in CSF protein or a lymphocytic pleocytosis; EEG is likewise not specifically indicated but can show generalized slowing, a non-specific pointer towards "organic" illness [732]. Cerebrospinal fluid oligoclonal bands are present in up to 50% of patients with CNS lupus [26]. A skin biopsy of any rash (together with a biopsy of normal skin) can be very useful [26].

Psychotropics that can cause **drug-induced lupus erythematosus** (DILE) include bupropion, chlorpromazine, lithium, olanzapine, and valproate. The drugs that are most liable to cause DILE, however, are hydralazine, procainamide, quinidine, isoniazid, diltiazem, and minocycline. In DILE, symptoms can appear between 3 weeks and 2 years following consumption of the drug, and clinical improvement is rapid following drug discontinuation, though serological parameters are slower to resolve. In DILE, antihistone antibodies are present in >95% of patients (compared to 50% with SLE), and anti-ssDNA is commoner (compared to anti-dsDNA in SLE). Drug-induced lupus erythematosus is less likely to cause CNS involvement than SLE, though it can occur. **Drug-induced exacerbation of existing SLE** is a different phenomenon and occurs faster [758, 759].

13.1.2 Antiphospholipid syndrome

Antiphospholipid (**Hughes'**) syndrome (APS) is an autoimmune thrombophilia characterized by antibodies against phospholipids or phospholipid binding proteins (antiphospholipid antibodies; aPL). It may be primary, or secondary to other autoimmune disease, most commonly SLE. The diagnostic criteria are vascular thrombosis (arterial, venous, or small vessel thrombosis, other than superficial venous thrombosis) or pregnancy morbidity (one spontaneous abortion of a normal fetus after the 10th week of gestation, three or more such miscarriages before the 10th week, or premature birth before the 34th week secondary to pre-eclampsia, eclampsia, or placental insufficiency) in the presence of an aPL (lupus anticoagulant, anticardiolipin antibody, or anti-β_2 glycoprotein-1 antibody) measured on two occasions at least 12 weeks apart [760, 761]. There may also be thrombocytopenia, sometimes mild. The presence of aPL alone is insufficient to diagnose APS: aPL can also occur in infections that are not associated with thrombosis (e.g. syphilis, Lyme disease, cytomegalovirus, Epstein–Barr virus), in infections that may be associated with thrombosis (e.g. varicella zoster virus, HIV, hepatitis C), in rheumatic disease, in response to drugs (such as chlorpromazine and other phenothiazines), in malignancy including lymphoma, and in the general population, with a prevalence of 2–5% [26, 760, 762–764].

There is debate about the association of APS and aPL with psychosis. Antiphospholipid antibodies are associated with neuropsychiatric manifestations of SLE [731]. Well-documented neurological manifestations of APS include cerebral thrombosis (strokes, TIAs, and more rarely acute ischaemic encephalopathy, moyamoya disease, and venous sinus thrombosis), but also non-thrombotic events including epilepsy (~6–14% of patients), headache including migraine, chorea (~1%), a multiple sclerosis-like syndrome, transverse myelitis, idiopathic intracranial hypertension, sensorineural hearing loss, Guillain–Barré syndrome, transient global amnesia, ocular syndromes including amaurosis fugax and optic neuropathy, dystonia with parkinsonism, cognitive dysfunction, and dementia [761]. Psychiatric manifestations including psychosis, delirium, catatonia, depression, anxiety, aggression, and mania have all been described in association with aPL and APS [764, 765]. The relationship to APS is not fully clear, but there is some evidence that aPL are primarily associated with psychosis [761, 766], with one study showing aPL in 32% of unmedicated patients with acute psychosis, compared to 0% of controls [767].

The triad of livedo reticularis, hypertension, and strokes (Chapter 6.1 ▶) may be seen in SLE (Chapter 13.1.1 ▶) and antiphospholipid syndrome; this is sometimes called **Sneddon's syndrome** [768].

13.1.3 Sjögren's syndrome

Sjögren's syndrome (SS) is an inflammatory disorder characterized by involvement of the salivary and lacrimal glands and synovial tissue. It is seen in 0.5–2.0% of the population, making it the second-most common collagen vascular disease after rheumatoid arthritis; 90% of patients are female. It may occur in isolation (primary SS), or in the context of RA, SLE, systemic sclerosis, or other connective tissue diseases. It is associated with RhF, ANA (Ro [SS-A] and La [SS-B] type), and antibodies to salivary duct antigens (which may in fact be SS-A or SS-B) [28, 769].

Typical clinical features follow from decreased tear and saliva production (the sicca syndrome), and primary SS is diagnosed in the presence of two of xerostomia, xerophthalmia, and arthritis. There may be associated extraglandular manifestations, including lymphadenopathy, hepatosplenomegaly, cutaneous vasculitis (non-thrombocytopenic purpura or urticaria), other vasculitis (usually involving the peripheral nervous system and muscle), small-joint arthritis (occurring in 80%), renal disease (in up to 40%, usually interstitial nephritis), pulmonary disease (pneumonitis or restrictive/obstructive changes in lung function), and lymphoproliferative disorders. Neurological manifestations may affect 25–80% of patients, sometimes as the presenting feature, and can include mild aseptic meningitis, focal neurological deficit, seizure, and occasionally eye signs, cerebellar signs, and other movement disorders. With CNS involvement, the EEG is abnormal in nearly 50%, MRI may show focal abnormalities, and there may be normal CSF or elevated CSF protein and/or cell counts [28]. Psychiatric dysfunction in Sjögren's syndrome is most commonly characterized by affective change (depression, hypomania), personality change, and mild cognitive dysfunction, but overt dementia may occur. Psychosis is relatively uncommon, occuring in 8% of one series of patients preselected for a high likelihood of CNS disease [770]. Diagnosis is clinical, serological, and sometimes by salivary gland biopsy showing lymphocytic infiltrates [771].

13.1.4 Systemic sclerosis

Systemic sclerosis (**progressive systemic sclerosis; scleroderma**) is a condition associated with skin thickening and tethering to subcutaneous tissues, along with fibrosis (gastrointestinal, pulmonary, cardiac, renal) and smooth muscle atrophy. There is increased collagen deposition and perivascular inflammation [28]. It has an annual incidence of ~14 per million [772], and usually affects women aged 40–60 (female:male ratio 3) [28]. Though terminology varies, it is often viewed as the diffuse, systemic form of scleroderma (of which the other forms are morphoea, confined to the skin, and limited scleroderma or CREST syndrome, characterized by calcinosis, Raynaud's syndrome, [o]esophageal dysmotility, sclerodactyly, and telangiectasia, and associated with anti-centromere antibodies). Systemic sclerosis is usually associated with ANA; antibodies to Scl-70 are specific but insensitive, and there may be anti-smooth muscle antibodies. Neurological involvement is uncommon, but may include global cognitive decline, focal neurological deficit, encephalopathy, migraine, seizures, and psychiatric changes [28]. Psychosis is rare in systemic sclerosis [773] but has been reported on several occasions [774–776].

13.1.5 Mixed connective tissue disease

Patients with mixed connective tissue disease have features of at least two connective tissue disorders, such as SLE, progressive systemic sclerosis, and polymyositis. Neurological involvement occurs in 10–55%. The CNS complications most closely resemble those of SLE [28], and likewise these include psychosis [777].

13.2 Vasculitis

There are many systems for classifying systemic vasculitis, but the dominant theme is classification according to the size of the dominant vessel involved, as follows [778, 779]:

- *Large arteries (aorta and major branches)*. Primary causes are *giant cell (temporal) arteritis*, *Takayasu's arteritis*, and *primary CNS angiitis*. Secondary causes are aortitis due to rheumatoid arthritis and infection (e.g. syphilis).
- *Medium-sized arteries*. Primary causes are *polyarteritis nodosa* and *Kawasaki's disease*. Secondary causes include infection (e.g. hepatitis B).

- *Small vessels (arterioles, venules, capillaries) and medium arteries.* Primary causes are *Wegener's granulomatosis, Churg–Strauss syndrome*, and *microscopic polyangiitis*. Secondary causes include vasculitis secondary to rheumatoid arthritis, SLE, and Sjögren's syndrome; drugs; and infection (e.g. HIV).
- *Small vessels (leukocytoclastic).* Primary causes are *Henoch–Schönlein purpura, essential cryoglobulinaemic vasculitis*, and *cutaneous leukocytoclastic angiitis*. Secondary causes include drugs (e.g. sulphonamides, penicillins, thiazides, and many others) and infection (e.g. hepatitis B, C).

Of the primary vasculitides, psychosis has not been reported in Henoch–Schönlein purpura, essential cryoglobulinaemic vasculitis, or cutaneous leukocytoclastic angiitis (which by definition has no systemic involvement). Kawasaki's disease (an acute febrile vasculitis predominantly affecting children and manifesting with conjuctivitis, strawberry tongue, oropharyngeal inflammation, skin changes with erythema then desquamation in the distal extremities, and coronary artery disease) has neurological manifestations in 0.4% including seizures, ataxia, facial palsy, subdural effusion, cerebral infarction, and acute encephalopathy [26, 780, 781], but psychosis has not been reported. Takayasu's arteritis ("pulseless disease", a granulomatous arteritis affecting primarily the aorta and the proximal portions of its major branches) can cause CNS involvement secondary to cerebral hypoperfusion [780] but psychosis has likewise not been reported.

Diagnosis of vasculitis may be based on a combination of biopsy-proven vasculitis or surrogate parameters, which are referred to below. Surrogate parameters for *glomerulonephritis* are proteinuria and haematuria with red blood cell casts. Surrogate parameters for *arteritis* are angiographic or ultrasonic demonstration of aneurysms or stenosis in arteries, provided the patient shows other signs of vasculitis. Surrogate parameters for *granulomatous inflammation in lower airways* are radiologically demonstrated pulmonary infiltrates or cavitations of >1 month's duration provided that all other causes (e.g. infections, malignancies) are ruled out. Surrogate parameters for *granulomatous inflammation in upper airways* are bloody nasal discharge and/or crusting of >1 month's duration; chronic sinusitis, otitis and/or mastoiditis (on X-ray, CT, or MRI); cranial bone or cartilage destruction; and acute hearing loss, without signs of traumatic disease [778].

No single investigation can confirm CNS vasculitis [782]. Serological markers, discussed below, are important. The ESR and CSF are often abnormal, but this is non-specific. MRI may show ischaemic areas, periventricular white matter lesions, haemorrhage, and focal parenchymal or meningeal enhancement, but this is neither specific nor sensitive. The use of MRA is controversial. Direct angiography may show abnormalities (dilatation, beading, occlusion, aneurysms) but has a false-negative rate of ~50% and significant risks of transient (~10%) or permanent (~1%) neurological deficit. Radiolabelled leukocyte imaging, examination of the ocular vessels, and functional imaging such as with SPECT may be useful [26, 47, 783]. Biopsy may sometimes be needed to distinguish primary vasculitis from infectious or malignant vasculopathies (q.v., Chapter 7, Chapter 8 ▶) [26].

Specific vasculitides that can cause psychosis are considered next.

13.2.1 Giant cell (temporal) arteritis

Giant cell (temporal) arteritis (GCA) is the most common primary systemic vasculitis. It is a granulomatous arteritis of the aorta and its major branches, and tends to affect preferentially the extracranial branches of the carotid artery, including the temporal artery. However, it can involve intracranial arteries. It is rare before the age of 50, chiefly affecting those aged 65–75, with an annual incidence of ~25:100 000 for women and ~10:100 000 for men [26, 780].

The onset may be dramatic and it develops fully within a few weeks. It may present with symptoms of temporal arteritis or other extracranial arteritis (headache, scalp sensitivity, tender thickened arteries, skin necrosis, jaw claudication, tongue pain and claudication, face and neck pain with nerve damage), symptoms of polymyalgia rheumatica (e.g. pain and stiffness in the shoulder and pelvic girdle, myalgia and peripheral synovitis), weight loss, malaise, fever, visual disturbance (blurred vision, amaurosis fugax, transient and permanent blindness, diplopia, visual hallucinations), headache (which may be overwhelming and generalized), anaemia, peripheral neuropathy, leg claudication, myocardial ischaemia, and occasionally brainstem stroke or aortic disease. Renal involvement is rare [26]. Isolated psychosis may be the presenting feature [780, 784].

Laboratory investigations typically show an acute phase response with an elevated ESR and CRP, often marked. A normal ESR occurs in 10% of patients. A mild hypochromic normocytic anaemia is common. Abnormal LFTs are typical, reflecting a mild hepatitis. Definite diagnosis is by temporal artery biopsy [26]. Urgent treatment with corticosteroids is required to reduce the risk of blindness [26].

13.2.2 Primary CNS angiitis

Primary angiitis of the central nervous system (PACNS, also known as isolated CNS angiitis or intracranial granulomatous arteritis/angiitis) may occur at any age but peaks in the fourth to sixth decade. The most common presentation is with a gradual-onset headache, encephalopathy, and multifocal neurological signs, though 11% have diffuse findings only [28, 780]. Behavioural and psychiatric symptoms are not uncommon [25, 780]. Systemic symptoms are typically absent. There may be subtypes, with "true" PACNS (characterized by a duration of >3 months and CSF features of chronic meningitis) being distinguished from "benign angiopathy" of the CNS (BACNS), in which there is an acute onset and normal CSF analysis [28]. Postpartum cerebral angiopathy has also been well described, and may be vasospastic [28]. Sometimes, PACNS is associated with immunosuppressive illness, such as lymphoma, leukaemia, drug-induced immunosuppression, or HIV [28].

The ESR is elevated in 66% of patients. Cerebrospinal fluid is abnormal in 81% (typically with a lymphocytosis and raised protein). The EEG is abnormal in 81%, typically showing diffuse slowing. A normal MRI is uncommon, and the combination of a normal MRI and normal CSF excludes most cases of CNS vasculitis. Angiography may show beading (although 13% of angiograms are normal), and a positive biopsy is definitive, though biopsy has only 74% sensitivity [28]. C-reactive protein, complement, cryoglobulins, immune complexes, ANCA, anti-Ro, anti-La, RhF, ACE, anticardiolipin, and protein electrophoresis should be normal/negative; ANA should be negative or in low titre only [780].

13.2.3 Polyarteritis nodosa

Polyarteritis nodosa (PAN) is a necrotizing vasculitis of small- and medium-sized arteries and can affect any organ. Its annual incidence is 3–4.5 per 100 000. Onset is most commonly in adults aged 40–60, with a male:female ratio of 1.6. It may be associated with streptococcal infection in childhood, and has been associated with hepatitis B, hepatitis C, CMV, and HIV infection in adults [785, 786].

Systemic symptoms occur in 50% of patients (fever, weight loss, malaise). Renal involvement occurs in 60% (renal failure, hypertension). Musculoskeletal symptoms (64%) include arthritis, arthralgia, and myalgia [785]. Central nervous system involvement most commonly presents with transient cerebral ischaemia, such as transient monocular blindness (amaurosis fugax). Cerebral arteritis occurs from the second or third year of the vasculitis, and may cause arterial thrombosis, intraparenchymal or subarachnoid haemorrhage, and myelopathy; sometimes there is encephalopathy, or seizures secondary to multiorgan failure. Peripheral neuropathy occurs in 60% of patients. Gastrointestinal involvement may cause abdominal pain, nausea and vomiting, bleeding, bowel infarction and perforation, cholecystitis, hepatic infarction, or pancreatic infarction. Skin signs (40%) include rash, purpura, nodules, cutaneous infarcts, livedo reticularis, and Raynaud's phenomenon. Cardiovascular consequences (35%) include congestive heart failure, myocardial infarction, and pericarditis. Genitourinary symptoms include testicular and ovarian pain [785]. Psychiatric manifestations occurred in 7.9% in one series (mainly severe depression), and psychosis has been reported [25, 785, 786].

There is typically an elevated ESR and a neutrophil leukocytosis. There is hypergammaglobulinaemia in 30%. Serology for p-ANCA is often positive but is not diagnostic. Diagnosis is typically by mesenteric angiography, showing microaneurysms; simultaneous biopsy may identify the vasculitis histologically. The EEG may show generalized slow-wave activity during encephalopathy. CSF is often normal. Approximately 30% of patients are positive for hepatitis B surface antigen [785].

13.2.4 ANCA-associated small-vessel vasculitides

The vasculitides associated with antineutrophil cytoplasmic antibodies (ANCA) are Wegener's granulomatosis, microscopic polyangiitis, and Churg–Strauss syndrome. Antineutrophil cytoplasmic antibodies bind to neutrophil cytoplasmic enzymes. They are typically screened for by indirect immunofluorescence, which can lead to a cytoplasmic pattern (c-ANCA), a perinuclear pattern (p-ANCA), or an atypical pattern. The ANCA is then typed by enzyme-linked immunosorbent assay (ELISA). The target antigen of the c-ANCA pattern is usually (90%) proteinase 3 (PR3-ANCA), whilst the p-ANCA pattern usually (70%) reflects anti-myeloperoxidase (MPO-ANCA) [26]. In Wegener's granulomatosis, the ANCA is PR3 in 75% of cases, MPO in 20%, and negative in 5%; thus, Wegener's granulomatosis typically gives the c-ANCA pattern. In microscopic polyangiitis, the ANCA is PR3 in 40%, MPO in 50%, and negative in 10%; thus, it often gives the p-ANCA pattern. In Churg–Strauss syndrome, the ANCA is PR3 in 10%, MPO in 60%, and negative in 30% [787]. The p-ANCA pattern may also be seen in idiopathic crescentic glomerulonephritis, inflammatory bowel disease, and Felty's syndrome, while the atypical ANCA pattern is also seen in HIV infection, endocarditis, and inflammatory bowel disease [788].

Wegener's granulomatosis (WG) is characterized by systemic necrotizing vasculitis, necrotizing granulomatous inflammation of the respiratory tract (upper and/or lower), and necrotizing glomerulonephritis. Its prevalence is ~8.5 per million; it can occur at any age, with a slight male preponderance (1.2:1). The ear, nose, and throat involvement may cause nasal obstruction, nosebleeds, sinusitis, central facial pain, hearing loss, and subglottic stenosis (hoarseness and stridor). Pulmonary involvement may cause cough, haemoptysis, and occasionally progressive dyspnoea. Renal involvement may produce haematuria and sometimes nephrotic syndrome. Skin involvement occurs in 14%, typically with a purpuric rash on the legs. Eye involvement (red or swollen eyes) occurs in 29%. Arthralgia is common, with non-erosive arthritis in 25%. Neurological involvement occurs in ~33% (including peripheral neuropathy, mononeuritis multiplex, cranial neuropathies, external ophthalmoplegia, seizures, cerebritis, and stroke) [28, 789, 790]. CNS involvement occurs in 2–8% [791], though neurological involvement at onset is rare [792]. There may be leukocytosis, thrombocytosis, elevated ESR and CRP, and normocytic normochromic anaemia. The ANCA is usually, but not always, positive [791]. Diagnostic criteria are (1) biopsy or surrogate parameter for granulomatous inflammation in the respiratory tract, (2) biopsy-verified necrotizing vasculitis in small- to medium-sized vessels or biopsy/surrogate parameter for glomerulonephritis or positive PR3-ANCA, and (3) lack of eosinophilia in blood and biopsy samples [778]. Psychosis has been reported in WG [791], though it is uncommon [793].

In the immunosuppressed, the differential diagnosis of WG includes lymphomatoid granulomatosis (Chapter 7 ▶).

Microscopic polyangiitis (MPA) is a necrotizing small-vessel vasculitis without granulomatous inflammation. It is distinguished from PAN (which is histologically identical) in that MPA typically involves vessels smaller than arteries (arterioles, venules, capillaries), and PAN does not. MPA produces a dermato-pulmonary-renal syndrome. It has an annual incidence of 3.6 per million, and a prevalence of 1–3 per 100 000 [794]. Symptoms can be constitutional (fever [55%], malaise, fatigue, flu-like symptoms, myalgia [48%], weight loss [72%]); rash (50%); pulmonary (haemoptysis [11%], dyspnoea, cough); cardiovascular (chest pain, heart failure); gastrointestinal (bleeding, abdominal pain); neurological (mononeuritis multiplex [57%], seizures [11%]); arthralgias (10–50%); testicular pain (2%); ocular (1%; red eye, eye pain, reduced visual acuity); and sinusitis (1%). Skin involvement may produce palpable purpura (41%), livedo reticularis (12%), ulcerations, digital ischaemia, necrosis and necrotizing nodules, urticaria. Cardiovascular signs include hypertension (34%), heart failure (17%), myocardial infarction (2%), and pericarditis (10%) [794].

There may be leukocytosis, normocytic anaemia, a raised ESR, renal failure, proteinuria, haematuria, and leukocyturia. There may be infiltrates on CXR. The diagnostic criteria are (1) biopsy-verified necrotizing vasculitis in small vessels and/or glomerulonephritis with few or no immune deposits, (2) involvement of more than one organ system as indicated by biopsy-verified vasculitis in small- to medium-sized vessels or surrogate parameter for glomerulonephritis, and (3) lack of biopsy and surrogate parameters for granulomatous inflammation in the respiratory system [778]. Psychosis is not common, but MPA has presented with the features of chronic schizophrenia [795].

Churg–Strauss syndrome is a rare small-vessel vasculitis involving the lungs, and often other organs; it is characterized by an association with asthma and by tissue and blood eosinophilia. Its onset is in the age range 15–69, with a male:female ratio of ~1.4:1. It begins with asthma, often with allergic rhinitis, nasal polyps, sinusitis, and recurrent respiratory infections. In a second phase, eosinophilia develops, often with eosinophilic pneumonia (sometimes with haemoptysis) and eosinophilic gastroenteritis; this phase relapses and remits, with fever during exacerbations. Sometimes there is myocarditis. After months to years, a systemic vasculitis develops (which may involve the heart, peripheral nerves, brain, gastrointestinal tract, skin, kidney, and testes). Rheumatoid factor may rise during exacerbations.

10–40 per 100 000 on average, but with wide variations, from 3 per 100 000 in Poland to 64 per 100 000 in Sweden. It is over-represented in black races (36 per 100 000 in the USA compared to 11 per 100 000 for white races) and almost unknown in Native American, Australian Aboriginal, or southern Asian races, in part related to HLA differences. It is more common in females. It can present at any age, but 70–90% of patients present aged 20–40 [26, 814, 815].

The frequencies of organ involvement are: lung (90%), liver (60–90%), pulmonary lymphatics (75%), peripheral lymphatics (60%), spleen (40%), bone marrow (30%), skin (25%), eyes (25%), upper respiratory tract (nose and tonsils; 20%), salivary glands (parotitis), joints (25%), CNS (5%), heart (5%); renal, endocrine, and gastrointestinal involvement may also occur. Features may include fever, night sweats, malaise, fatigue, weight loss, myositis, arthritis, uveitis, retinal vasculitis, keratoconjunctivitis, parotid enlargement, dry cough, exertional dyspnoea, haemoptysis, pleural effusion or pneumothorax (rare), lymphadenopathy, hyper- and hypopigmentation, keloid scarring, maculopapular rashes (involving the nares, lips, eyelids, and sites of previous trauma), lupus pernio (a violaceous plaque-like discolouration of the nose, cheeks, chin, and ears that is specific to sarcoid), erythema nodosum, subcutaneous nodules, cardiac conduction defects (such as ventricular tachycardia), myocarditis, pericarditis, cor pulmonale, hepatomegaly, splenomegaly, and renal stones secondary to hypercalcaemia [26, 814].

Non-psychiatric neurological manifestations include involvement of cranial and peripheral nerves (most commonly facial nerve palsy), visual deficits, lymphocytic meningitis, basal granulomatous meningitis (with involvement of the optic chiasm and nerve), hypothalamic/pituitary involvement (with diabetes insipidus and polydipsia, pituitary insufficiency, or optic chiasm compression), seizures, vasculitis, and stroke or TIA [26, 814]. Sometimes neurological or neuropsychiatric manifestations occur without obvious systemic involvement at presentation.

Psychiatric manifestations occur in 19% of patients with neurosarcoidosis [816]. They have included paranoid psychosis associated with meningeal and hypothalamic enhancement on MRI [817], progressive psychosis with non-specific subtle temporal lobe and white matter changes on MRI that proved to be granulomas on biopsy [818], initial presentation as first-episode schizophreniform disorder with subsequent cognitive decline and automatisms [819], psychosis and dementia in young patients [820, 821], first-episode psychosis with frontal granulomas [822], and major depression [823]. In one old series, sarcoid was implicated in 0.7% of cases of first-episode psychosis [824].

There is hypercalcaemia in 10–15% of cases, caused by 1,25-dihydroxycholecalciferol production by activated macrophages in the granulomas. Phosphate and alkaline phosphatase may be increased, and 24-hour urinary calcium excretion likewise. There may be an elevated ANA, RhF, immunoglobulins, and CK. Serum ACE is elevated in 75% of cases (note that ACE inhibitors may interfere with the assay) but elevation also occurs in other diseases. There may be a leukocytosis, and sometimes eosinophilia. The CXR is abnormal in 90% of cases at some point, typically with bilateral hilar adenopathy ± parenchymal involvement. Magnetic resonance imaging is most sensitive for identifying CNS lesions. Lumbar puncture may show a lymphocytic meningitis with raised protein; detection of ACE in CSF suggests but is not diagnostic of neurosarcoidosis. Diagnosis is by exclusion, but ideally requires biopsy demonstration of non-caseating granulomas in at least two organs, and exclusion of other causes of granuloma formation including tuberculosis (Chapter 8.1.6 ▶), fungal infections, foreign bodies, and malignancy [26, 814].

13.6 Scleromyxoedema

Scleromyxoedema (scleromyxedema, or generalized lichen myxoedematosus) is a rare cutaneous mucinosis. It usually affects patients aged 30–80 with an equal male:female ratio. There is mucin deposition, fibroblast proliferation, fibrosis, and monoclonal gammopathy. Clinically, there is a widespread eruption of small (2–3 mm), waxy, firm papules. The skin may be shiny. Mucin deposition outside the skin may cause multi-organ involvement (cardiovascular, GI, pulmonary, rheumatological, and neurological); the most common is dysphagia secondary to oesophageal dysmotility. Skin biopsy distinguishes between scleromyxoedema and systemic sclerosis. Central nervous system involvement may include encephalopathy, coma, stroke, seizures, and psychosis [825].

13.7 Thrombotic thrombocytopenic purpura

Thrombotic thrombocytopenic purpura (TTP), in its full-blown form, is the constellation of microangiopathic haemolytic anaemia, thrombocytopenic purpura, neurological disease, fever, and renal disease. Multiple platelet aggregates cause thrombi in the microvasculature. The incidence is approximately 6 cases per million per year. Thrombotic thrombocytopenic purpura, and the related haemolytic–uraemic syndrome (HUS), may be triggered by certain drugs, particularly cytotoxics, and by diarrhoeal illnesses (enterohaemorrhagic *Escherichia coli* and *Shigella*), though it may be spontaneous [826]. There is also an association with SLE (Chapter 13.1.1 ▶) [827].

A typical presentation is with an acute or subacute onset of neurological symptoms (change in mental status, seizures, sensorimotor deficits, aphasia), fatigue, or petechiae. Fever occurs in ~50%. There may be haemoglobinuria, but severe bleeding is unusual [826]. Neuropsychiatric features may be prominent, including headache, confusion, seizures, and coma, plus sensorimotor symptoms, reflecting small-vessel infarcts and haemorrhages [25]. Psychosis has been suggested to be part of this picture [828] and delirious psychosis has been seen in the overlap between TTP and the related haemolytic–uraemic syndrome [829], but this association has not been clearly established.

Investigations typically show a normal or slightly elevated white-cell count, anaemia, thrombocytopenia, schistocytosis (fragmented erythrocytes), an elevated D-dimer, a normal or high fibrinogen, normal or near-normal PT and APTT, evidence of renal impairment, and elevated indices of haemolysis (LDH and bilirubin).

13.8 Hyperviscosity and cryoglobulinaemia

Occasionally, hyperviscosity syndromes produce delirium [830], dementia [20], and psychosis. The key clinical features of hyperviscosity are oronasal bleeding, retinal haemorrhages, and variable neurological symptoms. The common causes are increased gamma globulins and increased red cell mass [831].

Polycythaemia rubra vera is a myeloproliferative disorder that elevates red cell mass and, usually, haemoglobin concentrations. There is an increased risk of thrombosis and the hyperviscosity reduces cerebral blood flow. The clinical manifestations include thromboses at unusual sites (e.g. splenic, portal, hepatic, and and mesenteric veins and inferior vena cava), thickening or vegetations on cardiac valves, haemorrhage (occurring in 30–40% of patients), peripheral vascular insufficiency, cardiac failure, and neurological abnormalities (60–80%). The neurological features include TIAs, cerebral infarcts (including small lacunar infarcts) and haemorrhage, confusion, fluctuating dementia, involuntary movements, dizziness, paraesthesiae, tinnitus, visual abnormalities, and headaches. Definitive diagnosis of polycythaemia rubra vera requires demonstration of an elevated red cell mass [26]. Depressive psychosis following TIAs has been reported in this context [25].

Hyperviscosity is also associated with **paraproteinaemia**, including macroglobulinaemia and multiple myeloma. Diagnosis of paraproteinaemia is by serum electrophoresis. Serum viscosity measurements do not always correlate well with symptoms, and fundoscopy is a better marker (retinal vein engorgement, haemorrhages) [26].

Cryoglobulins are immunoglobulins that precipitate reversibly at low temperatures. Cryoglobulinaemia is seen in lymphoproliferative disorders and chronic inflammatory disorders (such as connective tissue diseases, vasculitis, and chronic infections, particularly hepatitis C). Clinically, there is usually skin involvement, most typically with lesions in dependent areas (erythema, purpura, ulcers), livedo reticularis, Raynaud's phenomenon, and abnormal nailfold capillaries. Arthralgia and myalgia are common. There may be renal disease (glomerulonephritis, hypertension, proteinuria), pulmonary symptoms (dyspnoea, cough, pleurisy, effusions, bronchiectasis), abdominal pain, and neuropathy. The triad of purpura, arthralgia, and weakness is seen in up to 25–30% of patients [832]. Central nervous system involvement in cryoglobulinaemia is rare [832]; however, cryoglobulinaemia has presented with confusion and possible psychosis (not well described) [833]. The pathophysiology is varied but may include immune complex disease with vasculitis, cryoprecipitation, and hyperviscosity [26, 832]. Diagnosis requires blood taken to the laboratory at 37°C to be tested for cryoglobulins [26].

Chapter 14 Other autoimmune encephalopathies

14.1 Hashimoto's encephalopathy

Hashimoto's encephalopathy is a corticosteroid-responsive encephalopathy associated with autoimmune (Hashimoto's) thyroiditis [834, 835]. It is sometimes termed **steroid-responsive encephalopathy associated with autoimmune thyroiditis (SREAT)** [835]. It is diagnosed in the presence of an encephalopathy of unknown cause, having first excluded systemic connective tissue disorders and vasculitis, metabolic and toxic causes, overt hypothyroidism, and bacterial and viral infectious causes (including by CSF examination). In this situation, if antithyroid antibodies are present (with or without hypothyroidism), or the patient has a known history of autoimmune thyroiditis (even with corrected thyroid function), and the encephalopathy responds to steroid treatment, it is called Hashimoto's encephalopathy [834]. Clinically, there may be a relapsing–remitting course with multiple stroke-like episodes, or a diffuse progressive type with dementia and psychiatric symptoms; either may be accompanied by alterations of consciousness, tremor, seizures, or myoclonus [836]. There may be a raised ESR and altered LFTs, though in many cases there is no evidence of an inflammatory process, including by CSF examination and on neuroimaging [835]. The antithyroid antibodies may be antithyroglobulin or anti-thyroid peroxidase (also known as antithyroperoxidase, or antimicrosomal) antibodies. There is usually no relationship between the degree of thyroid dysfunction or the antibody level and the severity of neurological disease. The cause is debated; the encephalopathy may be related to a different antibody, with the antithyroid antibodies being a marker of generalized autoimmunity. Antithyroid antibodies are also common, occurring in 10% of the general population; it is therefore possible that autoimmune encephalopathy is more likely to be diagnosed simply because antithyroid antibodies are sought and found [834]. Encephalopathies of this type sometimes present with psychosis and/or a dementia-like syndrome [834, 837, 838], with psychosis occurring in 25–40% of patients with Hashimoto's encephalopathy [376, 835]. Encephalopathy associated with hypothyroidism that responds to correction of hypothyroidism alone [839] would not fall under this diagnostic label [834].

14.2 Autoimmune limbic encephalopathy, including paraneoplastic limbic encephalitis

Several types of autoimmune encephalitis or encephalopathy associated with psychosis have been described, which may be subdivided by the antigen concerned. These antigens include intraneuronal antigens, ion channels, and neuropil antigens not yet well defined. In some cases, syndromes are imperfectly associated with the autoantibody. The syndromes are often, but not always, paraneoplastic (**paraneoplastic limbic encephalitis**; PLE).

Paraneoplastic limbic encephalitis typically has a subacute onset (>80% of cases), with altered mental status including short-term memory loss (>80%); confusion (>40%); other cognitive impairment (~15%); psychiatric symptoms (>40%) including mood change (~15%), behavioural or personality change (~5%), and hallucinations (~10%); seizures (~50%, typically temporolimbic); signs of hypothalamic dysfunction (hyperthermia, somnolence, endocrine disturbance; >20%); other neurological signs (e.g. brainstem, cerebellar; 40–60%).

Paraneoplastic limbic encephalitis is usually (>60%) identified before the cancer is found. The CSF is abnormal in >80%, typically with mild pleocytosis (>50%) and/or a mildly elevated protein (>80%) only. The EEG is abnormal in >90%; typical EEG findings are focal or generalized slowing and/or epileptiform activity, maximal in temporal regions. Magnetic resonance imaging is abnormal in ~65%, typically with increased temporal lobe signal on T2WI and FLAIR imaging [385]. A normal MRI and EEG make PLE less likely [840], but by no means impossible [400]. Pathologically, there is a meningoencephalitis, predominantly in the medial temporal lobe [385]. Clear diagnosis of any form of autoimmune limbic encephalitis is by finding the autoantibody. The most common underlying cancer is small-cell lung carcinoma [840], but many other types of tumour can cause it, including thymomas and teratomas (gonadal or extragonadal germ cell tumours). Following identification of any autoantibody that may be paraneoplastic, a tumour "hunt" is required; if the source is not obvious, proceed to CT of the chest, abdomen, and pelvis, and if negative, whole-body FDG-PET [841, 842].

Complicating this process is the fact that the antigens are diverse and many patients with imaging or CSF evidence of limbic encephalitis have autoantibodies to currently unknown neuronal antigens [843]. These autoantibodies are detectable by immunohistochemistry to whole brain tissue (e.g. rat brain), which is a specialist test not always available in clinical settings, and such antibodies may be missed by currently available commercial tests [843]. One mechanism of autoantibody pathogenesis is by complement fixation. *In vitro* experiments have also suggested that antibodies to ion channels can cause dysfunction through complement-independent means such as by binding to channels and increasing their degradation [844]. The mechanism(s) of pathogenesis in the brain *in vivo* are unknown, and the degree to which blood–brain barrier compromise is required for disease is debated [752]. Likewise, it is not known whether any changes in inflammatory markers (e.g. ESR, CRP) are related to a mechanism of pathogenesis.

Some specific autoantibody syndromes are described below.

14.2.1 Antibodies against voltage-gated potassium channels

Morvan's syndrome is the combination of acquired neuromyotonia (known on its own as Isaacs' syndrome), autonomic hyperactivity, and fluctuating encephalopathy. There is muscle stiffness and twitching, with excessive sweating, and episodes of disorientation with prominent hallucinations, sleep disturbance (usually severe insomnia, circadian rhythm disturbance, and sometimes enacted dreams), and severe short-term memory dysfunction [748, 749]. Cognitive and behavioural abnormalities have included confusion, disorientation, memory impairment, behaviour change, delusions, hallucinations, confabulation, apathy, anxiety, panic attacks, disinhibition, agitation, and a syndrome clinically similar to frontotemporal dementia [845, 846]. In Morvan's syndrome, brain MRI is normal [748]. These conditions are associated with voltage-gated potassium channel (VGKC) autoantibodies. Neuromyotonia is due to peripheral nerve hyperexcitability.

A distinct syndrome of cognitive changes *without* peripheral nerve hyperexcitability in association with VGKC antibodies has also been described, usually called **limbic encephalitis**. It is normally not paraneoplastic [748, 749, 847]. It is much commoner in males. There may be cognitive and behavioural changes (as above) and temporal lobe epilepsy, with increased T2 and FLAIR MRI signal in the medial temporal lobes. A case having frontal lobe seizures with a normal structural MRI but abnormal SPECT has been described [848]. There is frequently hyponatraemia. It responds well to immunosuppression and/or plasma exchange (plasmapheresis).

VGKC autoantibodies are also observed in some cases of PLE (see above, Chapter 14.2 ▶) [749].

14.2.2 Antibodies against NMDA glutamate receptors

Autoantibodies against NMDA receptors (NR2 $NMDA_R$ autoantibodies) are associated with neuropsychiatric SLE (Chapter 13.1.1 ▶), though not very consistently [748, 749].

Paraneoplastic limbic encephalitis with psychosis has been described in association with $NMDA_R$ autoantibodies, often in young women with ovarian teratoma, who may be given a primary psychiatric diagnosis before seizures, autonomic instability, dyskinesia, or decreased consciousness occur [849–851]. It is potentially lethal. Psychiatric symptoms include changes in personality and behaviour, irritability, anxiety, aggressive behaviour, delusional thoughts, paranoia, and catatonia; short-term memory loss may occur. Other features include seizures, autonomic instability (such as hyper- or hypothermia, fluctuation in BP and heart rate, constipation or ileus), and abnormal movements (including orofacial dyskinesia, dystonic posturing, choreoathetoid movements, oculogyric crisis, myoclonus, and opisthotonus). Lumbar puncture may show elevated CSF protein with oligoclonal bands and IgG. The EEG may show focal or diffuse slow activity, or sometimes seizures. Magnetic resonance imaging may show small areas of FLAIR abnormalities but may be normal. $NMDA_R$ antibodies are found in serum and CSF, or sometimes only in CSF [849, 852].

In one series of patients with anti-NMDA-receptor encephalitis, 77% presented with prominent psychiatric disturbance (anxiety, agitation, bizarre behaviour, delusions or paranoid ideation, and visual/auditory hallucinations) and 23% with short-term memory impairment (with or without seizures and other psychiatric disturbance). Most (86%) had a prodrome including headache, low-grade fever, or symptoms suggesting viral infection within the two weeks before presentation; 91% were female, 88% had altered consciousness, 86% had dyskinesia, 76% had seizures within the first 3 weeks, 69% had autonomic instability, 66% had hypoventilation, and 59% of those assessed oncologically had tumours (most commonly ovarian teratoma). The EEG was abnormal in all those in whom one was performed; 55% had an abnormal brain MRI, and 95% had abnormal CSF [853]. In another series, an initial phase of neuropsychiatric symptoms, cognitive dysfunction, and/or seizures preceded (by medians of 10–20 days) a second phase of alteration in consciousness, movement disorder, and/or dysautonomia. Psychosis occurred in 45% of patients. CSF lymphocytosis occurred in 68% but generally disappeared by the 35-day point. CSF oligoclonal bands were initially present in 9% of patients but eventually appeared in 43%.

Magnetic resonance imaging was normal on the first scan in 89% and remained normal in 77%. Epileptiform activity was seen on EEG in 50%, mostly early in the disease, with slowing in 80%, mostly later in the disease course [854]. This case series included children and adults, 80% without identifiable tumours. The clinical features can overlap with encephalitis lethargica (Chapter 8.7.2 ▶), Hashimoto's encephalopathy (Chapter 14.1 ▶), and PANDAS (Chapter 8.7.1 ▶).

14.2.3 Other antibodies against neuropil and neuronal surface proteins

The neuropil is the mass of unmyelinated axonal and dendritic processes within grey matter. Antibodies against neuropil indicate antibodies to neuronal surface proteins [855]. Anti-VGKC and anti-$NMDA_R$ antibodies both fall into this category, but so do others.

Subacute limbic encephalitis secondary to hippocampal neuropil autoantibodies has recently been described [841]; in 5 out of 7 patients an underlying tumour was identified (teratoma, thymic tumours, thyroid carcinoma). Hyponatraemia was not seen. All had abnormal CSF (variously: pleocytosis, elevated protein, and oligoclonal bands), abnormal MRI, and abnormal EEG findings.

Antibodies to EFA6A, a neuropil protein, have been found in PLE [856]. Yet others include antibodies to mGluR1, GluRε2, voltage-gated calcium channels, and acetylcholine receptors (anti-AChR) [840, 842, 857].

In a survey in 2008 of antibodies in limbic encephalitis, neuronal surface antibodies were present in 64%, and of these, 45% were anti-VGKC, 17% were anti-$NMDA_R$, and 38% were to novel antigens [855]. There was often simultaneously antibody activity against intraneuronal and neuronal surface antigens. As discussed above, screening for unknown antineuronal antigens requires immunocytochemistry or immunohistochemistry, testing patient sera against (typically rat) brain tissue, and clinical testing is typically against identified specific antigens. The important message is that patients can have antibody-mediated limbic encephalitis/encephalopathy and test negative on standard screens. Yet others can have seronegative limbic encephalitis (none with PLE in this series, but 29% of those with idiopathic limbic encephalitis, for a total of 11% overall) [855].

14.2.4 Other antibodies against intraneuronal antigens

There are several other autoantibodies associated with PLE. Anti-neuronal nuclear antibodies include ANNA-1 (anti-Hu, also associated with peripheral neuropathy [858, 859]), ANNA-2 (anti-Ri), and ANNA-3. Anti-neuronal cytoplasmic antibodies include PCA-1 (anti-Yo, typically causing cerebellar dysfunction), PCA-2, PCA-Tr, and antibodies to CV2/CRMP-5 and amphiphysin. Other intraneuronal antigens include Zic4, Ma1, and Ma2 (Ta). Yet others include antibodies to BR serine/threonine kinase 2, CRMP3–4, adenylate kinase 5, and muscle cytoplasm [385, 840, 842, 857, 860].

Anti-GAD antibodies have been associated with non-paraneoplastic limbic encephalitis [861], though these antibodies may also be markers of multiple autoimmunity [862].

14.3 Nonvasculitic autoimmune inflammatory meningoencephalitis

Recently named as an entity, NAIM is characterized by acute, subacute, or chronic encephalopathy with fluctuating or increasing confusion and cognitive decline, and hallucinations, sometimes with paranoid delusions [863, 864]. Cerebrospinal fluid, EEG, and brain biopsy were consistent with a meningoencephalitis. In 4 of the 5 original cases described, there were identifiable autoimmune abnormalities (two with Sjögren's syndrome, one with antiphospholipid antibodies, and one with antithyroid antibodies and ANA/SS-A) [863]. In several but not all cases the ESR was raised [863–865]. Nonvasculitic autoimmune-mediated meningoencephalitides are associated with Sjögren's syndrome (Chapter 13.1.3 ▶), hypereosinophilic syndrome (Chapter 18.2 ▶), Hashimoto's encephalopathy (Chapter 14.1 ▶), and SLE (Chapter 13.1.1 ▶), and therefore NAIM might be an umbrella term for these autoimmune encephalopathies, or a distinct entity [864]. All cases in the original series were steroid-responsive [863, 864]. Sometimes the disease has mimicked Creutzfeldt–Jakob disease (Chapter 8.6 ▶), including its characteristic EEG findings [866], and sometimes it has mimicked a dementing process [865].

Chapter 15 Poisoning

15.1 Therapeutic drugs

Drugs that can cause psychosis are listed below. Drug categories are emboldened and italicized. For some drugs (e.g. anticholinergics, amphetamines, sympathomimetics, dopamine agonists, steroids) there is excellent evidence for psychotogenicity, whereas for others the evidence is based on *ad hoc* reporting. Brand names are given only for combination drugs where the causal agent is unclear. Side effect frequency is usually based on the classification of common (>1% of patients), infrequent (0.1–1%), and rare (<0.1%); the manufacturers' literature should be consulted for detailed frequency information, and absence of frequency information in the list below does not imply the effect is common or rare. Exact frequencies are given in parentheses in some cases. Note that the elderly are more vulnerable to many drug side effects, including hallucinations and delusions. Note also that diseases affecting drug clearance (e.g. renal failure [Chapter 12.4.1 ▶], hepatic failure [Chapter 12.4.2 ▶]) may predispose to drug-induced psychosis, as may hypoalbuminaemia (e.g. by increasing the free fraction of protein-bound drugs) [867].

Acamprosate, for maintaining alcohol abstinence (rare) [38].

ACE inhibitors (rarely) [15].

Acetylcholinesterase inhibitors: donepezil; galantamine (rarely); rivastigmine (very rarely); tacrine [27, 38].

Amiodarone, antiarrhythmic (rare) [38].

Aminocaproic acid, fibinolysis inhibitor [38].

Amphetamine: see dexamfetamine and Chapter 15.3 ▶.

Angiotensin receptor antagonists (rarely) [15].

Antibacterial antibiotics: ***cephalosporins*** (including cefaclor, cefalexin, cefepime, cefpodoxime, ceftibuten); clarithromycin (very rarely); colistin; co-trimoxazole (trimethoprim plus sulfamethoxazole) (very rarely); cycloserine; dapsone; daptomycin (<1%); ertapenem (very rarely); ethambutol (very rarely); ethionamide; gentamicin (rarely hallucinations); imipenem/cilastatin; isoniazid (rarely; see also Chapter 11.3 ▶); meropenem; metronidazole (particularly if combined with disulfiram); nitrofurantoin; piperacillin/tazobactam; procaine benzylpenicillin (a.k.a. procaine penicillin); ***quinolones*** and derivatives (cinoxacin, ciprofloxacin, enoxacin, gatifloxacin, gemifloxacin, grepafloxacin, levofloxacin, lomefloxacin, moxifloxacin, nalixidic acid, norfloxacin, ofloxacin, sparfloxacin, trovafloxacin); possibly rifampicin (rifampin); ***sulphonamides*** (e.g. sulfamethoxazole, sulfisoxazole) [15, 27, 38, 868]. Psychosis with procaine penicillin as part of a pseudoanaphylactic reaction is known as **Hoigne's syndrome** or **antibiomania**, and may be due to the procaine

[869, 870]. Very high-dose intravenous penicillins may also induce an encephalopathy with psychosis, particularly in patients with renal failure [38].

Anticonvulsants: carbamazepine; ethosuximide; felbamate; levetiracetam (sometimes with onset of psychosis several months after commencement [871, 872]); lamotrigine; methsuximide (mesuximide); oxcarbazepine; phenytoin (in overdose); tiagabine; topiramate; valproate (rarely); vigabatrin (in ~3% of patients); zonisamide [15, 27, 38, 873, 874]. See also barbiturates (below).

Antidepressants: possibly amoxapine; atomoxetine (0.2%); bupropion (see below); duloxetine (rarely); maprotiline; mirtazapine (may aggravate pre-existing psychosis); ***MAO inhibitors*** (isocarboxazid [rarely], phenelzine, and the combination of tranylcypromine and dextromethorphan [q.v.]); ***MAO inhibitor withdrawal***; nefazodone (withdrawn); ***SSRIs*** (citalopram, escitalopram, fluoxetine, fluvoxamine, paroxetine, sertraline: psychosis including hallucinations and delusions); trazodone (hallucinations, delusions); ***tricyclic antidepressants*** in general (amitriptyline, clomipramine, desipramine, dosulepin [dothiepin], doxepin, imipramine, lofepramine, nortriptyline, trimipramine: perhaps via anticholinergic activity); venlafaxine (rarely); venlafaxine withdrawal [15, 20, 27, 38, 875–878].

Antifungals: amphotericin; flucytosine; pentamidine; posaconazole; voriconazole; fluconazole (in overdose) [27, 38].

Antihistamines: hallucinations reported with the H_2 receptor antagonists (cimetidine, famotidine, nizatidine, ranitidine), particularly in the very ill; cetirizine and levocetirizine (very rarely hallucinations); desloratadine (very rarely hallucinations) [27, 38]. H_1 receptor antagonists including dimenhydrinate and pheniramine have been abused as hallucinogens [15]. ***Antihistamines with anticholinergic properties*** include chlorphenamine (chlorpheniramine), cyproheptadine, doxylamine, hydroxyzine, dimenhydrinate, diphenhydramine, meclizine, promethazine [879].

Antimalarials: possibly atovaquone/proguanil (Malarone®); chloroquine; hydroxychloroquine; mefloquine; quinidine (also an antiarrhythmic; first-dose psychosis reported but very rare); sulfadoxine/pyrimethamine (Fansidar®) [27, 38, 437, 438].

Antimuscarinics: all can cause a central anticholinergic syndrome with hallucinations [15, 27, 38, 879]; they include atropine, benzatropine (benztropine), biperiden, clidinium, cyclopentolate, darifenacin, dicycloverine (dicyclomine), duloxetine, ethopropazine, flavoxate, glycopyrronium (glycopyrrolate), homatropine, hyoscine (scopolamine), hyoscyamine (L-atropine), orphenadrine, oxybutynin, procyclidine, propantheline, propiverine, solifenacin, tolterodine, trihexyphenidyl (benzhexol), tropicamide, and trospium. (See also Chapter 15.4 ▶.)

Antipsychotics: obviously difficult to distinguish from the condition being treated, but hallucinations reported on olanzapine, quetiapine, risperidone; exacerbation of psychosis reported with haloperidol, phenothiazines (e.g. chlorpromazine, thioridazine, fluphenazine, perphenazine, prochlorperazine, trifluoperazine), thioxanthenes (e.g. flupenthixol, zuclopenthixol); rare side effects include catatonia (aripiprazole, risperidone) [20, 27, 38]. Bradyphrenia induced by antipsychotic overdose may resemble thought block. Bradykinesia in overdose may resemble catatonia, which can also occur as a drug reaction (e.g. phenothiazines) [38]. ***Antipsychotics with anticholinergic properties*** include chlorpromazine, clozapine, mesoridazine, olanzapine, quetiapine, and thioridazine [879]. ***Antipsychotic withdrawal***: **supersensitivity psychosis** ("tardive psychosis") is postulated to be psychosis occurring after chronic (>1 year) treatment with antipsychotics (dopamine antagonists) when the drug is reduced. The concept has been criticized as merely representing exacerbations of the underlying psychotic condition, though supporters point to cases triggered by reduction in long-term dopamine antagonists used for non-psychotic (e.g. gastrointestinal) conditions in patients with no history of psychosis [20, 880, 881].

Antivirals, including nucleoside analogues: possibly abacavir; aciclovir (very rarely); amantadine (see dopamine agonists); cidofovir; delavirdine; efavirenz (psychiatric side effects common); famciclovir (very rarely); foscarnet; ganciclovir; nevirapine; possibly oseltamivir; ribavarin (<1%); rimantadine (<0.3% at normal doses); ritonavir; saquinavir; valaciclovir; vidarabine; zalcitabine; zanamivir; zidovudine (azidothymidine, AZT); zidovudine with lamivudine [15, 27, 38, 882–885].

Baclofen, $GABA_B$ agonist and muscle relaxant. Both baclofen withdrawal, and baclofen itself, have caused psychosis [27, 886, 887].

Barbiturates: e.g. butabarbital, mephobarbital, pentobarbital (<1%), phenobarbitone [27, 38].

Barbiturate withdrawal may precipitate psychosis; typically, if hallucinations occur, they precede full-blown delirium, occuring 3–8 days after cessation of pentobarbital [22, 888].

Benzodiazepines and related GABA agonist hypnotics: e.g. alprazolam, chlordiazepoxide, clonazepam, estazolam, flurazepam, diazepam (rarely hallucinations, delusions), lorazepam, midazolam, temazepam (hallucinations in <0.5%), quazepam, triazolam, zaleplon, zolpidem, zopiclone (rarely hallucinations) [27, 38].

Benzodiazepine withdrawal may precipitate psychosis [22, 27, 33, 38], including Schneiderian first-rank symptoms [20]. The timing of onset depends on the half-life of the benzodiazepine.

Beta adrenoceptor blockers (such as propranolol): hallucinations and catatonia can occur [38].

Benzonatate, antitussive; rarely visual hallucinations [38].

Bisphosphonates: rarely, hallucinations with etidronate, pamidronate [27, 38].

Bretylium, antiarrhythmic, possibly (~0.1%) [38].

Brimonidine, alpha adrenoceptor agonist [15].

Bromide, largely obsolete group of compounds (e.g. potassium bromide) formerly used as sedatives and as antiepileptics, for which potassium bromide is still in use in some countries. It used to be a common cause of psychosis. Bromide can cause a neurotoxic syndrome known as **bromism**. Its effects may include a rash resembling acne vulgaris (bromoderma), cognitive and mnemonic impairment, personality change, paranoid delusions, hallucinations, pupillary dilation, ataxia, slurred speech, anorexia, constipation, fetor, decreased sensation, conjunctivitis, lacrimation, bradycardia, reduced reflexes, insomnia, restlessness, disorientation, apathy, stupor, seizures, coma, and death [889]. Psychosis can be the main feature. Diagnosis is by blood level, with intoxication usually occurring above about 150 mg/dl or 18.75 mM. Organic bromide compounds are also toxic, by different mechanisms (see bromomethane in Chapter 15.7.2 ▶).

Bupropion (amfebutamone), for smoking cessation or as an antidepressant (paranoia, delusions, auditory hallucinations all reported; bupropion is structurally related to amphetamines and inhibits dopamine and noradrenaline reuptake) [15, 27].

Buspirone, anxiolytic (hallucinations >1%, other psychosis <0.1%) [38].

Calcium channel blockers: diltiazem; verapamil (<2%) [38].

Cannabinoids: dronabinol (3–10%), nabilone [27, 38]. See also recreational drugs (Chapter 15.3 ▶).

Carisoprodol, central skeletal muscle relaxant in overdose [38].

Cevimeline, muscarinic ACh receptor agonist for Sjögren's syndrome [38].

Cisapride, withdrawn treatment for gastro-oesophageal reflux [38].

Chloral hydrate, sedative, either as a side effect (rare) or in withdrawal [38].

Clonidine, central antihypertensive that may rarely cause hallucinations and whose withdrawal has been reported to cause psychosis [38, 890].

Clopidogrel, antiplatelet (very rarely) [27].

COMT inhibitors: entacapone, tolcapone (used in Parkinson's disease) [27].

Contrast agents: transient psychosis reported following accidental intravenous administration of iodine-based oils, hallucinations after intravenous water-soluble iodine dyes (<1%), and hallucinations after gadoversetamide, a gadolinium-based contrast agent used in MRI [38].

Cyclobenzaprine, muscle relaxant [38].

Cyclosporin (ciclosporin), immunosuppressant [891].

Cytotoxic chemotherapeutic agents and other antineoplastic agents: aldesleukin (interleukin-2); asparaginase; bortezomib; busulfan (hallucinations in 5%); chlorambucil (rarely); ifosfamide; hydroxyurea; lenalidomide (a thalidomide analogue); procarbazine; temsirolimus (in high doses); thalidomide (also used in leprosy); vincristine (hallucinations occur in 5%) [22, 27, 38].

Cysteamine bitartrate, for cystinosis [38].

Dexamfetamine (dexamphetamine, D-amphetamine), monoamine releaser and uptake inhibitor used in ADHD [27]. It is sufficiently psychotogenic to be used for this purpose experimentally. See also Chapter 15.3 ▶.

Dextromethorphan, synthetic analogue of a morphine derivative; it is an $NMDA_R$ antagonist, used as an antitussive [892].

Digoxin, antiarrhythmic and Na/K-ATPase inhibitor (hallucinations usually at excessive dose) [27].

Disopyramide, antiarrhythmic [27].

Disulfiram, for alcohol dependence [27], perhaps because it inhibits dopamine-β-hydroxylase [893]; particularly psychotogenic when combined with metronidazole [27].

Dopamine agonists: amantadine, apomorphine, bromocriptine, cabergoline, lergotrile (obsolete ergot derivative), lisuride, quinagolide, pergolide, pramipexole, ropinirole, rotigotine [27, 33, 894]. In general, psychosis caused by direct dopamine agonists is less common than that caused by levodopa (q.v.; see also Chapter 5.3 ▶) [20].

Doxapram, respiratory stimulant [27].

Doxazosin, alpha-blocking antihypertensive [895].

Epoprostenol, prostaglandin for pulmonary hypertension; can cause psychotic depression [38].

Erythropoietin may induce visual hallucinations on occasion, possibly via posterior hypertensive leukoencephalopathy (Chapter 6.4 ▶) [896, 897].

Fenfluramine withdrawal: fenfluramine is a serotonin releasing agent and appetite suppressant (withdrawn for risk of valvular heart disease and pulmonary hypertension); fenfluramine withdrawal has been suggested to trigger psychosis on occasion [898].

Flecainide, antiarrhythmic [27].

Flumazenil, benzodiazepine antagonist, reported to trigger psychosis in the context of hepatic encephalopathy [689].

Gabapentin, used for neuropathic pain [27], and gabapentin withdrawal [899].

Glatiramer, for multiple sclerosis (rarely) [38].

Gold, injected for rheumatoid arthritis; toxicity may include hallucinations as well as depression, delirium, ataxia, blurred vision, tremor, and peripheral neuropathy [29].

Hydralazine, vasodilator antihypertensive [15].

Hydroxyzine, anxiolytic (it has anticholinergic activity and hallucinations have been reported) [38].

Immunosuppressants and immunomodulators *(other than cytotoxic or steroid immunosuppressants)*: anti-tumour necrosis factor alpha (TNF-α) drugs (examples include adalimumab, etanercept, and infliximab); mycophenolate; tacrolimus (neurotoxicity in up to 55%) [27, 38, 900].

Interferon; alpha-interferon is used for hepatitis C treatment, and for some tumours [901].

Isotretinoin, used for acne (psychosis rarely) [15, 902].

Ketamine, $NMDA_R$ antagonist used as a dissociative anaesthetic. It is sufficiently psychotogenic to be used experimentally for this purpose. Its effects include delusions, hallucinations, abnormal salience phenomena, and catatonia [7, 17, 22, 27]. It magnifies amphetamine-induced striatal dopamine release [903] and exacerbates symptoms in schizophrenia [see 17].

Leuprolide, LHRH agonist [38].

Levodopa (L-DOPA), dopamine precursor used for Parkinson's disease (Chapter 5.3 ▶) [27]. Psychosis may occur when treatment is started but more commonly occurs after 3–4 years, with a gradual progression beginning with hallucinations with insight [20].

Levothyroxine (thyroxine). See Chapter 9.1 ▶.

Lithium, mood stabilizer; although often used in the treatment of manic psychosis, toxicity has been associated with new delusion formation and hallucinations can occur [38, 904].

Local anaesthetics: e.g. lidocaine (lignocaine); ropivacaine; tocainide in intravenous doses for arrhythmia [38, 905, 906].

Memantine, $NMDA_R$ antagonist for Alzheimer's disease (psychosis rare) [27].

Methyldopa, central antihypertensive [27].

Methylphenidate, monoamine releaser and uptake inhibitor used in ADHD [27, 907]; methylphenidate is sufficiently psychotogenic to be used for this purpose experimentally [705].

Mepacrine, used for giardiasis and lupus [27].

Mercaptamine, for nephropathic cystinosis [27].

Methylergonovine (methylergometrine), ergot alkaloid [38].

Methysergide, semi-synthetic ergot alkaloid [908] (note that another report was retracted [909]).

Metirosine (metyrosine), for phaeochromocytoma [27].

Metoclopramide, rarely hallucinations [38].

Metrizamide, obsolete radiocontrast agent formerly used for myelography [910].

Mexiletine, antiarrhythmic (hallucinations 0.3%; other psychosis 0.2%) [38].

Modafinil, an atypical psychostimulant [911].

Monoamine oxidase inhibitors: e.g. rasagiline, selegiline (L-deprenyl) (both MAO-B inhibitors used for PD; hallucinations) [27, 38].

Montelukast, leukotriene receptor antagonist for asthma (very rarely hallucinations) [27].

Naltrexone, opioid antagonist (very rarely) [27].

Nefopam, non-opioid centrally acting analgesic [27].

Nitrous oxide, inhalational analgesic (see Chapter 11.4▶) [639]; can also cause hallucinations acutely in children (2%) [912].

NSAIDs, possibly as a class effect: aspirin (very rare); possibly choline magnesium trisalicylate; diclofenac; diflunisal (<1%); flurbiprofen; possibly ibuprofen; indomethacin; ketoprofen; ketorolac; mefenamic acid; naproxen; oxaprozin; piroxicam; rofecoxib (withdrawn); suldinac; valdecoxib (withdrawn) [27, 38, 913]. Salicylate poisoning has on rare occasions caused psychosis as part of its toxic profile [33, 913] and can worsen pre-existing psychosis [914].

Oestrogen receptor modulators: possibly clomiphene; tamoxifen (rarely delusions); toremifene (hallucinations in overdose) [22, 38].

Opioids: nearly all opioids, prototypically morphine, have been reported to cause hallucinations; also pentazocine (hallucinations and thought disturbances), and pethidine (meperidine; it and its metabolite norpethidine [normeperidine] also have significant anticholinergic activity) [22, 27, 915]. Benzomorphan opioids (e.g. cyclazocine and related compounds) are psychotogenic, perhaps by binding to the sigma-1 receptor (now classified as a non-opioid receptor) [916]. ***Opioid withdrawal*** has been suggested to cause psychosis in a few cases (buprenorphine, methadone) [917–919].

Pemoline, stimulant used for ADHD, now withdrawn [38, 907].

Pentoxifylline, for peripheral vascular disease [27]; auditory hallucinations reported [20].

Phenylacetate/benzoate (Ammonul®), for hyperammonaemia (<3%) [38].

Pilocarpine, cholinergic parasympathomimetic (rarely hallucinations, delusions) [38].

Prazosin, alpha-adrenoceptor-blocking antihypertensive [27].

Pregabalin, used for neuropathic pain [27].

Procainamide, antiarrhythmic [27].

Propafenone, antiarrhythmic [38].

Propofol, anaesthetic agent (hallucinations) [38].

Proton pump inhibitors: esomeprazole (rare), lansoprazole, omeprazole (reversible hallucinations reported in the severely ill), pantoprazole [27, 38].

Reserpine, central antihypertensive (rarely; it was itself used as an antipsychotic) [15]; reserpine withdrawal [920, 921].

Riluzole, for motor neuron disease (infrequent) [38].

Rimonabant, cannabinoid receptor antagonist (rarely hallucinations) [27].

Sodium oxybate, hypnotic [27].

Sodium nitroprusside, vasodilator antihypertensive; the drug is converted *in vivo* to nitric oxide and cyanide, and excess causes toxicity by cyanide poisoning and thiocyanate accumulation [26].

Steroids, particularly high-dose systemic corticosteroids [27]; the risk of psychosis is dose-related. For prednisone, which is metabolized to prednisolone and is roughly equipotent to it [922], the risk of psychosis is 1.3% at ≤40 mg/day, 4.6% at 41–80 mg/day, and 18.4% at >80 mg/day [923], with ~75% developing mania at >80 mg/day [20]. *Dehydroepiandrosterone (DHEA)* is an adrenal steroid available over the counter in some regions. It has produced manic psychosis at 25–50 mg/day [924]. See also anabolic steroids (Chapter 15.3▶).

St John's wort (Hypericum perforatum), herbal antidepressant [925].

Sympathomimetics, including the amphetamines (see above and Chapter 15.3▶), benzphetamine, diethylpropion (anorexigenic), ephedrine, methylphenidate (see above and toxin; others include the more potent 5-methoxy-dimethyltryptamine. Many toads in the genus *Bufo* secrete bufotoxins, including *Bufo alvarius* (Colorado River or Sonoran Desert toad) and *Bufo marinus* (cane toad) [991]; in Amazon and Atlantic rainforests, frogs in the *Osteocephalus* genus also secrete bufotenine [992]. Of the bufotoxins, 5-methoxy-DMT (notably from *Bufo alvarius*) is clearly hallucinogenic [991].

15.5.3 Fish poisoning (ichthyoallyeinotoxism)

Rarely, fish consumption can trigger hallucinations. Such poisoning is termed ichthyoallyeinotoxism, and the fish responsible have been collectively termed "dreamfish". Fish that can be hallucinogenic include *Acanthurus triostegus* (common names include convict surgeonfish), *Kyphosus* species (sea chub), *Mugil* and *Neomyxus* species (surmullet, goatfish), *Abudefduf septemfasciatus* (damselfish), *Epinephelus corallicola* (coral grouper), *Siganus* species (rabbitfish), and *Sarpa salpa* (saupe or sea bream). The causatory toxins are unknown but are probably heat-stable; they may be from algal contamination of the fish, but ichthyoallyeinotoxism (causing CNS effects) is distinct from ciguatera poisoning (due to a fish-borne algal toxin but causing peripheral nervous system toxicity with gastrointestinal symptoms). The first symptoms are typically incoordination and malaise. There are sometimes low-grade gastrointestinal symptoms. The hallucinations typically begin within minutes to 2 hours of consumption, may be visual and/or auditory, and are frequently terrifying, with frightening nightmares if the patient can sleep. There may be feelings of impending death, with reactive sympathetic arousal. The symptoms subside within 24–36 hours [993].

15.5.4 Plant and fungus poisoning

A large number of plants can cause anticholinergic psychosis (Chapter 15.4 ▶). Plants with anticholinergic activity include *Amanita muscaria* (fly agaric), *Amanita pantherina* (panther mushroom), *Arctium lappa* (burdock root), *Atropa belladonna* (deadly nightshade), *Brugmansia* species (angel's trumpet), *Cestrum nocturnum* (night blooming jessamine), *Datura suaveolens* (another type of angel's trumpet), *Datura stramonium* (jimson weed; thorn apple), *Hyoscyamus niger* (black henbane), *Lantana camara* (red sage), *Methysticodendron amnesianum* (culebra-borrachera), *Solanum carolinensis* (wild tomato), *Solanum dulcamara* (bittersweet), *Solanum pseudocapsicum* (Jerusalem cherry), and *Solanum tuberosum* (potato) [26, 29, 879].

Mushroom poisoning may cause psychosis via several means. *Inocybe* and *Clitocybe* species, and to a much lesser extent *Amanita muscaria* (fly agaric), contain muscarine and are thus anticholinergic, though hallucinations are not the commonest feature [26]. *Amanita pantherina* (panther cap), *Amanita muscaria* (fly agaric), and *Amanita strobiliformis* contain ibotenic acid, an $NMDA_R$ agonist, and muscimol, a $GABA_A$ agonist, and produce anxiety, mood elevation, and hallucinations [26, 933]. *Amanita muscaria* also contains the hallucinogen bufotenine (see also amphibian venom, Chapter 15.5.2 ▶) [933]. A range of "magic" mushrooms contain the hallucinogen psilocybin; these include *Psilocybe* species, *Conocybe* species, *Gymnopilus* species, *Panaeolina foenisecii*, *Panaeolus* species, *Pluteus* species, and *Stropharia* species [26].

Other plant hallucinogens include tetrahydrocannabinols in cannabis (*Cannabis sativa*), cocaine in coca (*Erythroxylum coca*), ibogaine in iboga (*Tabernanthe iboga*), cathinone (structurally related to amphetamine) in khat (qat; *Catha edulis*), LSD in morning glory (*Ipomoea* species and *Rivea*/*Turbina corymbosa*), mescaline in peyote (*Lophophora williamsii* and *diffusa*), myristicin in nutmeg (*Myristica fragrans*), and vincristine and vinblastine in periwinkle (*Vinca* and *Catharanthus* species) [26, 933] (see also Chapters 15.1, 15.3 ▶). Dimethyltryptamine (DMT) is present in species including jurema (*Mimosa hostilis*), *Psychotria viridis*, *Virola calophylla* (epená, which also contains bufotenine or 5-hydroxy-DMT), and many *Acacia* species and is hallucinogenic if inhaled as snuff or injected, or if taken with plants containing MAO inhibitors such as harmala alkaloids [22, 29, 933, 994, 995].

Other hallucinogenic plants include *Acorus calamus* (sweet flag), *Alchornea floribunda* (niando), *Argyreia nervosa* (silver morning glory), *Coleus* species, *Cytisus canariensis* (Canary Island broom), *Duboisia hopwoodii* (pituri), *Foeniculum vulgare* (fennel), *Heimia salicifolia* (sinicuichi), *Lobelia inflata* (Indian tobacco), *Mandragora officinarum* (mandrake), *Olmedioperebea sclerophylla* (rape dos indios), *Pancratium trianthum* (kwashi), *Sarcostemma acidum* (soma), and *Sophora secundiflora* (mescal bean) [29].

One plant containing a non-alkaloid hallucinogen is *Salvia divinorum* (salvia; diviner's sage; "magic mint"). This contains salvinorin A, a diterpene κ-opioid agonist often referred to as a powerful hallucinogen and suggested to be a trigger for acute and also persistent psychosis (e.g. [996–1000]). It sometimes causes hallucinations [1001]; however, its more typical subjective effects are depersonalization or psychedelic perceptual distortions [1000, 1002].

Some therapeutic drugs that can cause psychosis (Chapter 15.1 ▶) originate from plants, such as the cardiac glycosides (digoxin and digitoxin from the foxglove *Digitalis purpurea*), ephedrine (from *Ephedra sinica*), and vinca alkaloids (as above).

Cereal crop contamination by the ascomycete fungus *Claviceps purpurea* may lead to ergot poisoning. The commonest syndrome is of vasoconstriction (St Anthony's fire) but a syndrome of tremor, convulsions, and hallucinations can also occur [26]; this may reflect serotonin syndrome (Chapter 15.2 ▶) [1003]. Hallucinogenic ergot alkaloids include isoergine (lysergic acid amide) [933].

15.6 Metal and metalloid poisoning

15.6.1 Mercury (Hg) poisoning

Mercury poisoning was made famous in Victorian Britain by its occurrence amongst hatters, who used mercury compounds in the treatment of hat felt; hence "mad as a hatter" [1004]. Mercury exposure can be as the element (by contact, ingestion, vapour inhalation, or occasionally self-injection), as inorganic compounds (mercury salts), or as organic compounds (most commonly methylmercury). Elemental mercury poisoning typically occurs by exposure to vapour from spilled liquid mercury; this can be from industrial sources, from broken mercury-based devices including electrical switches, fluorescent bulbs, thermometers, and sphygmomanometers, and from some religious practices. Liquid mercury is poorly absorbed from the skin and GI tract, but small spills are very hard to identify and clean up and very small amounts of metallic mercury can produce dangerous levels of vapour, which can lead to chronic exposure. Mercury vapour is odourless, readily absorbed through the lungs, and toxic [1005]. The small amounts of mercury vapour released by dental amalgam appear not to be toxic to the owner, though dental staff may have higher exposure [1005]. Some old remedies for worms or teething disorders in children contained mercurous chloride [1005]. Methylmercury, used as a fungicide until the 1970s, is readily absorbed by ingestion and bioaccumulates, especially in large saltwater fish such as shark and swordfish [1005]; poisoning by it is known as Minamata disease, after mass poisoning by contaminated fish consumption in 1953 at Minamata, Japan [1006].

Clinical features. Acute poisoning typically causes cough, dyspnoea, and chest pain, with pneumonitis and in severe cases pulmonary oedema; hypertension and tachycardia; fatigue, fever, chills, and leukocytosis; and renal and sometimes hepatic damage. Stomatitis (inflammation of the oral mucosa) and gingivitis are classic signs of mercury poisoning (acute or chronic), sometimes with hypersalivation, and other GI symptoms such as nausea, anorexia, and a metallic taste are well described [1005, 1007]. Dermatological reactions include erythematous and pruritic rashes, heavy perspiration, and reddened and/or peeling skin on palms and soles [1005]. The terms acrodynia and "pink disease" describe irritability, photophobia, pink discolouration of the hands and feet, and polyneuritis in children secondary to chronic mercury poisoning [1008]. However, the CNS is the most sensitive target for mercury. Symptoms include tremor (usually beginning in the hands) and ataxia, personality change with emotional lability (typically with irritability, excessive shyness, loss of confidence, and nervousness), insomnia, memory loss, neuromuscular changes (weakness, muscle atrophy, twitching), headaches, polyneuropathy (paraesthesiae, glove and stocking sensory loss, brisk reflexes, reduced nerve conduction velocities), impaired cognitive function, hearing loss, visual field impairments (typically constriction), and hallucinations [1005]. The term erethism is used for the constellation of irritability, excitability, anxiety, insomnia, and social withdrawal [1009].

Mercury levels in urine (24 h collection) are used to test for exposure to elemental and inorganic mercury, but are not useful for methylmercury, for which blood or scalp hair levels are used [1005, 1008]. Blood levels are useful in acute exposure [1009]. Mercury inhibits a coenzyme necessary for COMT function, and hence blocks catecholamine breakdown, so elevated urinary catecholamines may be found whilst investigating hypertension [1007, 1010].

15.6.2 Arsenic (As) poisoning

Arsenic exposure may occur through smelting of ores (the main route of production), in wood preservatives, in arsenical pesticides, in the metallurgy and electronics industries, and occasionally in deliberate poisoning (including the use of Lewisite in World War I). Fish can accumulate arsenic, but usually in a relatively non-toxic organic form (arsenobetaine or "fish arsenic"). Most cases of human poisoning have been due to inorganic forms of arsenic [1011, 1012].

Systemic poisoning can cause GI irritation with abdominal pain, nausea, vomiting, and diarrhoea; anaemia and leukopenia; arrhythmias; easy bruising; peripheral neuropathy; and sore throat and respiratory tract irritation. The most characteristic feature is patches of hyperpigmented skin with interspersed spots of hypopigmentation, and hyperkeratosis on the palms, soles, and torso, typically with multiple hyperkeratinized corns or warts. Peripheral vascular disease may occur. Arsenic is also a carcinogen (lung, bladder, liver) [1011]. Arsenic encephalopathy can include confusion, hallucinations, impaired memory, and emotional lability. Other features have included fatigue, headache, lethargy, dizziness, insomnia, nightmares, seizures, and coma [1011].

Urinary arsenic measures are the most useful to measure recent exposure, with hair or nail arsenic levels being more sensitive to exposure months previously [1011].

15.6.3 Thallium (Tl) poisoning

Thallium is used in the manufacture of electronic devices, in glass manufacture, and in diagnostic imaging; it is produced in power plants, cement factories, and smelters. Historically, it was used as a rat poison, and it has been used homicidally. It may be absorbed orally or by inhalation.

Hair loss, and dark pigmentation of the hair roots, are characteristic of thallium poisoning. Neurological effects include ataxia, lethargy, painful peripheral neuropathy, confusion, disorientation, hallucinations, and memory impairment. Gastrointestinal effects include vomiting and diarrhoea; hepatic necrosis has also been observed. Renal function can be impaired [33, 1013–1015].

Thallium is cleared rapidly from blood, so measurement is usually of urinary thallium, and sometimes of thallium levels in hair [1013].

15.6.4 Lead (Pb) poisoning

Lead poisoning (plumbism) can occur through a wide variety of routes. These include direct industrial contact with lead (occupations at risk include painting, plumbing, shipbuilding, lead smelting and refining, brass founding, pottery glazing, vitreous enamelling, typesetting, and the manufacture of batteries, rubber, glass, pigments and lead products themselves); demolition of structures (e.g. railway bridges) previously painted with lead paint; in children with pica (chewing of lead-painted objects, direct ingestion of metallic lead, eating of contaminated soil); drinking from lead-glazed mugs; home-distilled ("moonshine") alcohol consumption; ingestion of lead-based paints; inadvertent food contamination; some "tonics" and herbal remedies; the use of lead-based cosmetics (particularly in Asian communities); retained lead bullets following gunshot wounds; and exposure to tetraethyl lead as an anti-knock agent in gasoline (industrially or by gasoline sniffing) [26, 33, 1016–1018]. Lead poisoning is commonest in children under 6 and in adults in high-risk occupations [1019]. Historically, lead poisoning has also occurred through mining, the use of lead compounds as wine sweeteners, and through lead water pipes, drinking vessels, and cosmetics. Perhaps the most dramatic series was an outbreak of psychosis and mania (and death) that occurred in factories that had begun to manufacture tetraethyl lead in the USA. Tetraethyl lead can be absorbed by inhalation, ingestion, and through the skin, and was known as "looney gas" [1020]. Lead has adverse neurological effects in children even at very low levels [1021].

Clinical features of lead poisoning can include intermittent colicky abdominal pains ("lead colic"); constipation; diarrhoea; nausea; vomiting; poor appetite; weight loss; weakness; muscle cramps; joint pains; headache; hypertension; neuropsychiatric abnormalities including irritability, lethargy or hyperactivity, insomnia, and psychosis; and peripheral neuropathy (motor and sensory). Sometimes a blue-tinged line in the gums is visible [1012]. Ataxia has been described [1022]. In severe poisoning, seizures and coma may occur. In mild poisoning, features such as mild cognitive impairment, poor concentration, depression, decreased libido, impotence, reduced fertility, nervousness, and lethargy occur [1021]. Lead poisoning may produce a clinical picture called **plumboporphyria** that mimics aminolaevulinate dehydratase deficiency porphyria (Chapter 10.2 ▶), since lead inhibits this enzyme [1023].

Gastrointestinal symptoms typically occur at blood lead levels of 100–200 μg/dl, but can occur above 40 μg/dl; anaemia typically occurs above 50 μg/dl in adults but children are more sensitive; cramps and joint pains occur above 40 μg/dl; severe lead encephalopathy is usually not seen unless levels are >300 μg/dl, but have sometimes been seen earlier in acute poisoning; mild symptomatic neurotoxicity and neuropsychological deficits have been observed at levels of 40–120 μg/dl after acute and chronic poisoning [1021].

Initial investigations may reveal a microcytic, hypochromic anaemia (which looks like an iron-deficiency pattern; iron deficiency frequently coexists, and ferritin should be measured). Lead can also produce an acute haemolytic anaemia. Basophilic stippling of red blood cells occurs (this should substantially raise the suspicion of lead poisoning), as does reticulocytosis. There may be renal impairment. Serum urate may be elevated. In children, abdominal radiography may reveal radio-opaque foreign bodies (the swallowed source of the lead), and long bone radiography may reveal "lead lines" (growth arrest lines). If measured, urinary porphyrins, coproporphyrins, and ALA are typically elevated, as are blood and plasma ALA and erythrocyte protoporphyrin [26, 1021, 1024].

Diagnosis is by a whole blood lead level. Treatment is by removal from exposure and chelation therapy.

15.6.5 Manganese (Mn) poisoning

Manganism initially presents with a neuropsychiatric syndrome known as locura manganica or "manganese madness". Details presented here are taken from [1025] unless stated. Manganese may have its actions via neurotoxicity to cholinergic systems.

Manganese exposure is usually occupational, from welding, mining, ferromanganese alloy manufacture, and battery manufacturing. Inhalation is probably the main method of exposure. Poisoning has also occurred through exposure to the pesticide maneb (manganese ethylene-bis-dithiocarbamate). High levels of manganese in drinking water have been associated with reduced intellectual function in children. Manganese is an enzyme cofactor and necessary micronutrient; it is therefore an ingredient in total parenteral nutrition formulae, and manganese poisoning via this route has been reported. Methylcyclopentadienyl manganese tricarbonyl (MMT) is an anti-knock compound added to petrol in some countries. The use of intravenous potassium permanganate as part of drug abuse has caused manganism [1026]. Serum manganese levels are also elevated in liver failure and hepatic encephalopathy [1027, 1028], as the liver excretes manganese, and manganese is likely to be responsible for a component of hepatic encephalopathy (Chapter 12.4.2 ▶) [686].

Typically, manganism begins with non-specific symptoms, such as anorexia, lassitude, fatigue, apathy, joint pains, and muscle cramps. This is followed by a psychotic syndrome including disorientation, impaired memory and judgement, acute anxiety, depression, emotional lability, compulsive behaviour, flight of ideas, visual hallucinations, illusions, and delusions. Later, psychomotor slowing and cognitive decline typically evolve. Subsequently, excessive salivation and an extrapyramidal gait disorder resembling Parkinson's disease evolve (often with little response to L-DOPA); this stage indicates irreversible CNS damage [1025, 1029]. The most characteristic gait abnormality (though present in a third of patients or fewer) is the "cock-walk", a dystonia in which patients walk on their metatarsophalangeal joints as if on high heels, sometimes with flexed elbows [20].

Diagnosis requires a high index of suspicion in at-risk groups, and measurement of serum manganese [1030]. Increased T1-weighted signal in the basal ganglia on MRI is supportive, and reflects brain manganese deposition [1028, 1031, 1032]. The disease is treatable with removal from exposure and chelation therapy [1033].

15.6.6 Copper (Cu) poisoning

Copper toxicity in Wilson's disease, which can cause psychosis, is considered above (Chapter 10.4 ▶). Psychosis following acute exogenous copper poisoning appears to be very rare; one case has been described incompletely [1034, 1035]. More typically, acute copper poisoning causes GI symptoms, usually nausea and vomiting [1036]. Chronic copper poisoning may be relatively common through water contaminated by copper piping or vessels, or sometimes through industrial exposure [1037–1039], but psychosis has not been described [1037]. A hypercupric state is diagnosed by showing high serum free copper or elevated copper levels in urine [1038]; exogenous chronic copper poisoning is differentiated from Wilson's disease by the finding of a normal caeruloplasmin and normalization when copper intake ceases [1039]. However, exogenous copper is of relevance in that individuals with Wilson's disease, their relatives, and those with similar copper metabolic abnormalities are more vulnerable to excess exogenous copper [1037].

15.6.7 Aluminium (Al) poisoning

Aluminium poisoning in chronic renal failure, through the use of dialysis fluids containing aluminium, leads to "dialysis dementia". It is a subacute, progressive disease that presents with dysarthria, dysphasia, apraxia, personality change, psychosis, myoclonus, seizures, dementia, and usually death within 6 months [678]. In renal failure, oral intake of aluminium may also contribute to its development [1040].

15.6.8 Bismuth (Bi) poisoning

Bismuth can induce an encephalopathy that includes psychosis [1041]. Poisoning is usually by ingestion, but identical neuropsychiatric features have followed the use of topical bismuth pastes and creams [1041]. Bismuth compounds are used in surgical dressings and in the treatment of gastric and duodenal ulcers. Tripotassium dicitratobismuthate is still used for this, but encephalopathy following ingestion has not been reported; older medications contained significantly higher levels of bismuth [27]. Alloys of bismuth are used in thermoelectric safety appliance manufacture but occupational exposure is rare [1041].

Acute poisoning typically leads to nausea, vomiting, and abdominal pain, followed by nephrotoxicity and neurotoxicity, sometimes after several days; there may be muscle cramps, weakness, blurred vision, hyperreflexia, and transient hepatitis. However, bismuth encephalopathy is more typical of chronic bismuth exposure. There may be an insidious onset of incoordination, paraesthesiae, behavioural change, memory deterioration, insomnia, fatigue, impaired concentration, delusions, hallucinations, and ataxia, progressing to overt encephalopathy with myoclonic jerks, confusion, dysarthria, and sometimes coma and seizures [25, 1041]. There may also be erythematous rashes, renal failure, thrombocytopenia, bone demineralization with spontaneous thoracic vertebral fractures, and paralytic ileus. The encephalopathy usually resolves when exposure ceases [1041]. Bismuth toxicity resembles CJD (Chapter 8.6 ▶).

Diagnosis is by blood bismuth level [1041].

15.6.9 Molybdenum (Mo) poisoning

Frank psychosis as the presenting syndrome has been reported as being due to molybdenum poisoning once, in the context of a dietary supplement [1042]; diagnosis was by blood molybdenum levels.

15.7 Poisoning by other organic and non-metallic substances

In addition to those listed below, see the inhalants in Chapter 15.3 ▶.

15.7.1 Carbon monoxide (CO) poisoning

Carbon monoxide (CO) can cause psychosis either during mild chronic poisoning or as part of the neuropsychiatric sequelae of severe acute poisoning. Carbon monoxide is generated by incomplete combustion of organic compounds. Typically, poisoning – accidental, suicidal, or homicidal – is from vehicle engine exhaust, accidental fires, or inadequately vented domestic gas, wood, or oil fires. Carbon monoxide poisoning causes hypoxia (by binding to haemoglobin) and cardiac depression (by hypoxia and binding to myoglobin) and arrhythmias [1043, 1044].

Mild chronic CO poisoning causes quite non-specific symptoms, which can include psychosis and emotional lability [1043]. When COHb is <10%, individuals are usually asymptomatic. As the CO level rises, symptoms may include a mild then progressive headache, progressive dyspnoea, provocation of existing angina, fatigue, poor judgement, dimness of vision, dizziness, nausea, vomiting, confusion, tachypnoea, tachycardia, syncope, seizures, coma, hypotension, respiratory failure, and death (usually when COHb levels are ~60% and more).

Survivors of severe CO poisoning may be left with neuropsychiatric sequelae including psychosis, personality deterioration (typically with irritability and impulsivity), memory impairment, and emotional lability. Cognitive sequelae occur in ~43% of acute poisoning survivors [1045]. Sometimes the onset of these sequelae is delayed by some days or even weeks after an apparent good initial recovery [1043, 1046]. This may reflect the more general syndrome of **delayed post-anoxic encephalopathy** (Chapter 12.1 ▶) rather than anything specific to carbon monoxide, though carbon monoxide is the most common cause of this condition [1047, 1048].

Diagnosis of active CO poisoning is by measurement of arterial COHb. The normal range is <2% in non-smokers and 5–13% in smokers [1044]. Symptoms typically begin to occur when the COHb level rises above 10% [1043], though there is wide variation in individual responses to similar levels of CO exposure [1044]. In chronic CO poisoning, the CO level may be normal if measured after some time spent outside the contaminated environment [1043], as CO is rapidly exhaled and the half-life of COHb is 4–5 hours [1044]. Environmental measurement may be required. Treatment is required as an emergency as soon as CO poisoning is suspected, with removal from exposure, immediate 100% oxygen, ventilation and intensive care support as required, and consideration of hyperbaric oxygen. Subsequent EEG abnormalities in survivors are common and have some relationship to the degree of encephalopathy [1043].

15.7.2 Poisoning by other organic compounds

Bromomethane (methyl bromide) is an odourless gaseous pesticide (also occasionally used as a refrigerant and fire extinguisher) that can cause psychosis as part of its acute neurotoxic effects, typically after inhalation [33, 1049], though rarely as the presenting feature [1050]. More commonly, it produces headaches, dizziness, nausea, vomiting, confusion, weakness, and visual disturbances; these are sometimes followed by mania, ataxia, tremor, seizures, paralysis, and coma. Inhalation usually causes pneumonitis [1049]. For inorganic bromide poisoning, see bromide (Chapter 15.1 ▶). Methyl bromide is toxic at lower levels than inorganic bromide.

Carbon disulphide (CS_2; carbon disulfide) is a liquid with a sweet odour used primarily in viscose rayon and cellophane manufacture. It is a neurotoxin and can cause psychosis with hallucinations at very high doses, usually at the severe end of an obvious poisoning syndrome [1051, 1052], but sometimes in isolation [25, 33, 1053].

Chlorinated insecticide poisoning. Endosulfan is a manufactured organochlorine insecticide. Acute exposure usually produces hyperactivity, tremors, hypoventilation, dyspnoea, salivation, and convulsions; psychosis has also been described [1054]. Other organochlorine pesticides that have produced hallucinations include hexachlorocyclohexane [1055] and chlordecone [1056].

Chlorphenoxy herbicides typically cause poisoning by ingestion. Acute exposure usually produces vomiting, abdominal pain, and diarrhoea, sometimes with GI bleeding. Cardiorespiratory features typically include hypoventilation (sometimes hyperventilation), and sometimes hypotension. Neurological features include hypertonia, hyperreflexia or hyporeflexia, fasciculation, ataxia, nystagmus, miosis, hallucinations, convulsions, coma, and paralysis. Other features have included fever, metabolic acidosis, rhabdomyolysis, renal failure, and deranged LFTs [1057].

Cyanide (–CN) may be encountered as gaseous hydrogen cyanide or as solid or dissolved cyanide salts (e.g. sodium or potassium cyanide); all have a faint almond odour. They occur naturally (e.g. in rotten fish) and are manufactured and used industrially in electroplating, metallurgy, organic chemical manufacture, fumigation, and some mining processes. Cyanide has been used homicidally. It is extremely toxic when consumed or inhaled, causing cellular hypoxia by inhibiting mitochondrial respiration, with subsequent neurological failure leading to apnoea and further hypoxia. Typically, acute poisoning causes rapid, deep breathing and dyspnoea followed by loss of consciousness (often with a scream) and seizures. Chronic exposure can cause neurological effects including headaches, weakness, changes in taste and smell, dizziness, paraesthesia, hallucinations, and paranoid psychosis [1058]. Hallucinations have also been reported as part of a cyanide poisoning syndrome following dermal acrylonitrile exposure [1059].

Ethylene glycol is a sweet-tasting antifreeze that is a relatively common cause of intentional and accidental poisoning. Poisoning causes severe metabolic acidosis, with a high serum anion gap (calculated as $[Na^+] + [K^+] - [Cl^-] - [HCO_3^-]$) and osmolar gap (measured serum osmolarity minus the osmolarity calculated as $2 \times [Na^+]$ + [glucose] + [urea]). Early on, the patient is likely to appear intoxicated but the absence of a smell of alcohol should raise suspicion. Typically, the initial phase involves neurological symptoms, worst 6–12 hours after ingestion (hallucinations, stupor, coma); subsequently, there is cardiac failure and sometimes respiratory compromise; next, there is acute tubular necrosis with renal failure (apparent 24–72 hours after ingestion). There is often hypocalcaemia. The urine may fluoresce and oxalate crystals may be seen microscopically within it, though these may take some hours to develop. There are also methods for direct detection. Early recognition is vital [1060–1062].

Hydrogen sulphide (H_2S) is a gas produced naturally (from volcanoes and other sulphurous sources) and in many industrial applications; it smells of rotten eggs. Psychosis with hallucinations has been reported as a consequence of high-dose H_2S exposure, and a long-term sequela of near-fatal H_2S poisoning, though the latter effect may be confounded with that of hypoxic brain damage [1063].

Methanol (methyl alcohol, wood alcohol) is used as a solvent and in antifreeze and may be consumed as a contaminant of home-distilled ethanol. It is oxidized to formaldehyde and formic acid, producing acidosis with a raised osmolar gap. Symptoms of poisoning may not develop for 12–48 hours after consumption, and may last for several days. Systemic features of poisoning include nausea, vomiting, weakness, abdominal pain, and in severe cases death from respiratory failure. Neurological features include headache, weakness, vertigo, incoordination, delirium, hallucinations, visual loss, stupor, parkinsonism, and seizures [28].

Methyltin has been reported to produce "psychotic behaviour" in acute intoxication [1064]; details were not given. This series resulted from accidental exposure in a plastics factory where dimethyltin chloride and trimethyltin chloride were being used in the production of polyvinyl chloride. Organic tin compounds are much more toxic than inorganic tin compounds. After a latent period of 1–3 days, symptoms included headache, tinnitus, deafness, memory impairment, disorientation, aggression, psychosis, syncope, coma, and in severe cases ventilatory failure. Leukocytosis, hypokalaemia, abnormal LFTs, and frontotemporal EEG abnormalities were common [1064]. Other organic tin compounds are also neurotoxic [20]. Diagnosis is by urinary tin levels [1064].

N,N-diethyl m-toluamide (DEET) is the most widely used insect repellent worldwide. It has a very low probability of serious toxicity. However, psychosis with hallucinations or delusions has been described in extremely rare cases following dermal application [1065–1067].

Organophosphates are used as insecticides (e.g. malathion), chemical warfare agents (e.g. sarin, VX), in ophthalmology, and as antihelminthics. They may be absorbed by ingestion, inhalation, or skin contact. They inhibit enzymes including acetylcholinesterase, leading to cholinergic toxicity, both muscarinic and nicotinic. The muscarinic effects include salivation, lacrimation, urination, diarrhoea, vomiting, diaphoresis, miosis, bradycardia, bronchospasm, and bronchorrhoea. Nicotinic effects include fasciculations, cramps, weakness, respiratory failure, hypertension, tachycardia, mydriasis, and pallor. CNS effects may include anxiety, emotional lability, restlessness, confusion, ataxia, tremors, seizures, and coma [1068]. Both acute and chronic exposure has been reported to cause psychosis [25, 1068, 1069]. Diagnosis is clinical but can be confirmed with measurement of red cell cholinesterase (or plasma pseudocholinesterase) activity, or toxicological studies.

Toluene is a colourless liquid with a distinctive smell used industrially as a solvent (e.g. in petrol, paint, paint thinner, nail polish, glue, and rubber). It may be sniffed recreationally (Chapter 15.3 ▶). High-dose industrial exposure and chronic sniffing at doses leading to narcosis and euphoria have caused permanent or recurrent paranoid or hallucinatory psychosis, in addition to diverse other neurological effects, including ataxia, tremor, epilepsy, nystagmus, cerebral atrophy, speech impairment, and sensory impairment [1070]. It may be detected by increased hippuric acid levels in urine [29]. Toluene produces a leukoencephalopathy [33].

Trichloroethylene is a liquid solvent used mainly as an industrial degreaser, but also in other solvents such as paint remover. Typical neurological effects of exposure are headache, mild or severe drowsiness, and impaired coordination – indeed, it has been used as a surgical anaesthetic – but psychosis has occasionally been reported [1071].

Vitamin A has very occasionally been reported to cause psychosis in acute intoxication [1072–1074]. Acute toxicity usually results from overconsumption of pharmaceutical vitamin A and related retinoid products, or of animal livers rich in vitamin A, such as polar bear and seal liver [1074, 1075]. There is muscle and bone tenderness, especially over the long limb bones, and neurological manifestations (drowsiness, lethargy, somnolence, irritability, headache, vomiting) with increased intracranial pressure. Sometimes there is desquamation [1075, 1076].

White phosphorus is a flammable substance used industrially in the manufacture of phosphoric acid and related compounds, militarily in smoke grenades, and as poisons. Neurological effects of ingestion have included lethargy, irritability, hyperaesthesia, fasciculations, tremor, delirium, psychosis, and coma [1077].

Chapter 16 Sleep disorders

Normal sleep-related hallucinations. Hallucinations upon falling asleep (hypnagogic hallucinations) are normal and common. Also normal, but less common, are hallucinations on waking (hypnopompic hallucinations). These hallucinations may occur in multiple modalities and may have emotional overtones, and can be extremely vivid and bizarre (including conversations with other people or beings); they may be combined with sleep paralysis, and may be taken for a psychotic illness [1078]. Usually they are short-lived (seconds to minutes) [212]. Hypnagogic hallucinations occurred in 24.8% of people in one large sample, and hypnopompic hallucinations in 6.6% [1079].

Night terrors. Night terrors are most common in children aged 3–12, with a median age of onset of 3.5 years, and they affect 1–6% of all children. The onset is during the transition from stage 3 to stage 4 non-REM sleep. The patient arises approximately 90 minutes after falling asleep, in terror with marked autonomic activation and crying or screaming, and may appear to be actively hallucinating. The episode usually lasts 1–2 minutes, but can last up to 30 minutes. There is usually complete amnesia for the episode, and if the child wakes during the night terror they typically do not recall dreams. Diagnosis is usually by history; occasionally nocturnal seizures or sleep apnoea enter the differential [1080].

Sleep deprivation. There are several case reports of psychosis requiring psychiatric treatment apparently induced by severe sleep deprivation [29, 1081], and perceptual distortions and hallucinations can be induced experimentally by sleep deprivation, showing a linearly increasing tendency plus a circadian component [1082].

Sleep apnoea and obesity hypoventilation. There is an association between diagnoses of sleep apnoea and psychosis [1083]. On one occasion, "hebephrenic schizophrenia" with auditory hallucinations was reversed with successful treatment of obesity hypoventilation (Pickwickian syndrome) [1084]. Hypnagogic hallucinations may also feature [33]. Breathing disorders during sleep are common, with sleep-disordered breathing of some form occurring in 4% of women and 9% of men, and sleep apnoea in about 2% of women and 4% of men. Sleep apnoea is usually obstructive in nature, though sometimes central. Obstructive sleep apnoea (OSA) is more common in the obese. It is suggested by loud snoring, witnessed apnoea, waking breathless at night, poor sleep, excessive daytime somnolence (with associated cognitive and attentional impairment), and, if severe, morning headaches (due to nocturnal hypercapnia). Obesity hypoventilation (OH) is defined as a BMI of >30 with sleep-disordered breathing and chronic daytime hypercapnia; its pathophysiology is multifactorial. Ninety percent of patients with OH also have OSA. The screening test for OSA is overnight sleep oximetry, with polysomnography in difficult cases and arterial blood gas measurement if hypercapnia is suspected [1078, 1085, 1086].

Narcolepsy. Narcolepsy (also called narcolepsy–cataplexy syndrome) is not uncommon, with a prevalence of 2–5:10 000. Its cardinal features are excessive daytime sleepiness, cataplexy, hypnagogic/hypnopompic hallucinations, and sleep paralysis. It results from REM sleep intrusion into wakefulness. It is strongly associated with HLA type (especially DR2 and DQB1*0602; MIM 161400) [1088]. It may be due to loss of orexin (hypocretin) neurons in the hypothalamus. A few cases are due to lesions of the pons or midbrain [212]. Frequent hypnagogic hallucinations occur in up to 50% of patients [33]. In addition to the possibility of misdiagnosing the psychotic form of narcolepsy, in which hallucinations are prominent (and they may persist beyond the sleep attack for many hours), the psychostimulants used to treat narcolepsy may induce psychosis (e.g. amphetamine, methylphenidate, modafinil; see Chapter 15.1, Chapter 15.3 ▶). There is no good evidence of an association between narcolepsy and schizophrenia [1087]. Diagnosis is by polysomnography and multiple sleep latency testing [1078, 1088].

Kleine–Levin syndrome. This rare syndrome begins in adolescence and is characterized by recurrent episodes of hypersomnia, lasting days to weeks, and occurring several times a year for up to 8 years. Sleep is normal in between these episodes. During the episodes, in addition to hypersomnia, patients may develop cognitive changes (96%, usually including derealization and sometimes confusion), compulsive overeating (80%), hypersexuality (43%), compulsions (29%), depressed mood (48%), hallucinations (e.g. hypnagogic), irritability, and behavioural changes including impulsivity. The syndrome may be precipitated by infections (38%), head trauma (9%), and alcohol (5%) [33, 1089].

Sleep disorders in intensive care. Hallucinations and delusions can be prominent and are common in patients with **Guillain–Barré syndrome (acute inflammatory demyelinating polyradiculoneuropathy)** on intensive care units [1090], and this appears to be a REM intrusion disorder (**status dissociatus**, an admixture of polysomnographically identified REM sleep, non-REM sleep, and wakefulness), distinct from "ICU [intensive care unit] delirium" and present in non-confused patients.

Fatal familial insomnia is discussed above (Chapter 8.6 ▶).

Other parasomnias. Other parasomnias have also been misdiagnosed as psychiatric disease. These include **sleepwalking** (in which motor behaviour can be very complex), **confusional arousals** and **sleep terrors**, **REM sleep behaviour disorder** (in which REM sleep paralysis is lost and dreams are acted out), and **nocturnal seizures** including nocturnal frontal/temporal lobe epilepsy (Chapter 6.2 ▶). Diagnosis is by a good sleep history, followed if necessary by investigation in a sleep laboratory [28, 1078].

Sleep disruption in psychiatric disorders. In addition, schizophrenia is associated with disturbed sleep architecture, particularly reduced REM sleep latency, which correlates with positive psychotic symptoms and may be related to increased dopaminergic tone [1091, 1092]. Acute psychosis, mood disorders, anxiety disorders, and alcoholism are other important causes of sleep disturbance [28].

Chapter 17 Sensory deprivation and impairment

Visual and auditory sensory impairment is associated with hallucinations. Being blindfolded is sufficient to induce visual hallucinations in 77% of subjects within 5 days, and mostly within 1 day [1093]. Visual hallucinations may occur after visual degeneration, and auditory hallucinations after deafness [213, 1094, 1095] (see also Chapter 6.1 ▶). Visual hallucinations in late paraphrenia (see Chapter 21.17 ▶) are associated with visual impairment [1096], and idiopathic musical hallucinations in the elderly are seen particularly in deaf females, many of whom are depressed [1097, 1098]. Complex auditory hallucinations have been associated with injury to superior temporal auditory association cortex [28]. Psychosis has been described in **Usher syndrome**, a congenital condition that causes retinitis pigmentosa, blindness, and deafness [1099]; in one series, psychosis occurred in ~25% (MIM 276900).

Amputations are frequently followed by phantom somatic sensations [15].

Charles Bonnet syndrome (complex visual hallucinosis) is characterized by complex visual hallucinations occurring in the context of visual deterioration, most commonly macular degeneration. It occurs in ~11% of those with severe visual loss, generally in the elderly. The hallucinations may be vivid and last for hours; there is usually good insight. The pathology is most commonly ocular but Charles Bonnet syndrome has also occurred following lesions of the optic chiasm, optic radiation, and occipital cortex [212, 1100, 1101]; see also [17]. Its diagnostic criteria are (1) complex, persistent, or repetitive visual hallucinations (typical operational criteria: at least one complex visual hallucination within the last 4 weeks and >4 weeks between the first and the last hallucination); (2) full or partial insight into the unreal nature of the hallucinations; (3) absence of hallucinations in other modalities; (4) absence of delusions. Commonly (in 67% of patients) the hallucinations disappear on eye closure [1100].

Solitary confinement has been reported to cause hyperresponsivity to external stimuli, perceptual distortions, hallucinations, derealization, affective disturbances, ideas of reference, and paranoia, with a rapid diminution of symptoms upon release [1102].

Deliberate **sensory deprivation** can produce psychotic symptoms during the period of deprivation, as well as severe discomfort and anxiety [1103–1107]. It has been used as an interrogation technique [1108].

Chapter 18 Miscellaneous

18.1 Coeliac disease

Coeliac disease (gluten-sensitive enteropathy) is an inflammatory disease of the small intestine induced by cereal products, namely gliadin in wheat, hordein in barley, and secalin in rye. Gliadin is the alcohol-soluble glycoprotein component of gluten, the predominant protein in wheat seed. There is a variable inflammatory phenotype in the small intestine. It is predominantly a disease of Caucasians, in whom the prevalence is 1:300. Most affected individuals possess HLA DQ2 or HLA DQ8.

The association between coeliac disease and neurological symptoms is unclear. Neurological features occur in about 10% of patients with coeliac disease and there is a high frequency of gluten sensitivity (as indexed by antibody testing) in patients with unexplained neurological dysfunction, particularly cerebellar ataxia [1109]. This "gluten ataxia" may be due to a direct cross-reactivity of antigliadin antibodies with cerebellar Purkinje cells, though some antibodies associated with cerebellar ataxia (e.g. anti-GAD) are also markers of multiple autoimmunity [862].

Coeliac disease has been associated with an increased risk of psychosis in some but by no means all large-scale population studies [1110–1113], and immunological markers for coeliac disease (antigliadin, antitransglutaminase, and antiendomysial antibodies) have been associated with schizophrenia [1114]. There have been some studies showing an improvement in psychotic symptoms in schizophrenia following introduction of a gluten-free diet [1115], and various mechanisms have been suggested, including altered gut permeability [1116], altered cytokine expression, and the observation that genetic susceptibility regions for coeliac disease overlap with susceptibility regions for schizophrenia [1115].

Coeliac disease can cause growth retardation in children and adolescents. In adults, the most common presentations are anaemia (usually iron deficient, but sometimes with B_{12} and folate deficiencies if severe) and variable symptoms of discomfort, bloating, excess flatulence, altered bowel habit, mouth ulcers, weight loss, and sometimes steatorrhoea and nutritional deficiencies resulting from malabsorption. Dermatitis herpetiformis is associated with subclinical coeliac disease. Often, coeliac disease is subtle, and diagnosis requires a high index of suspicion. As described above, CNS manifestations apparently unrelated to deficiency states occur in ~10% of patients. It is associated with other autoimmune diseases [26].

Definitive diagnosis is by duodenal or jejunal biopsy. The most useful screening test is to measure antiendomysial (anti-tissue transglutaminase) antibodies; these have a sensitivity any time [1134]. It typically progresses over 24–72 hours [929]. Other causes or risk factors include schizophrenia, mania, delirium, dementia, agitation, dehydration, thyrotoxicosis, phaeochromocytoma, alcohol abuse, liver disease, hypocalcaemia, encephalitis (possibly), a prior history of MC/NMS or of another movement disorder (including basal ganglia disease and drug-induced extrapyramidal side effects), and high doses and rapid dose increases of neuroleptic drugs [5, 31, 1345].

Serotonin syndrome (Chapter 15.2 ▶) has also been argued to be a malignant catatonic disorder [31].

19.3 Other catatonic syndromes

This area is replete with synonyms and the reader is referred to Fink & Taylor [31] for a full description.

Retarded catatonia, with the primary feature of retardation and stupor is sometimes termed **Kahlbaum syndrome** or **benign stupor**.

Excited catatonia, with prominent excitement and agitation, has been called **delirious mania, manic delirium, catatonic excitement**, and **Bell's mania**. When the predominant feature of excited catatonia is a dreamy, stuporous state, the terms **onirisme, oneiroid state, oneirophrenia**, and **oneiroid syndrome** are sometimes used; others consider these variants of delirious mania.

Mixed affective states in the context of rapid-cycling bipolar affective disorder may overlap with catatonia, but the evidence base is limited.

Periodic catatonia (a.k.a. **Gjessing's periodic catatonia**), in which catatonia alternates with normalcy, has been described as a syndrome. It is sometimes considered a form of **cycloid psychosis** (Chapter 21.8 ▶), and sometimes distinguished from insidiously progressive or "systematic" catatonia [31]. The overlap of the historical descriptions of periodic catatonia with conditions such as bipolar affective disorder and seizure disorders is unclear [31]. Susceptibility loci for periodic catatonia have been found on chromosomes 15q15 (MIM 605419) and perhaps 22q13.

Akinetic mutism (a.k.a. **apallic syndrome, coma vigil**) describes the syndrome, typically of acute onset, characterized by immobility, rigidity, and inability to move voluntarily except for eye movements. Identified neurological causes include brainstem (particularly pontine) lesions (e.g. **locked-in syndrome**), **stiff person syndrome** (a syndrome of progressive symmetrical rigidity of axial musculature with superimposed muscle spasms triggered by a variety of stimuli), encephalitis, orbitofrontal or cingulate cortex damage (including tumours and anterior cerebral artery lesions), lesions of the caudal hypothalamus, and tumours of the third ventricle. If none is found, then the diagnosis of **primary akinetic mutism**, a form of primary catatonia, should be considered.

19.4 Mimics and causes of catatonia

Catatonia must be distinguished from elective mutism, isolated stupor (induced e.g. by depression, metabolic disorders, sedatives, epilepsy, encephalitis, and midbrain/pontine lesions), psychomotor slowing in advanced dementia and hypoactive delirium, Parkinson's disease and related syndromes, obsessive–compulsive disorder, malignant hyperthermia, locked-in syndrome (after pontine lesions), and stiff-person syndrome (see Chapter 19.3 ▶ above) [22, 31]. Parkinson's disease with superimposed infection is a key differential of NMS. Aside from the clinical features, the EEG is usually normal in catatonic stupor [31].

The differential diagnosis of catatonia includes the following (see individual descriptions for many ▶):

Autoimmune disease including SLE, antiphospholipid syndrome, paraneoplastic limbic encephalopathy, cerebral vasculitides, and TTP [20, 31, 765].

Developmental and childhood disorders: autism, Prader–Willi syndrome, schizencephaly, some mental retardation syndromes [15, 31, 427].

Environmental: heat stroke [31].

Epilepsy: postictal states, complex partial seizures, and convulsive or non-convulsive status epilepticus [31], interictal psychosis, and perhaps psychosis of forced normalization [20].

Focal brain injury: brain trauma, frontal/temporal brain lesions (e.g. stroke, tumour, haematoma, multiple sclerosis); also reported after cerebellar, pontine, pallidal, thalamic, parietal, and periventricular lesions, familial cerebellopontine atrophy, and dementias predominantly affecting white matter. Stupor may follow brainstem lesions. Akinetic mutism may follow intraventricular tumours of the third ventricle compressing the diencephalon, direct hypothalamic damage, obstructive hydrocephalus, and anterior cingulate cortex damage. Mutism may of course follow stroke [20, 31].

Infection including AIDS dementia, CJD, FFI, infectious mononucleosis, malaria, viral encephalitis (particularly herpesviruses) and encephalitis lethargica, American trypanosomiasis (Chagas' encephalitis), neuroborreliosis (Lyme disease), malaria, PML, SSPE, syphilis, tuberculosis, and typhoid [31, 427, 458].

Malignancy including Langerhans cell histiocytosis, and paraneoplastic limbic encephalopathy [31].

Metabolic disease including acute porphyria, Addison's disease/adrenal failure, Cushing's syndrome, diabetic ketoacidosis, hepatic encephalopathy, homocystinuria, hypercalcaemia, hyperthyroidism, hyponatraemia, hypopituitarism, pellagra, renal failure, SIADH, Tay–Sachs disease, vitamin B_{12} deficiency, Wernicke–Korsakoff encephalopathy, and Wilson's disease [31, 427].

Neurodegenerative diseases including CBGD, DRPLA, and HD [427].

Parkinsonism, e.g. acute parkinsonism triggered by withdrawal of treatment for Parkinson's disease, and postencephalitic parkinsonism [31].

Pharmaceutical drug triggers of catatonia (including MC/NMS) include antipsychotics and dopamine receptor antagonists of all types (particularly high potency agents at high dose); antidepressant/antipsychotic combinations; anticholinergics; antihistamines; aspirin (in overdose); azithromycin; beta blockers; carbamazepine; ciprofloxacin; corticosteroids; cyclobenzaprine; disulfiram (the catatonia may appear up to months after administration); dopamine-depleting agents (e.g. reserpine, tetrabenazine); immunosuppressants; ketamine; levetiracetam; lithium toxicity and lithium/phenelzine combinations; MAOIs (and their combination with tricyclic antidepressants, SSRIs, and meperidine); opioids (in overdose); phenelzine/dosulepin combinations; metoclopramide; sibutramine; triptans; and valproate. *Akinetic mutism* has been triggered by cyclosporin and by the combination of whole-body irradiation and amphotericin B. *Withdrawal* of the following can trigger catatonia: anticholinergics; antihistamines; antipsychotic drugs;

benzodiazepines; dopaminergic agents (levodopa, amantadine, bromocriptine); and gabapentin [5, 20, 22, 31, 38, 427].

Poisoning: tetanus, strychnine, organic fluorides, salicylates, inhalational anaesthetics triggering malignant hyperthermia, carbon monoxide, lead [31, 427].

Primary psychiatric disease: mania, depression, schizophrenia; serine- and glycine-evoked psychosis; rarely Ganser's syndrome [31, 1124].

Recreational drug triggers include amphetamine, cocaine, ketamine, mescaline, opiates, MDMA, phencyclidine, and psilocybin [22, 31].

Other: narcolepsy, tuberous sclerosis [31].

Chapter 20 Agitation and bizarre behaviour

Agitated and bizarre behaviour can be very hard to assess, and the differential diagnosis is extremely wide, particularly if the patient cannot communicate clearly. Obviously, it does not of itself indicate psychiatric disease. It is important to exclude *pain and discomfort*, and other forms of *distress* with an inability to communicate, in addition to *delirium* (Chapter 3 ▶) and *catatonia* (Chapter 19 ▶). Psychotic hallucinations and/or delusions may cause agitation, as may mania. Chronic, sometimes episodic, abnormal behaviour is seen in a variety of mental retardation syndromes, whose differential diagnosis is covered elsewhere [22].

Chapter 21

Primary psychiatric disease

What follows is a set of disorders whose biological aetiology is not fully understood and for which no biological diagnostic tests presently exist. Diagnostic criteria for the primary psychiatric diseases presuppose that secondary causes have been excluded [4]. We refer the reader to other sources for consideration of the epidemiology and neurobiology of the diseases considered here [15, 22, 1135]. Reflecting the lack of aetiological knowledge, diagnosis using the ICD-10 classification is fuzzy, in that it recognizes that syndromes may be diagnosed that "confidently", "provisionally", or "tentatively" fulfil ICD-10 diagnostic criteria, and the wording of the clinical criteria is deliberately non-committal in places [4]. The corresponding research criteria (DCR-10) are necessarily precise and more restrictive [10]. In what follows, diseases will be referred to parenthetically by their ICD-10 codes. In general, disease categories are similar in DSM-IV-TR [5], though not identical.

21.1 Schizophrenia (F20)

Schizophrenia is the archetypal primary psychosis. No symptoms are pathognomonic, but ICD-10 groups the symptoms of schizophrenia into the following categories [4, verbatim]:

(a) thought echo, thought insertion or withdrawal, and thought broadcasting;
(b) delusions of control, influence, or passivity, clearly referred to body or limb movements or specific thoughts, actions, or sensations; delusional perception;
(c) hallucinatory voices giving a running commentary on the patient's behaviour, or discussing the patient among themselves, or other types of hallucinatory voices coming from some part of the body;
(d) persistent delusions of other kinds that are culturally inappropriate and completely impossible, such as religious or political identity, or superhuman powers and abilities (e.g. being able to control the weather, or being in communication with aliens from another world);
(e) persistent hallucinations in any modality, when accompanied either by fleeting or half-formed delusions without clear affective content, or by persistent over-valued ideas, or when occurring every day for weeks or months on end;
(f) breaks or interpolations in the train of thought, resulting in incoherence or irrelevant speech, or neologisms;
(g) catatonic behaviour, such as excitement, posturing, or waxy flexibility, negativism, mutism, and stupor;
(h) "negative" symptoms such as marked apathy, paucity of speech, and blunting or incongruity of emotional responses, usually resulting in social withdrawal and lowering

of social performance; it must be clear that these are not due to depression or to neuroleptic medication;

(i) a significant and consistent change in the overall quality of some aspects of personal behaviour, manifest as loss of interest, aimlessness, idleness, a self-absorbed attitude, and social withdrawal.

"Negative" symptoms of schizophrenia (deficits) are so named in contrast to "positive" symptoms (symptoms that are not present in the normal state).

Schizophrenia is diagnosed clinically if, in the absence of an identifiable cause for psychosis or "negative" symptoms, at least one very clear symptom (and usually two or more if less clear-cut) belonging to groups (a) to (d), or symptoms from at least two of groups (e) to (h), are present for most of the time during a period of ≥1 month. If these symptoms have been present for less than a month, acute schizophrenia-like psychotic disorder (F23.2; Chapter 21.8 ▶) is diagnosed, to be reclassified as schizophrenia if symptoms persist.

Retrospectively, a non-psychotic prodrome (such as loss of interest in work, social activities, and personal appearance and hygiene, generalized anxiety, mild depression, and preoccupation) may have preceded the onset of psychotic symptoms by weeks or months, but the assessment of prodromes is subject to recall bias effects.

Symptom (i) is characteristic of simple schizophrenia (F20.6), which is diagnosed if symptom (i) is present for at least a year with "negative" symptoms and a marked decline in social, scholastic, or occupational performance.

If mood symptoms (depression or mania) predominate and predated the psychosis, schizophrenia is not diagnosed (the diagnosis likely being a form of psychotic depression [Chapter 21.3 ▶] or manic psychosis [Chapter 21.2 ▶]). If schizophrenic symptoms clearly predated mood symptoms, schizophrenia can be diagnosed. If affective symptoms develop simultaneously with schizophrenia symptoms and there is no clear dominance, schizoaffective disorder (F25; Chapter 21.4 ▶) is diagnosed.

Schizophrenia may be further classified. Subtypes of schizophrenia recognized in ICD-10 [1136] are:

- **paranoid schizophrenia** (F20.0), the most common subtype, diagnosed in the presence of schizophrenia dominated by delusions or hallucinations, but not markedly flattened or incongruous affect, catatonia, or incoherent speech;
- **hebephrenic schizophrenia** (F20.1), known in DSM-IV [5] as disorganized schizophrenia, in which schizophrenia is dominated by affective changes (shallow, flat, incongruous, or inappropriate affect) and either pronounced thought disorder or aimless, disjointed behaviour is present, while hallucinations and delusions are not prominent;
- **catatonic schizophrenia** (F20.2), in which psychomotor disturbances dominate (such as stupor, mutism, excitement, posturing, negativism, rigidity, waxy flexibility, command automatisms, or verbal perseveration);
- **undifferentiated schizophrenia** (F20.3), in which schizophrenia is present with active psychosis but which do not fit any, or fit more than one, of the preceding three types;
- **post-schizophrenic depression** (F20.4), in which a depressive episode has developed for at least 2 weeks following a schizophrenic episode within the last 12 months and in which schizophrenic symptoms persist but are not as prominent as the depression;

- **residual schizophrenia** (F20.5), in which previous psychotic episodes of schizophrenia have given way to a chronic condition with "negative" symptoms of schizophrenia as described above;
- **simple schizophrenia** (F20.6), described above, in which "negative" symptoms develop for at least one year without any psychotic episodes;
- **other schizophrenia** (F20.8). This category includes **cenesthopathic schizophrenia** (F20.8), in which body image aberration (such as desomatization, loss of bodily boundaries, or feelings of body size change) or abnormal bodily sensations (such as numbness, stiffness, feeling strange, depersonalization, or sensations of pain, temperature, electricity, heaviness, lightness, or discomfort when touched) dominate [1137]; it also includes **"schizophreniform disorder or psychosis, not otherwise specified"**, which has no specific diagnostic criteria [4, 10].

The DSM-IV criteria for schizophrenia and its subtypes of schizophrenia (**paranoid, disorganized, catatonic, undifferentiated, residual**) [5] differ slightly from the ICD-10 criteria, and are shown in Section 2. Of note, DSM-IV requires the overall disturbance to last 6 months (with one month of "active phase" symptoms, unless these are successfully treated), with a slightly different definition of core symptoms of schizophrenia. Psychosis that otherwise meets the criteria for schizophrenia but has lasted less than 6 months is termed **schizophreniform disorder** by DSM-IV.

Schizophrenia has a lifetime prevalence of approximately 0.55% [1138]. It usually begins in the age range 15–35 [1139]. Following a prodrome, there is typically a relapsing course of psychotic episodes, often with additional cognitive impairment. It is the cognitive impairment and negative symptoms that more strongly predict poor functional outcome [17, 1140–1142]. Estimates of the frequency of hallucinations in schizophrenia range from 47–98% for auditory hallucinations, 14–69% for visual hallucinations, and 4–25% for tactile hallucinations, with estimates of 17–34.6% for olfactory hallucinations and 12% for gustatory hallucinations [17, 663].

There is considerable evidence that neurodevelopmental abnormalities predispose to schizophrenia. Risk factors for schizophrenia, in addition to familial and sociodemographic factors, include complications of pregnancy (bleeding, pre-eclampsia, diabetes, rhesus incompatibility), infections during pregnancy (including influenza, rubella, and respiratory infections), severe adverse maternal life events in the first trimester, maternal malnutrition, abnormal fetal growth and development (low birth weight, congenital malformations, small head circumference, rhesus incompatibility), complications of delivery (asphyxia, uterine atony, emergency Caesarean section), and subsequent abnormalities in childhood (early developmental delay in speech or motor function, impaired social and cognitive development). Childhood meningitis and tuberculosis may also predispose to adult schizophrenia. Schizophrenia is associated with changes in macroscopic brain morphology (grey matter volume loss without gliosis) and microscopic brain morphology (abnormalities in neuronal size, arborization, synaptic organization, and glia). It is also associated with minor physical abnormalities, such as constant exotropia (divergent strabismus). The point prevalence of schizophrenia in those with mild learning disability is raised at 3%, in comparison with about 1% in the general population (as above). Animal models have demonstrated that very early insults can have substantially delayed behavioural effects; for example, neonatal hippocampal lesions or perinatal DISC1 knockdown can have behavioural effects manifesting after puberty [17, 22, 29, 33, 326, 1143–1150].

A large number of schizophrenia susceptibility genes have been described, including COMT, DTNBP1 (dysbindin), NRG1 (neuregulin-1), RGS4 (regulator of G-protein signalling 4), DISC1 (disrupted in schizophrenia-1), G72, and others [17, 22, 29, 1146, 1147, 1151] (MIM 181500). It has been suggested that susceptibility genes fall into two broad classes: genes affecting associative learning, particularly via NMDA receptor functioning, and genes affecting mesolimbic dopamine functioning, and that their effect on the development of psychosis is interactive [1152]. The total burden of individually rare genetic structural variants (microdeletions and microduplications) is substantially increased in schizophrenia, and these variants disproportionately affect genes involved in neurodevelopmental pathways [1153].

The neurological examination may be abnormal in schizophrenia, with a proportion of patients showing exaggerated or diminished tendon reflexes, reduced gag reflex, and occasionally anisocoria, diminished corneal reflexes, hyposmia, mild abnormalities of saccadic or pursuit eye movements, mildly increased muscle tone, mild decreases in sensory acuity, and mild cerebellar signs. However, any focal neurological abnormality raises the probability of a secondary psychosis [see 17]. In addition, neurological "soft" signs (meaning signs that are less reliable at localizing a discrete brain lesion, and including abnormalities of sensory integration, motor coordination, and sequencing of complex motor acts) [1154, 1155] are present in excess in schizophrenia [1156].

21.2 Manic psychosis (psychotic mania)

Affective disorders are common causes of psychosis, and psychosis is associated with the more severe forms of both mania and depression (by definition in ICD-10 diagnostic criteria; [4]). Affective psychoses are diagnosed when the mood disorder precedes the psychotic symptoms. Manic symptoms are classified in ICD-10 by severity, from hypomania to mania to mania with psychosis [4]. Full diagnostic criteria are given in Section 2 (Chapter 28.2 ▶).

Hypomania is marked by a persistent mild elevation of mood for days, increased energy and activity, feelings of well-being and physical and mental efficiency, increased sociability, mild overspending, talkativeness, overfamiliarity, increased sexual energy, and decreased sleep, sometimes with impaired concentration and attention. Irritability, conceit, and boorishness may be present instead of euphoric sociability [4]. Hallucinations and delusions are absent.

Mania (without psychosis) is a more severe form, in which symptoms are severely disruptive to ordinary work and social activities. Mood is elevated out of keeping with the patient's circumstances, with elation, overactivity, pressure of speech, increased energy, decreased sleep, social disinhibition, poor attention, distractibility, inflated self-esteem, and grandiosity or over-optimism. Perception may be vivid (for example, sounds may seem louder, colours brighter, or textures more marked), but psychotic symptoms are absent. Sometimes the mood in mania is irritable and suspicious, rather than elated. Patients may embark on elaborate and impractical schemes, and may be aggressive, amorous, or facetious inappropriately as their mood dictates [4].

In manic psychosis, mania is severe. Inflated self-esteem and grandiose ideas develop into delusions, and irritability and suspiciousness become delusions of persecution. Hallucinations and delusions may be mood-congruent (i.e. affectively positive) or incongruent (neutral or negative), and may include Schneiderian first-rank symptoms [1157]. Clearly, it may be difficult to distinguish manic psychosis from schizophrenia (Chapter 21.1 ▶) when seen at a severe stage. There is an excess of neurological "soft" signs (see Chapter 21.1 ▶) in bipolar I disorder compared to controls [1158–1161].

If there has been a single episode of manic psychosis, this is classified as **mania with psychotic symptoms** (F30.2). If there has been more than one affective episode (depressive, manic, hypomanic, or mixed), then a current episode of manic psychosis is classified as **bipolar affective disorder, current episode manic with psychotic symptoms** (F31.2).

The DSM-IV criteria for affective episodes are similar; these and its diagnostic algorithm for affective psychosis [5] are shown in Section 2 (Chapter 28.5 ▶, Chapter 28.6 ▶). A significant classificatory difference is the distinction in DSM-IV, but not ICD-10, between bipolar I disorder (characterized by a history of mania) and bipolar II disorder (characterized by a history of hypomania [and depression] but not mania).

Bipolar disorder has a lifetime prevalence of approximately 1.5% [20], with a lifetime prevalence for psychotic bipolar I disorder of approximately 0.12% [1162]. A large number of candidate genes have been associated with bipolar affective disorder (MIM 125480).

21.3 Depressive psychosis (psychotic depression)

Likewise, when depressive symptoms precede the development of delusions or hallucinations, depressive psychosis is diagnosed. Typically, but not necessarily, the psychotic symptoms are mood-congruent (i.e. affectively negative; unpleasant).

Depression is marked by persistent low mood, loss of interest and enjoyment in usually pleasurable activities (anhedonia), reduced energy, fatigue and fatiguability, and diminished activity. Concentration, attention, self-esteem, and self-confidence are often reduced, and the patient may have ideas of guilt and unworthiness, bleak and pessimistic views of the future, ideas or plans or acts of self-harm or suicide, poor sleep, and poor appetite. Diurnal variation of mood is common (often worst in the morning), as is early-morning waking, psychomotor retardation or agitation, loss of appetite and weight, and loss of libido. Full diagnostic criteria are given in Section 2 (Chapter 28.2 ▶, Chapter 28.6 ▶). Psychomotor retardation and negative cognitive biases may affect cognitive function. In the elderly, significant reversible cognitive impairment accompanying moderate/severe depression is sometimes termed *depressive pseudodementia* [22], though this is also a strong predictor of subsequent dementia [1347].

Psychotic symptoms are typically mood-congruent, with delusions of guilt, sin, evil, poverty, death, or imminent disaster, and hallucinations such as of defamatory or accusatory voices or the smell of rot or decomposing flesh [4, 17]. Sometimes they are mood-incongruent [1163] or include Schneiderian first-rank symptoms [1164]. Psychotic symptoms are seen in ~15% of cases of major depression (the DSM-IV category) [20, 28], and major depression has a lifetime prevalence of at least 5% [20]; a direct survey found a lifetime prevalence of psychotic depression of 0.35% [1162]. Mood disorders in general have low prevalence until early teenage years. There is then a roughly linear increase in prevalence until late middle age, and a more gradual increase thereafter, with the median age of onset of mood disorders ranging between 29 and 43 across countries [1139].

A single episode of depressive psychosis is classified under ICD-10 as a **severe depressive episode with psychotic symptoms** (F32.3). A repeated episode, with no history of mania, is classified as **recurrent depressive disorder, current episode severe with psychotic symptoms** (F33.3); a similar episode in the context of bipolar affective disorder would be classified as **bipolar affective disorder, current episode severe depression with psychotic symptoms** (F31.5). Genetic predispositions to depression have been identified (MIM 608516).

The DSM-IV criteria for affective episodes are similar; these and its diagnostic algorithm for affective psychosis [5] are shown in Section 2. Appendix B discusses the changes proposed in the draft DSM-V, which include recognizing that depression with psychotic features is not always severe depression [1163].

Hypercortisolaemia is associated with depression (see Chapter 9.2 ▶), though the exact causal relationship between the two remains unclear [1165].

21.4 Schizoaffective disorders (F25)

If affective and schizophrenic symptoms are both prominent in the same psychotic episode(s) and develop simultaneously or within a few days of each other, and when this means that the patient meets diagnostic criteria for neither schizophrenia nor an affective disorder, then schizoaffective disorder is diagnosed. However, in a chronic episodic psychotic illness that predominantly has the features of bipolar affective disorder or recurrent depression, then occasional schizoaffective episodes would not alter the diagnosis. Note that mood-incongruent psychotic symptoms in affective disorders (manic psychosis, depressive psychosis) do not justify a diagnosis of schizoaffective disorder. Schizoaffective disorder may be categorized as **manic type** (F25.0), **depressive type** (F25.1), **mixed type** (F25.2), **other** (F25.8), or unspecified (F25.9). The comparable DSM-IV diagnostic algorithm is shown in Section 2. The exact prevalence of schizoaffective disorder is unknown but it is less common than schizophrenia [20, 1166], with the best estimate of the lifetime prevalence of schizoaffective disorder being 0.32% [1162]. There remains considerable debate as to its status between schizophrenia and bipolar affective disorder [1166]. Neurological "soft" signs are probably similar in prevalence to schizophrenia [1158, 1167].

21.5 Other affective psychoses

As one of ICD-10's categories of last resort, an affective psychosis that cannot be classified as a manic or depressive psychosis – or as a **mixed affective episode** (F38.00), in which a mixture of manic/hypomanic and depressive symptoms are present, or they alternate within hours – may be classified as **unspecified mood (affective) disorder** (F39).

21.6 Schizotypal disorder (F21)

This disorder is believed to be related to schizophrenia, being more common in relatives of those with schizophrenia [1168]. In DSM-IV it is called **schizotypal personality disorder** [5]. Its course is chronic with fluctuations of intensity, and there are features that overlap with simple schizophrenia and with schizoid and paranoid personality disorders. Typical features are:

(a) inappropriate or constricted affect (the individual appears cold and aloof);
(b) behaviour or appearance that is odd, eccentric, or peculiar;
(c) poor rapport with others and a tendency to social withdrawal;
(d) odd beliefs or magical thinking, influencing behaviour and inconsistent with subcultural norms;
(e) suspiciousness or paranoid ideas;
(f) obsessive ruminations without inner resistance, often with dysmorphophobic, sexual or aggressive contents;
(g) unusual perceptual experiences including somatosensory (bodily) or other illusions, depersonalization or derealization;

(h) vague, circumstantial, metaphorical, over-elaborate, or stereotyped thinking, manifested by odd speech or in other ways, without gross incoherence;
(i) occasional transient quasi-psychotic episodes with intense illusions, auditory or other hallucinations, and delusion-like ideas, usually occurring without external provocation.

For diagnosis under ICD-10, "three or four" of these typical features must have been present, continuously or episodically, for at least two years, without the patient ever having met criteria for schizophrenia [4]. The ICD-10 and DSM-IV criteria are shown in Section 2. Neurological "soft" signs relate to measures of schizotypy [1155].

21.7 Persistent delusional disorder (F22)

If patients have long-standing delusions as their only, or most prominent, symptom and the disease cannot be classified as organic, schizophrenic, or affective, then a persistent delusional disorder is diagnosed. In ICD-10, "long-standing" means at least 3 months (before which the diagnosis is likely to be an acute and transient psychotic disorder; Chapter 21.8 ▶); in DSM-IV's equivalent (delusional disorder), "long-standing" means at least one month.

The main subtype is **delusional disorder** (F22.0). The delusions are highly variable across patients. Intermittent depression and olfactory and tactile hallucinations do not invalidate the diagnosis, and nor do transient minor auditory hallucinations (particularly in the elderly), but clear and persistent auditory hallucinations, core schizophrenic symptoms (such as thought disorder, passivity phenomena, or thought broadcasting), or clear affective changes are incompatible with the diagnosis [4]. In ICD-10, this category subsumes **paranoia**, **paranoid psychosis**, and **late paraphrenia**. Paraphrenia was originally defined as a disorder of delusions without disorders of emotion or volition [1169], and late paraphrenia was defined as a schizophrenic disorder arising in those aged over 60 [1170, 1171], emphasizing the delusional rather than the hallucinatory nature of the condition [see 1172] (see also Chapter 21.17 ▶).

The label **other persistent delusional disorder** (F22.8) encompasses persistent delusional disorders that do not meet the criteria for F22.0, such as delusions accompanied by persistent hallucinatory voices or by schizophrenic symptoms that are insufficient to meet the criteria for schizophrenia.

Other disorders involving highly specific delusions or beliefs held with near-delusional intensity, with no other psychotic symptoms, include **somatization disorder** (F45.0), in which multiple physical symptoms are present with refusal to accept reassurance that there is no physical explanation for them, and the patient's emphasis is on seeking treatment for their symptoms, and **hypochondriacal disorder** (F45.2), in which the patient is preoccupied with having serious and progressive physical disorder(s) or deformity, requests investigations directed at the disease, and refuses to accept reassurance. The latter category includes **body dysmorphic disorder** [4]. The DSM-IV [5] distinguishes psychotic and non-psychotic variations of body dysmorphic disorder based on whether the belief is held with delusional intensity or not, but this may be an artificial distinction [1173]. Appendix B discusses the continuum of insight proposed in the draft DSM-V, and the proposed new **olfactory reference disorder** (characterized by a preoccupation with the belief that one emits a foul or offensive body odour, which is not perceived by others, which may also be held with delusional intensity).

The lifetime prevalence of delusional disorder is 0.01–0.18% [20, 1162].

21.8 Acute and transient psychotic disorders (F23)

Acute-onset psychotic disorders have an unsatisfactory classification [4]. They are defined as the onset of psychosis (a transition from a clearly non-psychotic to a clearly psychotic state) within 2 weeks, with the term "abrupt onset" referring to onset within 48 hours. All conditions in this group are defined by the exclusion of mood disorders (mania [Chapter 21.2 ▶] and depression [Chapter 21.3 ▶]) and organic causes [4]. The group of disorders is:

- **Acute polymorphic psychotic disorder without symptoms of schizophrenia** (F23.0). The diagnosis requires (a) an acute onset, as defined above; (b) several types of delusion or hallucination, changing in type and intensity from day to day or more rapidly; (c) a varying emotional state; and (d) no symptom being consistent enough to fulfil the criteria for schizophrenia or a manic or depressive episode, despite their variety [4]. This category subsumes the terms "**bouffée délirante** without symptoms of schizophrenia" and "**cycloid psychosis** without symptoms of schizophrenia". Bouffée délirante is a French term for an acute, florid psychotic illness with complete remission [1174–1176]. Cycloid psychosis is characterized by an acute onset of transient polymorphic symptoms (psychotic, cognitive, affective) [1177–1179]. Where used, diagnostic criteria [1178] are (1) acute-onset first-episode psychosis in a patient aged 15–50, having excluded organic causes; (2) onset of full-blown psychosis within hours or days; (3) at least four of: (i) confusion, (ii) mood-incongruent delusions, (iii) hallucinations, (iv) "pananxiety", i.e. anxiety not related to particular situations or circumstances, (v) deep feelings of happiness or ecstasy, (vi) motor disturbances such as akinesis or hyperkinesis, (vii) a particular concern with death, (viii) background mood swings insufficient to justify a diagnosis of affective disorder; (4) no fixed combination of symptoms, often with frequent changes of symptomatology. If the symptoms persist for >3 months, the diagnosis is changed (likely to persistent delusional disorder [Chapter 21.7 ▶] or other nonorganic psychotic disorder [Chapter 21.15 ▶]).
- **Acute polymorphic psychotic disorder with symptoms of schizophrenia** (F23.1). The diagnosis is as for F23.0, except that guideline (d) changes, so that symptoms that fulfil the criteria for schizophrenia must have been present for the majority of the time since psychosis was obviously present [4]. This category subsumes the terms "bouffée délirante with symptoms of schizophrenia" and "cycloid psychosis with symptoms of schizophrenia". If the schizophrenic symptoms persist for a month, the diagnosis is changed to that of schizophrenia (Chapter 21.1 ▶).
- **Acute schizophrenia-like psychotic disorder** (F23.2). In this condition, psychotic symptoms are stable and fulfil the criteria for schizophrenia, except they have lasted for less than a month. If this condition persists for a month, the diagnosis is changed to that of schizophrenia (Chapter 21.1 ▶). Some degree of emotional variability may be present, but not to the extent of acute polymorphic psychotic disorder. The criteria are (a) an acute onset; (b) symptoms that fulfil the criteria for schizophrenia have been present for most of the time since psychosis was obviously present; and (c) the criteria for acute polymorphic psychotic disorder are not fulfilled [4]. This category also subsumes the terms **acute (undifferentiated) schizophrenia** (equivalent to undifferentiated schizophrenia, F20.3, except with recent onset), **brief schizophreniform disorder/psychosis**, **oneirophrenia** (a dreamlike or "oneiroid" state of unreality characterized by amnesia, stupor, confusion, disorientation, illusions,

and hallucinations) [1180], and **schizophrenic reaction** (a term describing a self-limited schizophreniform psychosis after an emotionally traumatic event; see also Chapter 21.20.3 ▶) [see 1181].

- **Other acute predominantly delusional psychotic disorders** (F23.3). In these disorders, the main feature is of comparatively stable delusions or hallucinations that do not fulfil the criteria for schizophrenia (Chapter 21.1 ▶). Typically, hallucinations are second-person auditory (voices talking directly to the patient). Delusions of persecution or reference are common. The diagnostic criteria are (a) an acute onset; (b) delusions or hallucinations present for most of the time since the patient was obviously psychotic; and (c) neither the criteria for schizophrenia (F20) nor acute polymorphic psychotic disorder (F23.0) are fulfilled [4]. This category subsumes the descriptive terms **paranoid reaction** and **psychogenic paranoid psychosis**, in which persecutory delusions predominate. If delusions persist for >3 months, the diagnosis is changed to persistent delusional disorder (Chapter 21.7 ▶). If only hallucinations persist for >3 months, the diagnosis is changed to other nonorganic psychotic disorder (Chapter 21.15 ▶).
- **Other acute and transient psychotic disorders** (F23.8). Acute psychotic states not classifiable into any other category within F23 are classified here. Typically, these are acute psychotic states in which definite delusions or hallucinations occur but are only present for a small proportion of the time. "Undifferentiated excitement", which cannot be diagnosed because the patient's mental state cannot be assessed, is also classified here, having excluded organic causes [4].
- There is also a category for conditions not better specified: **acute and transient psychotic disorder, unspecified** (F23.9). This category subsumes the terms **brief reactive psychosis (not otherwise specified**) and **reactive psychosis**; the latter is a concept, widely used in Scandinavia, of psychosis following severe psychological stress (**psychogenic psychosis**) [29]. This concept originated in the 19th century as hysterical psychosis, and has also been termed **reactive dissociative psychosis** [1182]. Some have argued that atypical visual hallucinations closely conforming to the patient's fantasies and cultural background, or to what the patient considers characteristically psychotic, typify this disorder [30, 1183]. The relationship between stress and psychosis is discussed further in Chapter 21.20.3 ▶.

In DSM-IV, the dominant category for such psychoses is termed **brief psychotic disorder**, in which specifiers may be applied to indicate the presence or absence of marked stressors, or postpartum occurrence (having onset within 4 weeks postpartum; see also Chapter 9.6.2 ▶). See [17] for a discussion of the aetiology of acute brief psychosis.

21.9 Induced delusional disorder (F24)

In induced delusional disorder (also known as **folie à deux**, **induced paranoid disorder**, and **induced psychotic disorder**), a delusional disorder is shared by two or more people with close emotional links. One has a genuine psychotic disorder; the other(s) have an induced delusion, which usually disappears when they are separated [4].

21.10 Obsessive–compulsive disorder (F42)

Psychosis is not generally considered a feature of OCD itself [4], which is characterized by repetitive obsessional thoughts (stereotyped, distressing, recognized as the patient's own, and resisted), and compulsive acts that give no pleasure except relief from tension or anxiety. However, there is some overlap between OCD and psychosis. Obsessions are distinguished from delusions by the presence of insight into their abnormal character, so if insight is impaired, there may be diagnostic difficulty. For example, DSM-IV-TR [5] has the diagnostic category of "OCD without insight" [1184, see 1185], and insight might be best viewed as a continuum rather than a sharp psychotic/non-psychotic divide [1173]. Appendix B discusses the insight continuum for OCD proposed in the draft DSM-V. Compulsions have sometimes evolved into command hallucinations [1186]. Schizophrenia, and psychotic symptoms in general, co-occur with OCD more often than would be expected by chance, though the reasons are unclear and the degree to which there is a genuine overlap syndrome ("schizo-obsessive disorder") is debated [1184, 1187–1191]. Neurological "soft" signs occur in OCD more often than in controls [1192, 1193].

The lifetime prevalence of OCD is 2–5% [20].

21.11 Panic attacks with psychotic features

Psychotic features have been reported during severe panic attacks [1194, 1195], responding in some cases to conventional (benzodiazepine and SSRI) therapy [1194]. Panic attacks in adolescence are also associated with psychotic symptoms in young adulthood [1196].

21.12 Post-traumatic stress disorder (F43.1)

Post-traumatic stress disorder (PTSD) is characterized by an exceptionally distressing event followed by persistent re-experience of the event as repeated intrusive memories or dreams, persistent avoidance of activities and situations reminiscent of the trauma, and persistent hyperarousal (hypervigilance, enhanced startle reaction, insomnia). Although psychosis is not part of the definition of PTSD, PTSD appears to be associated with positive psychotic symptoms [1197, 1198]. The reason for this association is unclear. See also Chapters 21.8 ▶ and 21.20.3 ▶.

21.13 Psychosis in the context of eating disorders (F50)

Food-related hallucinations and other forms of psychosis have been reported in the context of severe eating disorders (**anorexia nervosa; bulimia nervosa**); see starvation (Chapter 11.8 ▶). There is some debate as to the aetiology of psychosis in the context of eating disorders [665, 1199]. One study suggesting a relationship between psychosis and both anorexia nervosa and bulimia nervosa found an association between these diagnoses and higher scores on the "psychoticism" and "paranoid ideation" dimensions of the SCL-90-R questionnaire, but no association with any individual symptom that would count under a conventional definition of psychosis (see Chapter 1 ▶). The associations were driven instead by endorsements of statements such as "never feeling close to another person" or "feeling that people take advantage of you" [1200]. In another series of patients with eating disorders, all psychotic symptoms were attributable to an alternative psychiatric disorder [1199].

21.14 Psychotic and near-psychotic phenomena in the context of personality disorder

Several personality disorders are associated with occasional psychotic symptoms, usually in response to psychological stress [5]. These are detailed below. Diagnosis of any personality disorder by ICD-10 requires all of the following criteria to be met: (A1) that the individual's enduring patterns of inner experience and behaviour deviate markedly from the cultural norm, manifest in more than one of cognition, affect, impulse control, and interpersonal relationships; (A2) that the deviation is pervasive, not situation-specific; (A3) that it causes personal distress or adverse social consequences; (A4) that it is stable and long-lasting, having its onset in late childhood or adolescence; (A5) that it is not a consequence of other adult mental disorders; (A6) that organic brain disease is excluded as a cause.

Note that schizotypal disorder (Chapter 21.6 ▶) is classified as a personality disorder in DSM-IV [5].

21.14.1 Paranoid personality disorder (F60.0)

Patients with paranoid personality disorder may exhibit extreme suspiciousness, a preoccupation with conspiratorial explanations, and a self-referential attitude [4], but not of delusional intensity [4, 5]. However, in response to stress, such patients may experience brief psychotic episodes (lasting minutes to hours) [5].

The ICD-10 criteria are all of A1–A6 above, plus four of (B1) excessive sensitivity to setbacks and rebuffs; (B2) a tendency to bear grudges persistently; (B3) suspiciousness and a pervasive tendency to distort experience by misconstruing the neutral or friendly actions of others as hostile or contemptuous; (B4) a combative and tenacious sense of personal rights out of keeping with the actual situation; (B5) recurrent suspicions, without justification, regarding the sexual fidelity of a spouse or sexual partner; (B6) persistent self-referential attitude, associated particularly with excessive self-importance; (B7) preoccupation with unsubstantiated conspiratorial explanations of events around the subject or in the world at large.

21.14.2 Schizoid personality disorder (F60.1)

Very brief psychotic episodes (minutes to hours) may also be seen in schizoid personality disorder [5]. The ICD-10 criteria are all of A1–A6 above, plus four of (B1) few, if any, activities provide pleasure; (B2) emotional coldness, detachment, or flattened affectivity; (B3) a limited capacity to express warm, tender feelings or anger towards others; (B4) appears indifferent to either praise or criticism of others; (B5) little interest in having sexual experiences with another person, taking into account age; (B6) almost always chooses solitary activities; (B7) excessive preoccupation with fantasy and introspection; (B8) neither desires, nor has, any close friends or confiding relationships, or has only one; (B9) marked insensitivity to prevailing social norms and conventions, with breach of them being unintentional.

21.14.3 Emotionally unstable personality disorder, borderline type (F60.31)

Patients with emotionally unstable personality disorder, borderline type [4], or **borderline personality disorder** [5], may exhibit hallucinations, body image distortions, ideas of reference, and hypnagogic phenomena (Chapter 16 ▶) during times of stress [5, 1201–1203].

The ICD-10 criteria are all of A1–A6 above; three of (B1) a marked tendency to act unexpectedly and without consideration of the consequences; (B2) a marked tendency to quarrelsome behaviour and to conflicts with others, especially when impulsive acts are thwarted or criticized; (B3) liability to outbursts of anger or violence, with inability to control the resulting behavioural explosions; (B4) difficulty in maintaining any course of action that offers no immediate reward; (B5) unstable and capricious mood; and two of (C1) disturbances in and uncertainty about self-image, aims and internal, including sexual, preferences; (C2) liability to become involved in intense and unstable relationships, often leading to emotional crises; (C3) excessive efforts to avoid abandonment; (C4) recurrent threats or acts of self-harm; (C5) chronic feelings of emptiness.

21.15 Chronic hallucinatory psychosis and other nonorganic psychotic disorders (F28)

Delusional or hallucinatory disorders that do not justify a diagnosis of schizophrenia (F20), persistent delusional disorders (F22), acute and transient psychotic disorders (F23), schizoaffective disorder (F25), manic psychosis (F30.2), or depressive psychosis (F32.3), are classified under F28 ("other nonorganic psychotic disorders"). This category includes chronic hallucinatory psychosis.

21.16 Unspecified nonorganic psychosis (F29)

The diagnostic category of last resort for psychosis in ICD-10 is F29 (unspecified nonorganic psychosis) [4]. In DSM-IV, the final category is psychotic disorder not otherwise specified [5]. The use of these categories (with F28, above) is by no means uncommon in first-episode psychosis [1346].

21.17 Late-onset psychosis

Current classificatory systems do not differentiate psychiatric causes of psychosis by age of onset [4, 5]. However, there are a number of issues for which age is particularly relevant. Amongst these is the view that schizophrenia is generally a disease of early onset, with late-onset schizophrenia-like psychosis representing a different entity or set of entities [1204]. Another is the relationship of psychosis to dementia: since dementia is a frequent syndrome and a frequent cause of psychotic symptoms, it comes increasingly to the fore in the diagnosis of psychosis as age increases, as do other secondary causes of psychosis.

Some historical background is worthwhile. Kraepelin subdivided psychosis into manic depression (later to be termed bipolar affective disorder), dementia praecox (using Morel's term of démence précoce, literally premature dementia), and paraphrenia (delusions and hallucinations, with a preponderance of paranoid symptoms, but without deterioration or disturbance of affective response) [1169, 1204, 1205]. Bleuler's concept of schizophrenia evolved from that of dementia praecox [1206], and his original work used an age cut-off of 40 years to define late-onset schizophrenia [1204]. The term "paraphrenia" was largely subsumed into the wider category of schizophrenic syndromes [1205]. The term "late paraphrenia" subsequently evolved as a description of schizophrenia-like psychosis in those over 55 or 60 (in later years, a schizophreniform non-affective psychosis arising in those aged over 60, emphasizing delusions rather than hallucinations, and the lack of dementia) [1170–1172], although Kraepelin's paraphrenia was never distinguished by age of onset [1204]. DSM-III's diagnostic criteria for schizophrenia required an onset before the age of 45. The concept of late paraphrenia was included in ICD-9 and a category was introduced in DSM-III-R for late-onset schizophrenia, having onset at age ≥45 [1204, 1205]. In ICD-10 and DSM-IV, age cut-offs for the diagnosis of schizophrenia (Chapter 21.1 ▶) were removed [1204]. Late paraphrenia is subsumed in ICD-10 within persistent delusional disorder (Chapter 21.7 ▶).

Although schizophrenia typically begins in the age range 15–35 [1139], psychosis increases again in frequency in the elderly. The one-year prevalence of schizophrenia for individuals aged 45–64 is 0.6%, and the prevalence of schizophrenia in those aged >65 is 0.1–0.5%. The annual incidence of schizophrenia in those aged >44 is 12.6:100 000, with the annual incidence of schizophrenia-like psychosis increasing by 11% for each 5-year increase in age in those over 60 [1204]. Schizophrenia begins later in women (Chapter 9.6.1 ▶), and in late-onset schizophrenia, a higher proportion of patients are women [1204, 1205]. Early reports stressed an association between late-onset schizophrenia and sensory deficits such as deafness, but this has been questioned; it may be a stronger association in very-late-onset (>60 years) schizophrenia-like psychosis. Premorbid schizoid or paranoid personality traits may be associated with the development of late-onset schizophrenia [1204, 1205].

Current consensus is that within the heterogeneous group of conditions categorized as schizophrenia, there is sufficient evidence to categorize separately **late-onset schizophrenia**, being schizophrenia after the age of 40 years, and **very-late-onset schizophrenia-like psychosis**, with onset after the age of 60 [1204].

Obviously, as already discussed (Chapter 5 ▶, Chapter 6.1 ▶), dementia frequently causes psychosis, and a high proportion of the elderly with psychosis will have dementia [1204]. In those developing hallucinations without dementia, the chance of subsequently developing dementia is increased. In a sample followed longitudinally from the age of 70–90, excluding individuals developing dementia, the cumulative incidence of first-onset psychotic symptoms was 4.8% (or 8.0% including reports from key informants), and 19.8% in those who survived to the age of 85 [1207]. Hallucinations predicted dementia (64% of those with hallucinations later developed dementia, compared to 30% of those with delusions and 25% of those without psychotic symptoms) [1207]. In another sample of 95-year-olds without dementia, the one-year prevalence of hallucinations was 6.7% and of delusions 0.6%. Cognitive differences were not detectable by the MMSE between this group and those without psychotic symptoms. The prevalence of schizophrenia was 2.4% [1208]. Examining the predictors of psychotic symptoms, in a community-based study of over-65s, persecutory symptoms and perceptual disturbance (prevalence 3.9%) were predicted by dementia and subjective memory loss, by alcohol use, and by visual impairment [1209].

21.18 Conditions labelled as "psychotic" historically

Some conditions have historically been labelled as involving "psychosis" without true psychotic symptoms in the sense described in Chapter 1. These include "hysterical psychosis" (dissociative [conversion] disorders, F44), "infantile psychosis" (childhood autism, F84.0), "atypical childhood psychosis" (atypical autism, F84.1), and "disintegrative psychosis" and "symbiotic psychosis" (other childhood disintegrative disorder, F84.3, sometimes associated with a well-defined neurological disease) [4, 30].

There is debate as to whether autistic spectrum disorders, including Asperger's syndrome, are genuinely associated with psychosis. The ICD-10 notes that psychotic episodes occasionally occur in early adult life in those with Asperger's syndrome (F84.5) [4], though such evidence as exists tends to suggest that autism and childhood psychosis are distinct [15, 1210]. However, catatonia appears to be over-represented in patients with autism [15].

In the very rare **Ganser's syndrome**, whose most typical syndrome is approximate answers (*vorbeireden*), hallucinations have been described, but there is debate as to the nature of the disorder (psychosis, dissociation, factitious, or malingering) [29, 1211]. ICD-10 classifies it as a dissociative disorder [4].

21.19 Bereavement

Bereavement commonly induces hallucinations of the deceased, occurring in 45–61% of widows and widowers, though less commonly in the young, and less commonly in surviving spouses of unhappy marriages [1212, 1213]. These hallucinations are often not disclosed spontaneously and are often felt to be helpful. See also Chapters 21.8 ▶ and 21.20.3 ▶.

21.20 Normal and prodromal symptoms

The lifetime prevalence of mild psychotic experiences is high. For example, in a large telephone survey, 38.7% of randomly selected participants reported having had hallucinations of some sort, and 27% had had daytime hallucinations [1079] (see also hypnagogic and hypnopompic hallucinations, Chapter 16 ▶), with another survey showing an annual prevalence of psychotic symptoms of 5.5% in the UK [1214]. They are not confined to adults, with another survey showing a 9% one-year prevalence of auditory vocal hallucinations in 7–8-year-old children [1215]. The vast majority of such people never become psychotic to a degree warranting a diagnosis of a psychotic disorder [1216–1218]. Likewise, self-reported schizotypy (conceptualized as proneness to psychosis) is relatively common [1219]. The Launey–Slade Hallucination Scale yields normally distributed scores in normal subjects [1220], supporting the view that hallucinations are on a continuum with normal mental experience [8], and scores on this scale are contributed to by a tendency towards hallucinatory experiences, subjective externality of thought, and vivid daydreams [1221]. A recent meta-analysis found that ~75–90% of developmental psychotic experiences are transitory but some persist, and thus subclinical psychotic experiences are a predictor of later psychotic disorders. These authors emphasize the continuum from subclinical psychotic experiences (prevalence ~8%) to subclinical psychotic symptoms (prevalence ~4%), associated with some distress and help-seeking, to clinical psychotic disorder (prevalence of the order of 1–3%) [1222].

21.20.1 Pseudohallucinations

A particular difficulty surrounds the concept of **pseudohallucinations**. This is a term that has been used variously to describe hallucinatory experiences occurring in those without significant other mental illness; hallucinatory experiences that the patient recognizes as unreal; hallucinations that are not very vivid; internal imagery or re-experienced memories that are very vivid; and the experience of hearing voices originating within the mind or head. Many of these concepts place the idea of pseudohallucinations somewhere on a continuum between normal mental imagery and vivid hallucinations occurring without insight; some definitions assume a syndromal diagnosis. It is not clear that the concept is useful or discriminatory [1223, 1224]; it is not used in ICD-10 [4, 10] or DSM-IV [5] and we have avoided it in this text. There is no evidence that the distinction between internally and externally experienced auditory hallucinations is relevant for psychiatric diagnosis [1225].

21.20.2 Personality and predisposition to psychosis

As described above, some personality disorders (and schizotypal disorder, considered to be a personality disorder in DSM-IV but not ICD-10) are associated with psychotic and near-psychotic experiences. Appendix B ▶ discusses the model of personality and personality disorders proposed in the draft DSM-V.

Patients with first-episode psychosis differ in several ways from controls on dimensional measures of personality (having higher neuroticism, openness to experience, and agreeableness, and lower extroversion and conscientiousness [1226]), with personality factors remaining stable despite fluctuation in psychotic symptoms. However, no personality profile is a clear predictor of psychosis.

Despite its name, Eysenck's personality factor of *psychoticism (P)* does not describe psychotic symptoms, but instead "tough-mindedness"; it primarily measures antisocial, impulsive, non-conforming, callous, and sadistic traits, and secondarily paranoid ideation and anhedonia [1227, 1228]. It is not a normally distributed factor. It is a predictor of personality disorder dimensions (schizotypal and paranoid), and psychotic-like experiences (e.g. aberrant beliefs and aberrant visual experiences), rather than frank psychosis [1228, 1229].

21.20.3 Stress and psychosis

Many retrospective studies have suggested that highly traumatic events can be the trigger for a major psychotic illness, though there are methodological problems with many; for a review, see [1230].

Early adverse experiences such as childhood physical or sexual abuse may increase the predisposition to psychosis in women [1231] or regardless of sex [1232], and to schizotypal psychotic-like experiences (paranoia, suspiciousness, unusual perceptual experiences) regardless of sex [1232, 1233].

Psychological stress has been demonstrated experimentally to exacerbate paranoia in people with subclinical psychotic symptoms [1234]. Chronic or recurrent psychosocial stress probably increases the risk of major psychotic illness [1235]. As discussed above, psychological stress may trigger psychotic symptoms in some personality disorders (Chapter 21.14 ▶), bereavement may cause hallucinations (Chapter 21.19 ▶), correlative studies suggest stress may trigger recurrence of psychostimulant-induced psychotic experiences (Chapter 15.3 ▶, amphetamine), and there is an association between PTSD and psychotic symptoms (Chapter 21.12 ▶).

21.20.4 Prodromes and prediction of serious mental illness

Distinguishing normality from symptoms that represent a prodrome preceding a serious psychosis is not an exact process, but prediction is possible. Prodromal or prepsychotic symptoms include a disturbance in the perception of self; overvalued (attenuated delusional) ideas; extreme preoccupation with and withdrawal to overvalued ideas (including philosophical and mystical or religious themes); disturbances of simple perception (such as unusually vivid perception, and distorted body perception); attenuated (brief or mild or simple) hallucinations; mild thought disorder (difficulty with concentration and memory or the flow of thought); emotional disturbances (depression, suicidal ideation, anxiety, panic, mood instability, social anxiety, sleep disturbance, a feeling of tension or restlessness, irritability or rage); a feeling of loss of inner control; and coping responses (such as alcohol or drug use, social isolation, or trying to socialize to cope) [1236]. Frequent and distressing symptoms are obviously of greater concern [1216]. Behavioural indications of a prodromal state include leaving or truanting from school, university, or a job; marked and lasting shift of interests; marked and lasting social passivity, withdrawal, or isolation;

and a marked and lasting change in global appearance or behaviour [1236]. Some cognitive impairment may already be present [1237]. The Ultra High Risk (UHR) criteria, assessed by the Comprehensive Assessment of At Risk Mental States (CAARMS) tool, had a sensitivity of 83–92% and a specificity of 62–74% for the prediction of psychosis in recent studies of young adults [1238, 1239]. This system classifies patients as "UHR+" if they have attenuated psychosis within the previous 12 months (either of subthreshold intensity or subthreshold frequency for the diagnosis of a psychotic disorder), have brief limited intermittent psychotic symptoms (BLIPS) that spontaneously resolved within the previous 12 months, or have a "trait" vulnerability (a presumed genetic vulnerability to psychosis, such as a first-degree family history of a psychotic disorder) plus persistent low general functioning for at least 1 month within the previous 12 months [1238, 1239].

Appendix B ▶ discusses the **psychosis risk syndrome** or **attenuated psychotic symptoms syndrome** proposed in the draft DSM-V.

Chapter 22 Factitious disorder and malingering

It is obvious that psychotic symptoms can also be feigned. In factitious disorder (F68.1), illness is feigned without obvious motivation, or sometimes produced by self-harm, often in the context of disorders of personality or relationships. In malingering (conscious simulation) (Z76.5), there is a clear motivation for feigning illness (e.g. [1240]).

Chapter 23 Multiple simultaneous causes of psychosis, and questions of causality

Finally, multiple causes of psychosis may coexist, including simultaneous primary psychiatric and medical/neurological conditions, which undoubtedly make clear diagnosis difficult (e.g. [17, 1241]). This point raises the general question of how a given condition can be said to *cause* psychosis, in general and in a particular patient.

Causality itself is a complex topic [1242]. Claims about causality may be general ("smoking causes lung cancer") or singular ("John's smoking caused his lung cancer"). Though oversimplified and incomplete, a very basic theory of general causation is that an event C is said to cause another event E if the probability of E is higher if C occurs than if C does not occur, i.e. $P(\mathrm{E} \mid \mathrm{C}) > P(\mathrm{E} \mid \text{not-C})$, and if C precedes E in time.

Establishing general causality may be done reliably in an appropriately controlled experiment, in which C is directly manipulated. Examples of causes of psychotic symptoms that have been established experimentally in this fashion include amphetamine, ketamine, methylphenidate, and THC (Chapter 15.1 ▶, Chapter 15.3 ▶).

General causality may also be established epidemiologically; in this method, associations between C and E are observed, though this approach requires careful attempts to avoid confounds that are absent in a well-designed controlled experiment. The appropriate criteria for epidemiological causality are debated [1243] but perhaps the most commonly used set are Hill's criteria [1244]. These measures by which to judge whether an association might be causal are: (1) the strength of association between the proposed cause and the effect in question; (2) the consistency of that association; (3) the specificity of the association, which can add weight to the proposal; (4) temporal order, or whether the proposed cause precedes the proposed effect; (5) a biological gradient, or dose–response curve between the proposed cause and the effect, adds weight; (6) biological plausibility contributes to belief in causality, though what is implausible in one era of science may be plausible in another; (7) likewise, coherence with existing knowledge about the disease is helpful; (8) experimental intervention, if possible, can provide the strongest support for a causal role; (9) analogy to similar causes or effects. By these measures, velocardiofacial syndrome and Alzheimer's disease are well-established causes of psychosis (Chapter 4.1 ▶, Chapter 5.1 ▶), while for other diseases (particularly for rare ones), the association is less certain (e.g. Chapter 4.8 ▶, Chapter 4.9 ▶, Chapter 5.12 ▶, Chapter 5.15 ▶, Chapter 5.16 ▶).

Such studies also indicate the potentially varied temporal relationship between neurological insults and psychosis. For example, neurological insults during development can increase the risk of psychosis many years later (see e.g. the discussion of schizophrenia, Chapter 21.1 ▶). Even in adults, there also is some evidence that psychosis induced by an acute insult may sometimes outlast that insult (examples including drug-induced psychosis persisting beyond clearance of the drug, Chapter 15.3 ▶), perhaps in part because delusions become systematized and harder to eradicate the longer they are present (e.g. [1245]).

Establishing causality in an individual patient, therefore – singular causality – can be particularly difficult if not theoretically impossible. Retrospectively, clinicans may attempt a "best guess" based on knowledge of general causation, i.e. by establishing the presence, in a given patient, of potential causes of psychosis (be those causes long-standing risk factors or acute insults) and by knowing the risk, in general, of developing psychosis given each cause. Beyond that, further information may be gleaned in some circumstances from observing the temporal relationship between potential causes and psychosis. For example, if one thinks a patient's psychosis is due to hypercalcaemia, then this assertion is supported if successful treatment of the hypercalcaemia is followed by resolution of the psychosis (with some temporal caveats concerning psychosis as described above), or if a subsequent episode of hypercalcaemia re-provokes psychosis. Nonetheless, absolute certainty in an individual patient may be elusive.

Section 2 A clinical approach to the diagnosis of psychosis

In Section 2 we outline a clinical approach to the diagnosis of psychosis. We begin with clues from the history, mental state and physical examination (Chapter 24 ▶) and initial or routine special investigations (Chapter 25 ▶). In Chapter 26 ▶, we present an aide-mémoire to causes of psychosis indexed by groups of symptoms and signs. In Chapter 27 ▶, more unusual special investigations are given, with an indication as to when these may be required (often in consultation with specialists in the relevant fields). Finally, we present classificatory systems for primary psychosis, based on ICD-10 and DSM-IV (Chapter 28 ▶). Section 2 is based on the review of causes presented in Section 1 and other sources as indicated, but the exact approach to the diagnosis of psychosis is not fixed in stone, with different authors giving slightly different approaches, and our approach should not be seen as prescriptive.

(2) General mental state examination (appearance, behaviour, speech, mood and affect, thought form and content, perception, cognition, insight, risks to self and others). The mental state examination is conducted throughout the interview, through questioning and observation.

The background and other clues from the history

(3) Past psychiatric history.
(4) Past medical history.
- Be comprehensive (and prepared to re-visit this should further information arise). Re-check: any heart, lung, liver, kidney, gut, skin, joint, nerve, thyroid, or eye disease? Hypertension? Diabetes? Seizures? Head injury? Stroke? Any unexplained symptoms? "… And anything else?"

(5) Systems review. Points to cover include:
- *Sleep history*. Problems sleeping, total duration of sleep, sleep pattern, hallucinations occurring at sleep/wake transitions, daytime tiredness or sleeping.
- *Cognitive function*. Difficulty concentrating, thinking, or remembering.
- *Movement*. Weakness, stiffness, difficulty moving, unwanted or involuntary movements, problems with coordination.
- *Sensation*. Numbness, tingling, change in vision, hearing, taste, or smell.
- *Paroxysmal limbic phenomena*. Micropsia, macropsia, metamorphopsia, déjà/jamais vu/écouté, forced thoughts or emotions, depersonalization, derealization, autoscopy, paranormal experiences (e.g. clairvoyance, telepathy) [22].
- *Other CNS*: headache, neck stiffness, photophobia, seizures, dizziness or vertigo, loss of consciousness, problems with bladder or bowel control, problems with speech.
- *General*. Fevers, malaise, sweats, change in weight, change in temperature sensitivity, pain anywhere.
- *Dermatological/rheumatological*. Rashes, itch, change in pigmentation, change in hair quality or quantity, photosensitivity, joint pains/swelling/stiffness, dry mouth or eyes.
- *Cardiorespiratory*. Breathlessness (at rest, on exercise, upon lying flat, at night), palpitations, chest pain, ankle swelling. Cough (productive?), haemoptysis, wheeze.
- *Abdominal/gastrointestinal*. Mouth ulcers, sore throat, change in appetite, swallowing problems, nausea or vomiting, change in bowel habit (constipation, diarrhoea), blood in stool.
- *Genitourinary*. Urinary frequency, dysuria, haematuria, urethral/vaginal discharge. Menstrual cycle.

(6) Drug history (prescribed, over-the-counter, and recreational drugs including alcohol). *Might this patient have a drug-induced psychosis or a poisoning syndrome?*
(7) Personal history, including developmental history. *Any suggestions of a neurodevelopmental disorder, or of other risk factors for psychosis* (e.g. Chapters 21.1, 21.20.3 ▶)?
(8) Personality. *Does the patient have features of any of the personality disorders associated with psychotic symptoms* (Chapter 28.4 ▶, Chapter 28.8 ▶)? *Any change in personality?*
(9) Occupational history. *Might this patient have a poisoning syndrome?*
(10) Travel history. *Unusual infections?*

(11) Family history. *Might this patient have a heritable psychotogenic condition?* Draw a family tree and ask about:
- psychotic illness
- mood disorders
- movement disorders or other neurological problems
- dementia and problems with memory
- medical illnesses
- consanguinity, particularly if an autosomal recessive genetic disorder is suspected

Pen-and-paper tests

(12) Cognitive/neuropsychological testing:
- 10-point Abbreviated Mental Test (AMT) [1247] or 30-point Mini-Mental State Examination (MMSE) [1248].
- Consider more thorough cognitive evaluation, e.g. 100-point Addenbrooke's Cognitive Evaluation (ACE-R) [1249] (which incorporates the MMSE) ± formal neuropsychological testing, particularly for tests of "lobar" function [33].

(13) Consider scoring with rating scales relevant to psychosis (e.g. BPRS, PANSS, SAPS/SANS) to monitor progress [22, 1250–1252].

To the examination couch

(14) Physical examination (general, cardiovascular, respiratory, abdominal, neurological) [1246]. Do not forget:
- The very basics (e.g. temperature, blood pressure, respiratory rate).
- Movement disorders: these can be subtle (e.g. chorea masked as fidgeting).
- The skin and joints.
- To look at the patient as a whole (e.g. endocrinopathies, dysmorphism).

(15) Incorporate focused examination relating to any abnormalities found or suspected from the history [1246].

(16) Examine for catatonia [31, 1130] (Chapter 28.9 ▶).

With informants

(17) Detailed collateral history.
- Discuss with the patient first regarding consent, i.e. what you may or may not discuss with others such as family or friends, distinguishing what the patient's family may choose to tell you from what you are allowed to tell the patient's family.
- Obtain a collateral history about the patient's reported symptoms and behaviour (not forgetting recreational drug use).
- Obtain collateral history regarding the background (as above). Check medical and drug histories with the patient's general practitioner.

Sit and think

Consider **risk factors** for different diseases apparent from the history and examination, and the disease **time course**. For example, extreme chronicity (decades) can be a feature of schizophrenia but not of frontal lobe tumours [28]. Gradual progression (e.g. neurodegenerative diseases), an acute onset (e.g. delirium, drug-induced psychosis), and a relapsing course (e.g. schizophrenia, bipolar affective disorder, porphyria) are other temporal patterns. Be alert to the possibility of a medical emergency presenting as psychosis (Chapter 24.4 ▶).

Consider **non-psychiatric symptoms** by group:

- Is there cognitive dysfunction?
- Are there localizing central sensorimotor symptoms or signs, such as:
  - pyramidal tract dysfunction (upper motor neuron pattern weakness with hyperreflexia and increased tone in a spastic pattern – disproportionately increased tone in upper limb flexors and lower limb extensors),
  - basal ganglia dysfunction (e.g. hypokinesia, bradykinesia, dystonia, dyskinesia, rigidity [increase in tone equal in flexors and extensors], akathisia, tremor, chorea, athetosis, ballismus),
  - cerebellar signs (e.g. limb ataxia, intention tremor, truncal ataxia, gait ataxia, dysarthria, nystagmus),
  - other motor abnormalities (e.g. myoclonus, asterixis, tics),
  - sensory loss in any modality, or
  - focal seizures [28]?

  Beware attributing extrapyramidal signs exclusively to psychotropic drugs.
- Is there evidence of diffuse neurological dysfunction (e.g. alteration in consciousness, generalized seizures)?
- Is there evidence of neuropathy of cranial or peripheral nerves (e.g. lower motor neuron pattern weakness with atrophy, fasciculation, and hyporeflexia; sensory loss or change in an appropriate distribution, or neuropathic pain; features of autonomic neuropathy) [28]?
- Are there features of systemic disease (e.g. fever; cardiovascular or other autonomic dysfunction; respiratory disease; gastrointestinal disease; skin or musculoskeletal abnormalities)?
- Is there evidence of developmental abnormality (e.g. developmental delay, dysmorphism)?
- Do symptoms fall into clusters explained by endocrine disturbance (e.g. hypothyroidism, hyperthyroidism, adrenal failure, Cushing's syndrome)?
- Are there symptoms or signs in many organ systems that suggest a widespread process such as vasculitis or another systemic inflammatory state?
- Do the symptoms fit any other well-known pattern of disease?

In Chapter 26 ▶, causes of psychosis from Section 1 are indexed by these categories.

Consider the **psychiatric symptoms**. Sometimes these may give very direct clues to aetiology in secondary psychosis (e.g. in simple visual hallucinations, consider visual pathway defects; in complex visual hallucinations, consider brainstem pathology or a cholinergic deficit [17, 1253]). The symptoms are the basis for psychiatric diagnosis: in Chapter 28 ▶, flowcharts and formal diagnostic criteria are given for primary psychiatric diagnoses.

Investigations and rethink

Consider which investigations to perform (Chapter 25 ▶, Chapter 27 ▶), then rethink with the results (Chapter 26 ▶).

24.2 Probe questions for psychotic symptoms

From the Present State Examination, ninth edition [1254], reproduced with permission from the Medical Research Council.

Introduction

- **To begin with, I should like to get an idea of the sort of problems that have been troubling you during the past month. What have been the main difficulties?**

Means of exploration, if subject gives inadequate information:

If subject's statement too brief	Can you tell me more about that?
If subject has no more to add	What else has been troubling you?
If statements are difficult to understand	Can you explain what you mean by...?
If subject is vague	Could you give an example of...?
If no other response forthcoming	Why did you come to the (hospital)?

General

Ask for explanations of symptoms:	How do you explain it?

Hallucinations

- **I should like to ask you a routine question which we ask of everybody. Do you ever seem to hear noises or voices when there is no one about, and nothing else to explain it?**
- **Have you had visions, or seen things other people couldn't see?**
- **Is there anything unusual about the way things feel or taste or smell?**

If auditory...

- Do you hear noises like tapping, or music? (What is it like?)
- Does it sound like muttering or whispering?
- Can you make out the words?
- What does the voice say?
  - *(If accusatory: Do you think that it is justified? Do you deserve it?)*
- Do you hear your name being called?
- Do you hear several voices talking about you?
  - *Do they refer to you as "he" ("she")?*
  - *What do they say?*
  - *Do they seem to comment on what you are thinking, or reading, or doing?*
- Do they speak directly to you?
  - *Are they threatening or unpleasant?*
  - *Do they call you names?*
  - *Do they give you orders? (Do you obey?)*
- Can you carry on a two-way conversation with —?
  - *(You can reply, and then — replies to you, and you reply again, just as in an ordinary conversation?)*
  - *Do you see anything, or smell anything at the same time as you hear the voice?*
  - *Who is it you are talking to?*
  - *What is the explanation? Do you know anyone else who has this kind of experience?*
- Are these voices in your mind or can you hear them through your ears?

If visual...

- With your eyes or in your mind?
- What did you see?
- Were you half asleep at the time?
- Has it occurred when you were fully awake?
- Did you realise you were "seeing things"?
- Did the vision seem to arise out of a pattern on the wallpaper or a shadow?
- How do you explain it?

If other...

- Do you sometimes notice strange smells that other people don't notice?
- Do you seem to think that you yourself give off a smell which is noticed?
- Do you ever feel that someone is touching you, but when you look there is nobody there?
- Have you noticed that food and drink seems to have an unusual taste recently?
- [... Any other unusual experiences?] (Temperature, pain, etc.)

Perceptual abnormalities other than hallucinations

- **Do you ever get the feeling that something odd is going on which you can't explain?**
- **Or that familiar surroundings seem strange?**
- **Does your imagination sometimes play tricks on you?**
- **Is there anything unusual about the way things look or sound, or smell, or taste?**
- **Does your body function normally? Is your own appearance normal?**

Thinking and thought reading, insertion, echo, broadcast

- **Can you think clearly or is there any interference with your thoughts?**
- **Are you in full control of your thoughts?**
- **Can people read your mind?**
- **Is anything like hypnotism or telepathy going on?**

If positive responses:

- Are thoughts put into your head which you know are not your own?
  - *How do you know they're not your own? Where do they come from?*
- Do you ever seem to hear your own thoughts spoken aloud in your head, so that someone standing near might be able to hear them?
- Are your thoughts broadcast, so that other people know what you are thinking?
- Do you ever seem to hear your own thoughts repeated or echoed?
  - *What is that like? How do you explain it? Where does it come from?*
- Do you ever experience your thoughts stopping quite unexpectedly so that there are none left in your mind, even when your thoughts were flowing freely before?
  - *How often does that occur? (etc.)*
- Do your thoughts ever seem to be taken out of your head, as though some external person or force were removing them?
- Can anyone read your thoughts?

Delusions

- **Do you feel under the control of some force or power other than yourself?**
  - As though you were a robot or zombie without a will of your own?
  - As though you were possessed by someone or something else?
  - What is that like?

- Does this force make your movements for you without your willing it, or use your voice, or your handwriting? Does it replace your personality? What is the explanation?
- **Do people seem to drop hints about you or say things with a double meaning, or do things in a special way so as to convey a meaning?**
  - Does everyone seem to gossip about you?
  - Do people follow you about or check up on you or record your movements?
  - How do they do it? Why?
  - Are there people about who are not what they seem to be?
- **Do things seem to be specially arranged?**
  - Is an experiment going on, to test you out?
  - Do you see any reference to yourself on TV or in the papers?
  - Do you ever seem to see special meanings in advertisements, or shop windows, or in the way things are arranged?
  - How do you explain this?
- **Is someone deliberately trying to harm you, such as trying to poison you or kill you?**
  - How? Is there an organisation like the Mafia behind it?
  - Is there any other kind of persecution? How do you explain this?
- **Do you think that people are organising things specially to help you?**
- **Is there anything special about you? Do you have special abilities or powers?**
  - Can you read people's thoughts?
  - Is there a special purpose or mission to your life?
  - Are you especially clever or inventive? How do you explain this?
  - Are you a very prominent person or related to someone prominent, like royalty?
  - Are you very rich or famous?
  - How do you explain this?
- **Are you a very religious person?**
  - Specially close to Christ or God?
  - Can God communicate with you? How?
  - Are you yourself a saint?
  - How do you explain this?
- **How do you explain the things that have been happening? (SPECIFY)** Is anything like hypnotism, telepathy, or the occult going on? What is the explanation?
- **Is anything like electricity, X-rays, or radio-waves affecting you?** (In what way? What is the explanation?)
- **Do you have any reason to be jealous of anybody?**
- **Have you had any unusual experience or adventure recently?**
- **Do you have committed a crime, or sinned greatly, or deserve punishment?** (Have you felt that your presence might contaminate or ruin other people?)
- **Do you think your appearance is normal? Is there anything the matter with your brain? Is there anything the matter with your body?**
- **Do you have the feeling that something terrible is going to happen?** What?

To differentiate full delusions and partial (overvalued ideas):

Even when you seem to be most convinced, do you really feel in the back of your mind that it might well not be true, that it might be imagination?

For a likely delusion:

How did it come into your mind that this was the explanation? (Did it happen suddenly? How did it begin?)

Insight

- **Do you think there is anything the matter with you?**
  - What do you think it is? Could it be a nervous condition? What do you think the cause is? Why did you need to come to hospital?
- **Do you think *(specify delusions or hallucinations)* were part of a nervous condition?**

Ending

- **Have there been any other things lately that I haven't covered?**

24.3 Probe questions for depression and mania

Adapted from the PSE (ninth edition) [1254], reproduced with permission from the Medical Research Council, and ICD-10 criteria [10].

Depression

- **Do you keep reasonably cheerful or have you been very depressed or low-spirited recently?**
  - Have you cried at all?
  - When did you last really enjoy doing anything?
- **How do you see the future?**
  - Has life seemed quite hopeless?
  - Can you see any future?
  - Have you given up or does there still seem some reason for trying?
- **Have you lost interest or pleasure in things you typically enjoy?**
- **How has your energy been recently?**
- **Have you been getting exhausted or worn out during the day or evening, even when you haven't been working very hard?**

If core symptoms of depression:

- **Have you had any trouble sleeping recently?**
  - Establish bedtime, time of falling asleep, sleep pattern across the night, whether the patient wakes early (and why).
- **What is your opinion of yourself compared to other people?**
  - Do you feel better, or not as good, or about the same as most?
  - Do you feel inferior or even worthless?
- **What has your appetite been like recently?**
- **Has your weight changed during the past few months?**
  - ... by how much?
- **Do you feel guilty or that you are to blame for something?**
  - Do you tend to blame yourself at all?
  - If people are critical, do you think you deserve it?
- **What has your concentration been like recently?**
  - Can you read an article in the paper or watch a TV programme right through?
  - Do your thoughts drift off so that you don't take things in?
- **Have you felt agitated, or worried, or more irritable than usual recently?** How do you show it?

- **Have you felt slowed down in your thoughts or movements?** Do things seem to be moving too fast for you?
- **Have you felt that life wasn't worth living?**
  - Did you ever feel like ending it all?
  - What did you think you might do?
  - Did you actually try?
  - Have you been thinking of ending your life recently?
  - Are you thinking about it now?
  - Have you thought about specific ways to end your life?
  - Do you have plans to do so?
  - Have you made any preparations?
  - Are there things that would prevent you from acting on those plans?
  - Do you want to end your life?
- **Have you been having other thoughts about death recently?**

The rest of the somatic syndrome, and menstrual variation:

- **Is the depression worse at any particular time of day?**
- (if applicable) **Does the depression or tension vary with your menstrual period?**
- **Do you feel that you have lost your emotions in some way?**
  - That you are empty of all feeling, incapable of reacting emotionally?
  - Is this a definite change, or have you always been like that?
- **Has there been any change in your interest in sex?**

Mania

- **Have you sometimes felt particularly cheerful and on top of the world, without any reason?**
  - Too cheerful to be healthy?
  - How long does it last?
- **Have you felt more easily irritated lately?**
- **Have other people commented on a change in you?**

- **Have you had difficulty concentrating lately, or felt easily distracted?**
- **Have you felt particularly full of energy lately, or full of exciting ideas?**
  - Do things seem to go too slowly for you?
  - Have you felt your thoughts racing?
  - Do you find yourself extremely active but not getting tired?
  - Have you felt specially healthy?
  - Have you felt restless?
- **Do you need less sleep than usual?**
- **Have you been buying any interesting things lately?**
- **Have you developed any new interests recently?**
- **Have you been reckless or taken any risks lately?**
- **Have you become more sociable recently?**
- **Has there been any change in your interest in sex?**
- **Have you seemed super-efficient at work, or as though you had special powers or talents quite out of the ordinary?**

24.4 Rapid exclusion of medical emergencies presenting as psychosis

Some treatable medical emergencies may present with psychosis and these must be rapidly excluded. Consideration should always be given to:

Intracranial emergencies:

- *Intracranial infection*. Fever and altered consciousness must prompt consideration of encephalitis (particularly in the presence of headache, meningeal signs, focal neurological signs, or focal seizures). The most common infectious cause of limbic encephalitis is HSV (Chapter 8.2.1 ▶); this is destructive to brain tissue and treatable.
- *Cerebral infarction*. An acute onset of focal neurological signs warrants immediate imaging and assessment, including regarding the need for thrombolysis in the case of ischaemic stroke [1255].
- *Epilepsy*. Consider in particular non-convulsive status epilepticus (Chapter 6.2 ▶), which needs to be terminated rapidly. Consider this particularly in the presence of confusion and psychosis with fluctuating consciousness (which may be accompanied by episodic hallucinations, marked mood changes, bizarre behaviour, and complex automatisms).
- *Intracranial mass lesions*, heralded by localizing neurological signs and/or red-flag features described in Chapter 6.7 ▶.

Systemic emergencies:

- *Systemic causes of delirium*. Altered consciousness and cognition (including confusion and/or drowsiness) is the hallmark of delirium. The history, examination, and tests described in Chapter 3 ▶ should give a good indication as to the most likely cause. Delirium is not a final diagnosis and a cause must be sought urgently. Some causes (e.g. hypoxia, hypotension, hypoglycaemia) are immediately life-threatening; see Chapter 3 ▶.
- *Endocrine disease*. Consider in particular severe hypothyroidism, severe hyperthyroidism (Chapter 9.1 ▶), and adrenal insufficiency (Chapter 9.3 ▶).
- *Nutritional deficiency*. Consider in particular thiamine deficiency (Wernicke's encephalopathy, particularly in the presence of cognitive impairment, eye signs, or ataxia; Chapter 11.1 ▶) and niacin deficiency encephalopathy (background malnutrition or alcoholism, recent catabolic state, delirium or dementia, neuropathy, extrapyramidal signs, glossitis/stomatitis, diarrhoea, dermatitis; Chapter 11.2 ▶).
- *Poisoning*. Consider categories: (a) recreational drugs, including alcohol; (b) therapeutic drugs; (c) environmental exposure. For drug poisoning, consider withdrawal as well as intoxication. Consider also serotonin syndrome (recent use of serotonergic agents; tremor, rigidity, or hyperreflexia; fever, sweating, agitation; Chapter 15.2 ▶), anticholinergic poisoning ("blind as a bat, mad as a hatter, red as a beet, hot as a hare, and dry as a bone"; Chapter 15.4 ▶), and NMS/MC (autonomic instability including fever, tachycardia, labile blood pressure; rigidity, dyskinesia, other abnormal movements or catatonic features; altered consciousness; Chapter 19.2 ▶).

Either:

- *Unexplained inflammatory states* should prompt early consideration of the infectious (Chapter 8 ▶) and autoimmune (Chapter 13 ▶, Chapter 14 ▶) causes of psychosis.

Chapter 25

Initial investigations relevant to psychosis

Suggested initial investigations are given in Chapter 25.1 ▶.

Following these initial investigations, any abnormalities should be pursued (Chapter 25.2 ▶), both from a general medical stance and for their value in providing clues to the cause of psychosis.

25.1 Suggested initial investigations in psychosis

The basic set of investigations is debated (e.g. [1256, 1257]), and we could find no good evidence as to which tests should be performed; this area is one dominated by a range of opinions. We suggest one initial set of investigations below, divided into "always do" and "always consider", and then discuss the rationale for the tests. Tests have been included in this list only if they might be expected to yield an identifiable cause for psychosis or contribute substantially to general medical management or the drug treatment of psychosis.

Always do:

- *Bedside*: pulse oximetry, ECG*
- *Urine testing*: urine screen for common drugs of abuse (typically, cannabinoids, opiates, cocaine, amphetamines, MDMA, PCP, benzodiazepines, barbiturates); urinary βHCG in females who could be pregnant*
- *Haematology*: FBC, ESR
- *Biochemistry*: U&E, BFT, LFT, CRP, TSH (with free T4 ± T3 if TSH abnormal), CK, vitamin B_{12}, red cell folate, random or fasting glucose*, random or fasting lipid profile*
- *Microbiology*: syphilis serology

Always consider from the outset:

- *Bedside*: fingerprick capillary glucose, urine dipstick
- *Haematology*: clotting (PT and APTT)
- *Biochemistry*: Mg
- *Immunology*: ANA (with subtyping if positive)
- *Radiology*: MRI brain (T1, T2, and FLAIR sequences)
- *Neurophysiology*: EEG

Investigations marked (*): rationale

These investigations are infrequently relevant to the diagnosis of psychosis without suggestive features in the history or examination, but have significant implications for choice of antipsychotic treatment [1256].

glucose 6.1–6.9 mM with a 2-h glucose of <7.8 mM defines impaired fasting glucose [1279]. Glucose <3 mM defines hypoglycaemia [26].

ECG. The main indications for an ECG in psychosis are to measure the QT interval, and to help exclude clozapine-induced myocarditis. However, myocarditis and pericarditis may be associated with unusual inflammatory causes of psychosis (e.g. Churg–Strauss, sarcoid, SLE, microscopic polyangiitis, polyarteritis nodosa) and sometimes serious cardiac disease may result in delirious psychosis (e.g. MI).

Urine testing

Urine dipstick: protein. Proteinuria has many causes; think of infections (UTI), diabetes mellitus, renal inflammatory disorders (in the context of psychosis, e.g. SLE), intrinsic renal disorders (e.g. aminoaciduria, many causes of renal failure), malignancy (e.g. myeloma).

Urine dipstick: blood. Think of infection, trauma, stones, urinary tract cancer, nephritic syndrome, very prolonged exercise. Think also of other pigments (porphyria, myoglobinuria, drugs).

Urine dipstick: leukocytes. Pyuria (neutrophils in the urine) is commonly due to urinary infection, though it may also be drug-induced or seen in renal inflammatory disease (e.g. SLE).

Urine dipstick: nitrites. Nitrites (not nitrates!) are a specific indicator of bacteriuria. Humans don't make urinary nitrites. Nitrites imply bugs in the urine. This may be colonization (is the patient catheterized?) or, commonly, infection (symptoms? systemic inflammatory response?). Urinary infections are a common trigger for delirious psychosis, particularly in the elderly.

Urine drug screen. Consider drug-induced psychosis.

Haematology

FBC: WBC and differential. Consider not just the total white cell count but, more importantly, the differential (the absolute values of subtypes of leukocytes). In particular [673, 1280–1283]:

- *Neutrophilia.* Most commonly due to infection (typically bacterial), but also to other inflammatory disorders (including infarction); it can also be due to other alterations in neutrophil release from marrow, margination, or egress from circulation (e.g. steroids, trauma and severe pain, afebrile seizues, hypoxia), and much more rarely due to malignancy (myeloproliferation and as a paraneoplastic reaction) and other causes.
- *Neutropenia.* A feature of some bacterial infections (e.g. typhoid, brucellosis, *Staphylococcus aureus*, rickettsia, TB), infection being the commonest kind of acquired neutropenia, but also bone marrow failure, a range of unusual haematological disorders, nutritional deficiencies (B_{12}, folate, copper), splenomegaly, and in response to a large number of drugs and toxins (including, in the context of psychosis, most notably clozapine but a number of other commonly used psychotropic drugs). Neutropenia of whatever cause is a very significant risk factor for bacterial infection; in addition to a "standard" examination, examine the skin, oral mucosa, lymph nodes, and perineum carefully.
- *Lymphocytosis.* Consider in particular viral infection (though also protozoal and intracellular bacterial infection), lymphoproliferative disorders (leukaemia, lymphoma), and occasionally primary immunodeficiencies. In viral infection, there may or may not be neutrophila as well.
- *Lymphopenia.* Consider acute infection of any cause (the lymphocytes have migrated out of the blood to be of more use elsewhere), but also HIV (broadening the infectious

differential diagnosis substantially), renal failure, marrow failure, steroid therapy, cytotoxic chemotherapy and radiotherapy, SLE, primary immunodeficiencies.

- *Eosinophilia.* Consider in particular helminth infection (in the context of psychosis most notably neurocysticercosis), allergic and hypersensitivity reactions, during convalescence from infection, adrenal insufficiency, and rarer causes such as neoplasia (e.g. lymphoma, paraneoplastic eosinophilia), Churg–Strauss syndrome/idiopathic hypereosinophilic syndrome, PAN, and sarcoidosis.
- *Monocytosis.* Consider viral infections (e.g. EBV), bacterial infections (e.g. tuberculosis, endocarditis, brucellosis, syphilis, rickettsial infections), and protozoal infections; recovery from neutropenia or acute infection; malignancies (haematological and paraneoplastic); autoimmune disease (e.g. SLE, sarcoidosis).

FBC: Hb and MCV/MCH. A few potentially psychotogenic conditions are specifically associated with anaemia (see neuroacanthocytosis; several of the infectious causes; hypothyroidism; Wilson's disease; mitochondrial encephalopathies; deficiencies of B_6, B_{12}, and folate; SLE; giant cell arteritis; ANCA-associated vasculitides; Reiter's disease; TTP; arsenic; lead; atrial myxoma; see also coeliac disease). More generally, divide into [1284, 1285]:

- microcytic, hypochromic anaemia (consider iron deficiency [the most common reason, so confirm with iron studies and consider why], chronic disease [and consider why], thalassaemias, lead poisoning, sideroblastic anaemia);
- macrocytic anaemia: check for megaloblastosis (megalocytes and segmented neutrophils) and divide into:
  - megaloblastic (B_{12} and folate deficiencies, other [e.g. drug-induced] impairment of DNA synthesis), and
  - non-megaloblastic (alcohol abuse, liver disease, myelodysplasia, hypothyroidism and hypopituitarism, reticulocytosis, hypoplastic/aplastic anaemia, bone marrow infiltration);
- normochromic anaemia: divide into
  - hyperproliferative (reticulocytes raised >2%) (haemorrhage and haemolytic anaemia), and
  - hypoproliferative (leukaemia, aplastic anaemia, pure red cell aplasia).

Erythrocytosis or polycythaemia is relatively uncommon, and rarely relevant to psychosis (see polycythaemia rubra vera). Secondary polycythaemia is typically due to hypoxia or inappropriate erythropoietin production [1286].

FBC: Platelets. Thrombocytosis is either primary (myeloproliferation) or reactive, the latter often being secondary to inflammation (platelets are acute-phase reactants) and therefore non-specific. Hyposplenism (failure to destroy old platelets) may also elevate the platelet count, as may bleeding and iron-deficiency anaemia [1287]. Thrombocytopenia may be due to decreases in production (vitamin B_{12} or folate deficiency, liver disease, systemic infection, drug-induced myelosuppression, some hereditary platelet disorders) or increases in consumption (idiopathic thrombocytopenia purpura, TTP, HIV, excessive clotting, drug-induced autoimmune platelet destruction) [1288].

Clotting: PT/INR. Elevated in conditions including liver synthetic failure, disseminated intravascular coagulation, and by warfarin. The INR is simply the ratio of the patient's PT to the normal PT, corrected for the local lab's assay.

Clotting: APTT. Elevated by liver synthetic failure (though in this context concentrate on the PT instead), by warfarin (likewise), by heparin (leaving the PT unchanged), and by a number of coagulopathies (e.g. disseminated intravascular coagulation, haemophilia, lupus anticoagulant). The APTT may be lowered in an acute phase reaction (i.e. by inflammation).

ESR. Often elevated in inflammatory conditions; therefore a key screening test. See also the CRP. If the ESR is markedly elevated and the CRP is not, consider in particular SLE and HIV. The ESR is slower to go up and slower to go down than the CRP .

Biochemistry

U&E: Na. Severe hyponatraemia causing psychosis. Other conditions associated with psychosis and hyponatraemia (e.g. tuberculosis, hypothyroidism, hypoadrenalism, porphyria, hepatic failure, SLE, anti-VGKC encephalopathy). Other causes of hyponatraemia are legion (see text); think particularly in this context of psychotropic drugs. Very rarely, hypernatraemia causing psychosis. (Hypernatraemia nearly always indicates dehydration.)

U&E: K. Hypokalaemia: consider renal losses, gastrointestinal loss, drugs, a shift into cells, and malnutrition. Hypokalaemia causing psychosis is very rare. Check also Mg (especially if hypokalaemia appears refractory). Hyperkalaemia: think of renal failure, adrenal failure, rhabdomyolysis, and haemolysis (potassium that's leaked out of red cells after taking the sample). No specific association of hyperkalaemia with psychosis is known.

U&E: Urea and creatinine. Consider renal failure, and think why. (For an isolated or disproportionately raised urea, consider also dehydration, and protein breakdown or protein loads including gastrointestinal haemorrhage.) If the urea is low, think of urea cycle disorders.

Mg. Hypomagnesaemia is rarely an isolated cause of psychosis. Check for associated abnormalities of K, Ca, PO_4. Consider alcohol and diuretics, GI loss or malabsoroption, renal or adrenal disease, and thyroid disease. Hypermagnesaemia is very rare and suggests renal failure with excessive magnesium intake.

BFT: Calcium (corrected). If low: relating to psychosis: hypocalcaemia causing psychosis; hypocalcaemia in the context of velocardiofacial syndrome; malignant catatonia. More generally: first consider hypoparathyroidism and vitamin D deficiency (check PTH, and look also at PO_4 and alkP). If high: hypercalcaemia causing psychosis; hypercalcaemia associated with other causes (e.g. hyperthyroidism, sarcoid).

BFT: Phosphate. Unlikely to be specifically helpful regarding psychosis, but consider together with Ca and alkP (q.v.).

LFT: albumin. Reduced in liver synthetic failure (check PT and clinically), inflammatory states as part of the acute phase response, malnutrition, protein loss (e.g. nephrotic syndrome, enteropathy). Unlikely to be very helpful in the diagnosis of psychosis.

LFT: Bilirubin. Remember prehepatic, hepatic, and posthepatic causes of jaundice. Isolated mild elevated unconjugated bilirubin is often due to Gilbert's syndrome, which is benign, but remember also haemolysis (check FBC and if there is anaemia, check lactate dehydrogenase, haptoglobin, reticulocytes). If other LFTs are abnormal, the more likely things to consider are hepatitis (if ALT raised disproportionately to alkP), cholestasis (if alkP raised disproportionately to ALT), liver synthetic failure (check PT, glucose, and clinically), and other causes of hepatocyte injury (see ALT).

LFT: ALT. Elevated following hepatocyte damage of any cause (ALT and the similar aspartate aminotransferase or AST are made in hepatocytes; ALT is more specific to the liver). Always remember viral hepatitis, non-alcoholic steatohepatitis, alcohol, and other drugs as causes, but consider also cholestasis (typically the alkP is more markedly raised), liver tumours, coeliac disease, autoimmune/metabolic liver disease, hepatic congestion in right ventricular failure, and strenuous exercise [1289].

LFT: AlkP. Alkaline phosphatase primarily comes from liver and bone. Within the liver, it is found in the bile duct epithelium. Therefore, consider patterns: ALT and alkP markedly raised, but ALT disproportionately so: think of hepatocellular injury. ALT and alkP raised, but the alkP disproportionately raised (and particularly with elevated bilirubin): think of cholestasis. AlkP raised but normal ALT: think of bone disease (e.g. metastasis? osteomalacia? fracture? hyperparathyroidism?). Consider also benign causes (pregnancy, adolescents, benign/familial) [1289]. A few of these diseases have a connection with psychosis, but the alkP is not a key indicator with regard to psychosis.

CRP. A key screening test, as the CRP is often elevated in inflammatory conditions. The commonest cause of an elevation is infection, and delirium is a common cause of psychosis; check clinically to find the likely source (and consider urinalysis, blood cultures, CXR, ± echocardiography, LP).

Thyroid function: TSH ± free T4 ± free T3. Consider hyperthyroidism or hypothyroidism causing psychosis; Hashimoto's encephalopathy with autoimmune thyroiditis. Consider also whether adrenal and pituitary function are normal. Causes of hypo-/hyperthyroidism and the interpretation of TFTs are described in Section 1.

CK. Neuroacanthocytosis; hypothyroidism; mitochondrial disease. Myopathy secondary to antipsychotic drugs. Neuroleptic malignant syndrome/malignant catatonia (markedly raised). Other myopathy or strenuous exercise.

Vitamin B_{12}. Vitamin B_{12} deficiency causing psychosis.

Red cell folate. Folate deficiency causing psychosis.

Microbiology

Syphilis serology. Syphilis. Check also the laboratory's method: syphilis serology may be performed using methods specific to treponemes (e.g. TPHA, ELISA methods) or not (e.g. VDRL), and these differ in their sensitivity, their specificity, and their response to late-stage infection or previously eradicated infection [336].

Immunology

ANA. SLE, Sjögren's syndrome, systemic sclerosis, sarcoidosis, NAIM.

Radiology

MRI head. Any brain structural abnormality within the scanner's spatial and contrast resolution (e.g. ischaemia, certain epileptogenic foci, tumours, demyelination, other white-matter disease), many of which are relevant to psychosis. The sensitivity to different abnormalities is adjustable according to the type of imaging sequence. MRI is markedly better than CT for detection of white-matter disease, encephalitis, and a number of other disorders [47, 1290, 1291]. Note that high-signal white-matter abnormalities on T2-weighted/FLAIR imaging are common: in one study they were present in 11% of those <39 years old, 31% of those aged 40–49, 47% aged 50–59, 60% aged 60–69, and 83% of those aged ≥70 [47]; however, their burden is of psychiatric significance [1292].

CT head. As for MRI, except CT is less sensitive for most conditions, excepting fresh blood and calcification, for which CT is superior [47]. Use as an investigation for psychosis when MRI is not available or cannot be tolerated (implanted metals sensitive to high-strength magnetic fields, claustrophobia).

Section 2 A clinical approach to the diagnosis of psychosis

Chapter 26

Putting it together: clinical and paraclinical clues

Given that the differential diagnosis of psychosis is so broad, it may be difficult to recall all relevant disorders when faced with an individual patient. Here, as an aide-mémoire, we list disorders from Section 1 with their common symptoms and signs given in groups, to assist answering questions such as "in what disorders that cause psychosis is cerebellar dysfunction also commonly seen?" We also list salient risk factors and clinical features. In what follows, **standard type** indicates non-psychiatric symptoms, signs, or laboratory abnormalities that are commonly observed in the disorder. ***Italic* type** indicates uncommon occurrences. **Absence** indicates symptom groups that are very rare, absent, or not frequently documented (so absence does *not* necessarily exclude the presence of a symptom group in a disorder). The list is based primarily on Section 1, though at times on the wider medical literature. There are often few detailed studies of symptom frequencies in rare diseases, or studies comparing symptom patterns between diseases, so each line is intended to be useful as a synopsis of individual diseases rather than a starting point for comparison of symptoms between diseases. For major references, see Section 1.

Key

Cog	cognitive dysfunction
Pyr	pyramidal motor dysfunction (upper motor neuron pattern weakness with hyperreflexia and increased tone in a spastic pattern – disproportionately increased tone in upper limb flexors and lower limb extensors)
BG	basal ganglia motor dysfunction (e.g. hypokinesia, bradykinesia, dystonia, dyskinesia, rigidity [increase in tone equal in flexors and extensors], akathisia, tremor, chorea, athetosis, ballismus)
Cer	cerebellar dysfunction (e.g. limb ataxia, intention tremor, truncal ataxia, gait ataxia, dysarthria, nystagmus)
Sen	sensory disturbance (beyond peripheral neuropathy)
NF	relatively non-focal non-psychiatric neurological disease, e.g. disturbance of consciousness, diffuse encephalopathy, seizures
MR	structural brain abnormalities detectable
PN	peripheral or cranial neuropathies, including lower motor neuron signs
Aut	autonomic dysfunction
CV	cardiovascular involvement
Resp	respiratory tract involvement
Hep	liver involvement
GI	other gastrointestinal involvement (including nausea/vomiting)
Ren	renal involvement or basic electrolyte disturbance
Sk	skin involvement
MSk	musculoskeletal (e.g. myalgia, myositis, myopathy, arthralgia, arthritis, skeletal deformity)
Hae	haematological disturbance
End	endocrine abnormality
Infl	inflammation and related systemic symptoms (e.g. fever, acute phase response)
Dev	developmental abnormalities, including dysmorphism
Key points	important risk factors and clinical features

DELIRIUM	Cog	Pyr	BG	Cer	Sen	NF	MR	PN	Aut	CV	Resp	Hep	GI	Ren	Sk	MSk	Hae	End	Infl	Dev	Key points
Delirium (depends on specific cause; can include any of these features, except by definition acute in onset and involves cognitive disturbance)	Cog	*Pyr*	*BF*	*Cer*	*Sen*	*NF*	*MR*	*PN*	*Aut*	*CV*	*Resp*	*Hep*	*GI*	*Ren*	*Sk*	*MSk*	*Hae*	*End*	*Infl*		Cognition and consciousness disturbed acutely. Multiple causes.
NEURODEVELOPMENTAL DISORDERS AND CHROMOSOMAL ABNORMALITIES	**Cog**	**Pyr**	**BG**	**Cer**	**Sen**	**NF**	**MR**	**PN**	**Aut**	**CV**	**Resp**	**Hep**	**GI**	**Ren**	**Sk**	**MSk**	**Hae**	**End**	**Infl**	**Dev**	**Key points**
Velocardiofacial syndrome	Cog									CV								End		Dev	Cardiac, palatal, facial, parathyroid abnormalities.
Trisomy 21	Cog				Sen	NF				CV			GI				*Hae*	End		Dev	Characteristic dysmorphism, strong predisposition to Alzheimer's disease, plus hypothyroidism, malabsorption, autoimmunity.
XXY (Klinefelter's syndrome)																		End		*Dev*	Hypogonadal men, features often subtle.
XXX (triple X)	*Cog*					*NF*	MR							*Ren*				*End*		*Dev*	Females, tall stature, epicanthic folds, clinodactyly.
XXYY	Cog									CV								End		Dev	Tall hypogonadal men.
Trisomy 8	Cog						MR			CV				Ren		MSk				Dev	Skeletal malformations (marfanoid), developmental delay.
Fragile X	Cog															MSk		*End*		Dev	In males, macroorchidism, facial dysmorphism, flat feet, lax joints, learning disability. Milder in females.

NEURODEVELOPMENTAL DISORDERS AND CHROMOSOMAL ABNORMALITIES	Cog	Pyr	BG	Cer	Sen	NF	MR	PN	Aut	CV	Resp	Hep	GI	Ren	Sk	MSk	Hae	End	Infl	Dev	Key points
45,X karyotype (Turner's syndrome)	Cog				Sen					CV				Ren		MSk		End		Dev	Females with short stature, webbed neck, cubitus valgus.
Agenesis of the corpus callosum							MR														—
Agenesis of the corpus callosum with peripheral neuropathy						NF	MR	PN												Dev	Mild facial dysmorphism, learning disability, seizures, sensorimotor neuropathy.
Acrocephalosyndactyly							MR									MSk				Dev	Skull abnormalities, syndactyly.
Prader–Willi syndrome	Cog						MR			*CV*								End		Dev	Hyperphagia, mild learning disability, mood swings, obsessional, skin-picking, hypogonadal, depigmentation.
Phenylketonuria	Cog					NF	MR								Sk					Dev	Mouse-like odour, learning disability, epilepsy.
X-linked mental retardation: PAK3	Cog																				Learning disability.
X-linked mental retardation: PPM-X	Cog	Pyr	BG																	Dev	Learning disability, parkinsonian, pyramidal, macroorchidism.
X-linked mental retardation: Coffin–Lowry	Cog				Sen	*NF*										MSk				Dev	Skeletal malformations, growth retardation, hearing deficit, paroxysmal movement disorders, drop attacks, cognitive impairment.
X-linked mental retardation: marfanoid (inc. Lujan–Fryns syndrome)										*CV*						MSk				Dev	Marfanoid.

NEURODEVELOPMENTAL DISORDERS AND CHROMOSOMAL ABNORMALITIES	Cog	Pyr	BG	Cer	Sen	NF	MR	PN	Aut	CV	Resp	Hep	GI	Ren	Sk	MSk	Hae	End	Infl	Dev	Key points
Bardet–Biedl syndrome	Cog				Sen							Hep		Ren		MSk		End		Dev	Retinitis pigmentosa, obesity, hypogonadism, polydactyly or syndactyly, learning disability, renal dysfunction.
Darier–White disease (keratosis follicularis)															Sk						Warty papules and plaques in seborrhoeic areas.
DIDMOAD (Wolfram's syndrome)					Sen													End			Diabetes insipidus, diabetes mellitus, optic atrophy, deafness.
Lafora disease	Cog					NF															Progressive myoclonic epilepsy, often occipital seizures.
Landau–Kleffner syndrome						NF															Aphasia and epilepsy in young children.
Myoclonic dystonia			BG																		Tremulous/jerky dystonia, sometimes with a dramatic response to alcohol.
Norrie disease	Cog				Sen	*NF*															Early childhood blindness, sometimes deafness.
Oculocutaneous albinism					Sen										Sk					Dev	Decreased pigment, other eye abnormalities.
Sjögren–Larsson syndrome	Cog	Pyr			Sen	NF									Sk					Dev	Hyperkeratosis with diplegia or quadriplegia, learning disability, frequently seizures.
Succinic semialdehyde dehydrogenase deficiency	Cog		*BG*			NF	*MR*														Developmental delay, abnormal eye movements, hyporeflexia and hypotonia, seizures.

NEURODEVELOPMENTAL DISORDERS AND CHROMOSOMAL ABNORMALITIES	Cog	Pyr	BG	Cer	Sen	NF	MR	PN	Aut	CV	Resp	Hep	GI	Ren	Sk	MSk	Hae	End	Infl	Dev	Key points
Neurocutaneous melanosis							MR								Sk						Large or multiple congenital melanocytic naevi, melanocytic meningeal tumours.
NEURODEGENERATIVE DISORDERS	**Cog**	**Pyr**	**BG**	**Cer**	**Sen**	**NF**	**MR**	**PN**	**Aut**	**CV**	**Resp**	**Hep**	**GI**	**Ren**	**Sk**	**MSk**	**Hae**	**End**	**Infl**	**Dev**	**Key points**
Alzheimer's disease	Cog	*Pyr*	*BG*	*Cer*	Sen		*MR*														Progressive cognitive decline in ≥2 domains including memory; motor neurological features are typically late. Anosmia.
Parkinson's disease			BG		Sen																Resting tremor, rigidity, bradykinesia, and (later) postural instability. Anosmia.
"Parkinson's plus" syndromes	Cog	Pyr	BG	Cer				PN	Aut												Parkinsonism with prominent other features (e.g. pyramidal signs, autonomic instability, supranuclear ophthalmoplegia).
Dementia with Lewy bodies	Cog		BG			NF			Aut												Visual hallucinations, dementia with fluctuating cognition, spontaneous motor features of parkinsonism.
Asymmetric cortical degeneration syndromes (inc. FTD, Pick's)	Cog	*Pyr*	*BG*		*Sen*				*Aut*												In FTD, personality change, abulia or disinhibition, relatively preserved memory, sometimes parkinsonism.
Motor neuron disease	*Cog*	Pyr			*Sen*		*MR*	PN													Mixture of upper and lower motor neuron signs, sometimes also FTD.

NEURODEGENERATIVE DISORDERS	Cog	Pyr	BG	Cer	Sen	NF	MR	PN	Aut	CV	Resp	Hep	GI	Ren	Sk	MSk	Hae	End	Infl	Dev	Key points
Huntington's disease	Cog		BG		Sen		MR														Family history with anticipation; chorea, dementia, OCD, depression. Caudate atrophy on MRI. Anosmia.
Dentatorubropallidoluysian atrophy	Cog		BG	Cer		NF	MR														Some combination of movement disorder, epilepsy, dementia. Characteristic MRI findings.
Spinocerebellar ataxia	*Cog*	Pyr		Cer	Sen			PN													Ataxia with pyramidal, extrapyramidal, and/or sensory signs.
Neuroacanthocytosis	Cog		BG	Cer		NF		PN		*CV*						MSk	Hae				Movement disorder, cognitive deterioration, seizures, neuropathy, myopathy. Sometimes lip/tongue-biting.
Basal ganglia calcification	Cog		BG			NF	MR														Parkinsonism/chorea, subcortical dementia, sometimes stroke-like events/ syncope. Calcification on CT.
PKAN	Cog	Pyr	BG	*Cer*		NF	MR	*PN*													Progressive dementia, pyramidal and extrapyramidal signs. Characteristic MRI findings.
Neuroferritinopathy	*Cog*		BG				MR														Autosomal dominant, progressive movement disorder. BG abnormalities on MRI.
Thalamic dementia	Cog	*Pyr*	*BG*			*NF*	*MR*														Dementia ± apathy, somnolence, emaciation, myoclonus.
Familial British/Danish dementia (psychosis	Cog			Cer	Sen	*NF*															Cataracts, hearing loss, cerebellar ataxia, psychosis and

NEURODEGENERATIVE DISORDERS	**Cog**	**Pyr**	**BG**	**Cer**	**Sen**	**NF**	**MR**	**PN**	**Aut**	**CV**	**Resp**	**Hep**	**GI**	**Ren**	**Sk**	**MSk**	**Hae**	**End**	**Infl**	**Dev**	**Key points**
Hereditary endotheliopathy with retinopathy, nephropathy, and stroke (HERNS)	Cog				Sen	NF								Ren							Retinopathy, frequent migraine, stroke-like episodes and dementia. Resembles CADASIL.
Leptomeningeal amyloidosis	Cog	*Pyr*			Sen	NF															Dementia, seizures, strokes, visual deterioration.
Pelizaeus–Merzbacher disease	Cog	Pyr		Cer			MR		Aut												In late-onset form, cerebellar and pyramidal signs, autonomic dysfunction, dementia. Progressive cortical and subcortical white matter abnormalities on MRI.
PLOSL	Cog	*Pyr*				*NF*										MSk					Early dementia, bone cysts in the wrists and ankles.
OTHER FOCAL NEUROLOGICAL DISEASE	**Cog**	**Pyr**	**BG**	**Cer**	**Sen**	**NF**	**MR**	**PN**	**Aut**	**CV**	**Resp**	**Hep**	**GI**	**Ren**	**Sk**	**MSk**	**Hae**	**End**	**Infl**	**Dev**	**Key points**
CVAs and vascular dementia	Cog	*Pyr*	*BG*	*Cer*	*Sen*	*NF*	MR						*GI*								Typically atherosclerotic (vascular risk factors e.g. age, smoking, hypertension, hyperlipidaemia, diabetes). Stepwise neurological deterioration. Infarcts on MRI. In atypical cases, or stroke in the young, see rare causes (see text) including:
… CADASIL	Cog	*Pyr*	*BG*	*Cer*	*Sen*	*NF*	MR														Early strokes, white-matter infarcts/dementia, migraine.

OTHER FOCAL NEUROLOGICAL DISEASE	**Cog**	**Pyr**	**BG**	**Cer**	**Sen**	**NF**	**MR**	**PN**	**Aut**	**CV**	**Resp**	**Hep**	**GI**	**Ren**	**Sk**	**MSk**	**Hae**	**End**	**Infl**	**Dev**	**Key points**
… Moyamoya disease	Cog	Pyr	BG		Sen	NF	*MR*														Transient exercise-or hyperventilation- induced neurological deficit, seizures, or headaches (children), or intracranial haemorrhage (adults).
… Thromboangiitis obliterans	*Cog*	*Pyr*	*BG*	*Cer*	*Sen*	*NF*	MR			CV											Smokers, peripheral ischaemia, TIA/CVA, seizures, migraine, lack of inflammation.
… Cerebral venous and sinus thrombosis	*Cog*	Pyr	BG	Cer	Sen	NF	MR						GI								Triggers: thrombophilia, pregnancy/Pill, intracranial infection. Headache, seizures, focal signs. Signs on MRV.
Subdural haematoma	Cog	Pyr			Sen	NF	MR						GI								History of head trauma; old age, coagulopathy, alcoholism. Signs due to compression, particularly hemiparesis, headache, confusion, personality change, drowsiness [1293, 1294]. Psychosis very rare.
NEURODEGENERATIVE DISORDERS	**Cog**	**Pyr**	**BG**	**Cer**	**Sen**	**NF**	**MR**	**PN**	**Aut**	**CV**	**Resp**	**Hep**	**GI**	**Ren**	**Sk**	**MSk**	**Hae**	**End**	**Infl**	**Dev**	**Key points**
Epilepsy	Cog	Pyr			Sen	NF	*MR*														Recurrent seizures. Hallucinations with sensory cortical involvement; other psychotic features with temporal/frontal seizures. Postictal/interictal psychosis may occur.

NEURODEGENERATIVE DISORDERS	Cog	Pyr	BG	Cer	Sen	NF	MR	PN	Aut	CV	Resp	Hep	GI	Ren	Sk	MSk	Hae	End	Infl	Dev	Key points
Migraine	*Cog*	*Pyr*		*Cer*	Sen	NF			*Aut*				GI								Simple hallucinatory aura common, then headache. More rarely, more complex psychotic features or altered consciousness.
Hypertensive encephalopathy and posterior reversible encephalopathy syndrome	Cog	Pyr			Sen	NF	MR			CV			GI								Often severe hypertension. Early headache, nausea, visual loss and/or hallucinations, confusion. Progressive. Oedema on MRI.
Head injury (traumatic brain injury)	*Cog*	*Pyr*	*BG*	*Cer*	*Sen*	*NF*	MR														Immediately preceding head injury. (Longer-term risks for psychosis debated, though dementia pugilistica resembles Alzheimer's disease.)
Normal-pressure hydrocephalus	Cog	*Pyr*	BG				MR		Aut												Dementia, urinary incontinence, gait abnormalities.
Intracranial mass lesions (tumours) and obstructive hydrocephalus	*Cog*	*Pyr*	*BG*	*Cer*	*Sen*	*NF*	MR						GI								Focal clinical and imaging findings (see main text). Sometimes headache, nausea/vomiting, seizures, papilloedema.
Multiple sclerosis	Cog	Pyr	*BG*	Cer	Sen	NF	MR		Aut												Focal lesions separated in time and space. Internuclear ophthalmoplegia, optic atrophy (disc pallor), Lhermitte's symptom, Uhthoff's phenomenon all relatively specific. Demyelination on MRI.

NEURODEGENERATIVE DISORDERS	**Cog**	**Pyr**	**BG**	**Cer**	**Sen**	**NF**	**MR**	**PN**	**Aut**	**CV**	**Resp**	**Hep**	**GI**	**Ren**	**Sk**	**MSk**	**Hae**	**End**	**Infl**	**Dev**	**Key points**
Central pontine and extrapontine myelinolysis	Cog	Pyr	*BG*				MR	PN						Ren							Neurological deterioration following rapid correction of hyponatraemia, MRI shows pontine demyelination.
Tuberous sclerosis	Cog					NF	MR			*CV*	*Resp*			*Ren*	Sk	*MSk*				Dev	Multiple hamartomas. Early-onset epilepsy, some learning disability, skin lesions (hypopigmented macules, "shagreen" plaque, café au lait patches, fibromas, angiomas).
MALIGNANCY	**Cog**	**Pyr**	**BG**	**Cer**	**Sen**	**NF**	**MR**	**PN**	**Aut**	**CV**	**Resp**	**Hep**	**GI**	**Ren**	**Sk**	**MSk**	**Hae**	**End**	**Infl**	**Dev**	**Key points**
See tumours above and PLE below. Also:																					Be suspicious if there are systemic features or focal signs of cancer (e.g. weight loss, cough, haemoptysis, change in bowel habit, blood in stool).
Phaeochromocytoma	*Cog*					NF			Aut	CV					Sk						Paroxysmal headache, sweating, palpitations, hypertension.
Carcinoid	*Cog*								Aut	CV	Resp		GI		Sk						Diarrhoea, flushing, fatigue, wheeze and dyspnoea, palpitations, hypotension.
Lymphomatoid granulomatosis	Cog	Pyr		Cer		NF	MR	PN			Resp			Ren	Sk	MSk	Hae		Infl		Immunosuppressed patients, lung disease, polyfocal neurological abnormalities.
Intravascular large-B-cell lymphoma	Cog	Pyr	BG	Cer	Sen	NF	MR								Sk		Hae	End			Multifocal or non-specific abnormalities (clinical and on MRI); mimics MS and CNS vasculitis.
Leptomeningeal carcinomatosis	Cog	Pyr		*Cer*	Sen	NF	MR	PN													Infiltration of meninges by pre-existing carcinoma.

INFECTIOUS AND POSTINFECTIOUS SYNDROMES	Cog	Pyr	BG	Cer	Sen	NF	MR	PN	Aut	CV	Resp	Hep	GI	Ren	Sk	MSk	Hae	End	Infl	Dev	Key points
Pyogenic bacterial meningitis						NF	MR			*CV*			*GI*		*Sk*		Hae		Infl		Fever, headache, nausea, vomiting, irritability, photophobia, nuchal and back rigidity, Kernig's sign, Brudzinski's sign.
Intracranial abscess	Cog	*Pyr*	*BG*	*Cer*	*Sen*	NF	MR			*CV*			*GI*				Hae		Infl		Fever, mass effect, focal signs.
Neurosyphilis	Cog	*Pyr*			*Sen*	NF		PN		CV		Hep	GI	Ren	Sk	MSk	Hae		Infl		Tertiary syphilis, more common in the immunosuppressed. Argyll–Robertson pupils and tabes dorsalis relatively specific. Facial, dental, and skeletal abnormalities in congenital syphilis.
Lyme disease	Cog	*Pyr*		*Cer*		NF	MR	PN		CV		Hep			Sk	MSk			Infl		Travel to an endemic area. Erythema migrans, arthritis, fatigue, neuropathies, carditis (AV block).
Bartonella infection		*Pyr*			*Sen*	NF		*PN*		*CV*					Sk	*MSk*			Infl		Cats, lice. In the immunosuppressed, multi-organ involvement including skin nodules.
Leptospirosis	Cog					*NF*		PN		*CV*	Resp	Hep		Ren	*Sk*	MSk	Hae		Infl		Rat urine. Fever, 'flu-like illness, confusion, jaundice, renal involvement, abnormal LFTs, low platelets, raised CK.
Tuberculosis			*BG*			NF	MR	PN			Resp	*Hep*		*Ren*				*End*	Infl		Previous non-CNS TB, immunosuppression. TB meningitis with headache, fever, meningism, basal cranial nerve palsies.

INFECTIOUS AND POSTINFECTIOUS SYNDROMES	Cog	Pyr	BG	Cer	Sen	NF	MR	PN	Aut	CV	Resp	Hep	GI	Ren	Sk	MSk	Hae	End	Infl	Dev	Key points
Brucellosis						NF	*MR*	PN		*CV*	Resp	Hep	GI		Sk	MSk	Hae		Infl		Animal exposure. Fever, joint/abdominal/testicular pain, rashes, hepatosplenomegaly, varied neurological picture.
Whipple's disease	Cog	Pyr	*BG*	Cer	Sen	NF	*MR*	PN		*CV*	*Resp*		GI		*Sk*	MSk	*Hae*	End	Infl		Middle-aged white males. Arthralgia; later weight loss, diarrhoea (malabsorption), abdominal pain, CNS involvement. Oculomasticatory myorhythmia pathognomonic.
Typhus	Cog					NF				CV	Resp	Hep		Ren	Sk		Hae		Infl		Lice, ticks. Fever, lymphadenopathy, rash, multi-organ involvement.
Typhoid	Cog					NF						Hep	GI	Ren	Sk		Hae		Infl		*Salmonella*. Fever, constipation then diarrhoea; cough, sore throat, abnormal LFTs.
Rocky Mountain spotted fever	Cog				*Sen*	NF					Resp	Hep	GI	*Ren*	Sk	MSk	Hae		Infl		Travel to endemic area. Fever, headache, rash.
Mycoplasma pneumoniae	*Cog*					NF					Resp								Infl		Pneumonia, pharyngitis/otitis/conjunctivitis.
Legionnaire's disease	Cog			Cer		NF				CV	Resp		GI	Ren		MSk	Hae		Infl		Pneumonia, diarrhoea, confusion.
Q fever	*Cog*					NF					Resp	Hep	GI	Ren			Hae		Infl		Pneumonia, headache, nausea/vomiting, diarrhoea.
Chlamydophila pneumoniae	*Cog*					NF					Resp								Infl		Pharyngitis, then pneumonia.
Psittacosis	Cog					NF				CV	Resp								Infl		Pneumonia, haemoptysis, headache, relative bradycardia.

INFECTIOUS AND POSTINFECTIOUS SYNDROMES	**Cog**	**Pyr**	**BG**	**Cer**	**Sen**	**NF**	**MR**	**PN**	**Aut**	**CV**	**Resp**	**Hep**	**GI**	**Ren**	**Sk**	**MSk**	**Hae**	**End**	**Infl**	**Dev**	**Key points**
Viral encephalitis	Cog	Pyr	*BG*	Cer	*Sen*	NF	MR	PN	Aut								Hae	End	Infl		Fever, headache, altered consciousness, some meningeal signs, focal signs (inc. seizures), inflammation on MRI.
HIV seroconversion encephalitis						NF					*Resp*		*GI*		Sk	MSk	Hae		Infl		Risk factors for HIV (e.g. intravenous drug abuse, risky sexual practices). 'Flu-like illness with fever and rash, sometimes weight loss and oral ulceration.
AIDS dementia	Cog	Pyr	BG	Cer	*Sen*		MR	PN									Hae				Established HIV infection, progressive cognitive and neurological decline, exclusion of other intracranial infections.
Rabies						NF		PN	Aut										Infl		Bite from infected mammal. Local pain/paraesthesiae, then spread to CNS and encephalopathy (hydrophobia and aerophobia virtually pathognomonic).
SSPE	Cog	Pyr	*BG*	*Cer*		NF	MR														Personality change and intellectual decline 7–12 years after measles infection (or more quickly in the immunosuppressed). Multiple lesions on MRI.
PML	Cog	Pyr	BG	Cer	Sen	NF	MR														Immunosuppressed patients. Focal neurological deficits, seizures, memory impairment, psychomotor retardation, and inattentiveness.

INFECTIOUS AND POSTINFECTIOUS SYNDROMES	Cog	Pyr	BG	Cer	Sen	NF	MR	PN	Aut	CV	Resp	Hep	GI	Ren	Sk	MSk	Hae	End	Infl	Dev	Key points
Malaria						NF				CV	Resp	Hep	GI	*Ren*		MSk	Hae		Infl		Travel to an endemic area. Fever, anaemia, thrombocytopenia, jaundice.
Toxoplasmosis	Cog	Pyr				NF	MR												Infl		Large proportion of humans infected. Overt encephalitis typically in the immunosuppressed.
Trypanosomiasis		*Pyr*	BG	Cer	Sen	NF				CV					Sk		Hae		Infl		Narrow geographical distribution; fly bite. Systemic haemolymphatic disease followed by encephalitis.
Fungal infection	Cog					NF	MR	PN											Infl		Typically immunosuppressed patients. Fever, malaise, headache, and altered cognition, behaviour, and/or level of consciousness. Dilated Virchow–Robin spaces or miliary enhancing lesions on MRI.
Neurocysticercosis	Cog	Pyr			Sen	NF	MR			*CV*					Sk				Infl		Infected pork. Epilepsy, headaches, intracranial hypertension, eosinophilic meningitis, stroke.
CJD	Cog	Pyr	BG	Cer	Sen	NF	MR														*Sporadic CJD*: rapidly progressive cognitive impairment, cerebellar dysfunction, or both, then rapid neurological progression. Myoclonic jerks (limb or whole body) develop early.

INFECTIOUS AND POSTINFECTIOUS SYNDROMES	Cog	Pyr	BG	Cer	Sen	NF	MR	PN	Aut	CV	Resp	Hep	GI	Ren	Sk	MSk	Hae	End	Infl	Dev	Key points
																					Variant CJD: Sensory symptoms (limb pain), psychiatric abnormalities earlier; myoclonus later.
GSS	Cog			Cer																	Autosomal dominant. Slowly progressive ataxia with dementia.
FFI	Cog	Pyr							Aut												Autosomal dominant. Severe insomnia, autonomic dysregulation, dementia, and motor paralysis
Sydenham's chorea and PANDAS	Cog	*Pyr*	BG							CV					Sk	MSk			Infl		Streptococcal infection (e.g. sore throat) followed by rheumatic fever (arthritis, carditis, chorea, erythema marginatum, and/or skin nodules) and subsequent autoimmunity; neurological features may lag the others. More common in children and pregnant women.
Encephalitis lethargica			BG			NF		PN													Pharyngitis followed by hypersomnolence, postencephalitic parkinsonism, cranial nerve palsies.
Postinfectious encephalomyelitis and acute disseminated encephalomyelitis		Pyr	*BG*	*Cer*	Sen	NF	MR	PN											Infl		Autoimmune response up to 2 weeks following infections or some vaccines. Resembles severe MS, sometimes encephalopathic. MRI becomes abnormal 5–14 days after symptom onset.

ENDOCRINE DISEASE	Cog	Pyr	BG	Cer	Sen	NF	MR	PN	Aut	CV	Resp	Hep	GI	Ren	Sk	MSk	Hae	End	Infl	Dev	Key points
Hypothyroidism	Cog			*Cer*	*Sen*	*NF*			Aut	CV		Hep	GI	Ren	Sk	MSk	Hae	End			Fatigue, cold intolerance, dry skin/hair, weight gain, constipation, carpal tunnel, menstrual disturbance, bradycardia, diastolic hypertension, hoarseness, goitre, periorbital and peripheral oedema, hyporeflexia, depression or mania, cognitive impairment.
Hyperthyroidism	*Cog*		*BG*			*NF*			Aut	CV		Hep	GI		Sk	MSk	Hae	End			Hyperactivity, irritability, heat intolerance, tachycardia/AF, insomnia, fatigue, weakness, weight loss, diarrhoea, oligomenorrhoea, fine tremor, alopecia, proximal myopathy, hyperreflexia, eye signs.
Cushing's syndrome	Cog								Aut	CV			GI	*Ren*	Sk	MSk		End			Myopathy, weight gain, depression, obesity, plethora, moon face, hypertension, diabetes, infections, bruising, gastric ulceration.
Adrenal failure	Cog					NF			Aut	CV			GI	Ren	Sk	MSk		End			Postural hypotension, weakness, tiredness, weight loss, nausea, vomiting, abdominal pain, diarrhoea or constipation, malaise, muscle cramps, ± pigmentation. Low Na, high K, low glucose.
Hypopituitarism	Cog					NF	*MR*		Aut	CV		Hep	GI	Ren	Sk	MSk	Hae	End			Multiple hormone deficiencies (e.g. thyroid and adrenal failure). Sometimes pituitary adenoma on MRI.

ENDOCRINE DISEASE	Cog	Pyr	BG	Cer	Sen	NF	MR	PN	Aut	CV	Resp	Hep	GI	Ren	Sk	MSk	Hae	End	Infl	Dev	Key points
Hypoparathyroidism	Cog	Pyr	BG		Sen	NF				CV	Resp		GI	*Ren*		MSk		End			Features of hypocalcaemia (q.v.).
Hyperparathyroidism	Cog	Pyr				NF				CV			GI	Ren		MSk		End			Features of hypercalcaemia (q.v.).
Postpartum psychosis																					Psychosis after childbirth (the risk extends to at least 90 days).
INBORN ERRORS OF METABOLISM	**Cog**	**Pyr**	**BG**	**Cer**	**Sen**	**NF**	**MR**	**PN**	**Aut**	**CV**	**Resp**	**Hep**	**GI**	**Ren**	**Sk**	**MSk**	**Hae**	**End**	**Infl**	**Dev**	**Key points**
Hyperammonaemia and urea cycle disorders	Cog	Pyr		Cer		NF	*MR*					Hep	GI								Congenital disorders, Reye's syndrome, hepatic failure, and following drugs (e.g. valproate). Can be intermittent presentation with confusion and/or psychosis, triggered by high protein intake or catabolism.
Porphyria	Cog					NF	*MR*	PN	*Aut*	CV			GI	Ren		MSk					Neurovisceral attacks: abdominal pain (or other GI, urinary, or cardiovascular disturbance), neuropathy, psychiatric symptoms. May be hyponatraemia.
Hereditary tyrosinaemia				*Cer*		*NF*		PN					GI								Usually diagnosed in infancy. Can exhibit crises resembling porphyria.
Hyperhomocysteinaemia and homocystinuria	Cog	Pyr	BG	Cer			*MR*	PN		CV										*Dev*	Vitamin B_{12} or folate deficiency (e.g. dietary), or inborn errors of metabolism. Variable neurological picture, thromboembolism. Marfanoid appearance in some congenital forms.

INBORN ERRORS OF METABOLISM	**Cog**	**Pyr**	**BG**	**Cer**	**Sen**	**NF**	**MR**	**PN**	**Aut**	**CV**	**Resp**	**Hep**	**GI**	**Ren**	**Sk**	**MSk**	**Hae**	**End**	**Infl**	**Dev**	**Key points**
Hartnup's disease	Cog	*Pyr*		Cer		*NF*		PN					GI		Sk						Congenital. Resembles pellagra (niacin deficiency) ± ataxia.
Maple syrup urine disease				Cer		NF															Intermittent form has normal development but ataxia, lethargy, seizures ± coma triggered by catabolic stress.
Wilson's disease	Cog	Pyr	BG	Cer			MR					Hep		Ren	*Sk*	MSk	Hae				Movement disorder, liver disease, Kayser–Fleischer rings, cataracts, abnormalities on MRI.
Neuronal ceroid lipofuscinosis	Cog	Pyr	BG	Cer	*Sen*	NF	*MR*														Adult-onset form exhibits seizures and myoclonus or dementia with extrapyramidal or cerebellar signs.
Niemann–Pick disease, type C	Cog		*BG*	*Cer*		*NF*						Hep					*Hae*				Usually neurologically normal if presenting with psychosis. Vertical supranuclear ophthalmoplegia in 80%, though may be subtle. Movement disorders, dementia may occur. Splenomegaly, hepatomegaly.
Hexosaminidase deficiency	*Cog*	Pyr	BG	Cer				PN		*CV*											Lower motor neuron disease, cerebellar ataxia, or dystonia. Cherry-red macular spots. Acute psychotic episodes.
Mucopolysaccharidosis					Sen		MR			CV	Resp	Hep				MSk	Hae			Dev	Short stature, facial and skeletal abnormalities, hepatosplenomegaly, mild cardiac abnormalities, frequent respiratory infections.

INBORN ERRORS OF METABOLISM	Cog	Pyr	BG	Cer	Sen	NF	MR	PN	Aut	CV	Resp	Hep	GI	Ren	Sk	MSk	Hae	End	Infl	Dev	Key points
Fabry's disease		*Pyr*			Sen			PN	Aut	*CV*			GI	*Ren*					Infl		More severe in males. Lancinating pain in the extremities from childhood. Angiokeratomas. Diarrhoea after eating, febrile attacks with abdominal pain. Other features of autonomic neuropathy.
Aspartylglucosaminuria	Cog															MSk	Hae			Dev	Severe mental retardation, thick sagging skin of the cheeks, broad nose and face, short neck, cranial asymmetry, scoliosis, periodic hyperactivity, recurrent infections, vacuolated lymphocytes.
Metachromatic leukodystrophy	Cog	*Pyr*	*BG*			*NF*	MR	*PN*													Psychiatric features, cognitive impairment, motor involvement usually late in adult-onset forms. White matter abnormalities on MRI.
X-linked adrenoleukodystrophy	Cog	Pyr		Cer	Sen	NF	MR	PN	Aut	CV			GI	Ren	Sk	MSk		End			Adrenal insufficiency, testicular failure, neurological involvement.
Cerebrotendinous xanthomatosis	Cog	Pyr	BG	Cer			MR	PN		CV			GI			MSk					Tendon xanthomas, diarrhoea, atherosclerosis, cataracts. Cerebellar ataxia, pseudobulbar palsy, ± other neurological features. Low-normal serum cholesterol.

INBORN ERRORS OF METABOLISM	Cog	Pyr	BG	Cer	Sen	NF	MR	PN	Aut	CV	Resp	Hep	GI	Ren	Sk	MSk	Hae	End	Infl	Dev	Key points
Alpha-mannosidosis	Cog	Pyr		Cer	Sen	NF						Hep				MSk	Hae			Dev	Mild learning disability, progressive sensorineural hearing loss, immunodeficiency, dysmorphism, ± hepatosplenomegaly, progressive neurological dysfunction. Episodic psychosis or confusion followed by somnolence.
Krabbe's disease	*Cog*	Pyr					MR	PN													Pes cavus, optic disc pallor, progressive spastic tetraparesis, sensorimotor demyelinating neuropathy, demyelination on MRI.
Gaucher's disease	Cog	Pyr		Cer		NF	*MR*			CV	Resp	Hep			Sk	MSk	Hae				CNS involvement, bone disease, visceral disease (inc. hepatosplenomegaly), cytopenia, skin changes.
Vanishing white matter leukoencephalopathy	*Cog*	Pyr		Cer	*Sen*	*NF*	MR														Predominantly cerebellar ataxia and spasticity. Diffuse cystic degeneration of white matter on MRI.
Diffuse sclerosis	Cog	Pyr	*BG*	Cer	Sen	*NF*	MR														Cognitive impairment, mental state changes, deafness, other brainstem and cerebellar signs. Pseudotumoural demyelinating lesions on MRI; histologically like MS.

INBORN ERRORS OF METABOLISM	**Cog**	**Pyr**	**BG**	**Cer**	**Sen**	**NF**	**MR**	**PN**	**Aut**	**CV**	**Resp**	**Hep**	**GI**	**Ren**	**Sk**	**MSk**	**Hae**	**End**	**Infl**	**Dev**	**Key points**
Mitochondrial encephalopathies	Cog	Pyr	BG	Cer	Sen	NF	*MR*	PN		CV				Ren		MSk	Hae	End		Dev	Ptosis, ophthalmoplegia, retinopathy; diabetes, deafness, short stature, cardiac involvement, renal involvement, sideroblastic anaemia; dementia, ataxia, myoclonus, seizures, and stroke-like episodes; myopathy and peripheral neuropathy. Lactic acidosis during episodes.
Glucose-6-phosphate dehydrogenase deficiency																	Hae				Haemolysis triggered by infections, oxidative drugs, or broad beans.
NUTRITIONAL DEFICIENCY	**Cog**	**Pyr**	**BG**	**Cer**	**Sen**	**NF**	**MR**	**PN**	**Aut**	**CV**	**Resp**	**Hep**	**GI**	**Ren**	**Sk**	**MSk**	**Hae**	**End**	**Infl**	**Dev**	**Key points**
Thiamine (vitamin B_1) deficiency	Cog			Cer	*Sen*	*NF*	*MR*	PN	*Aut*	*CV*			GI			MSk					Common in alcoholism, malnutrition, malabsorption, hypermetabolic states. Tachycardia, weakness, decreased deep tendon reflexes, peripheral neuropathy. Wernicke's encephalopathy: mental state changes, ± eye signs, ataxia.
Niacin (vitamin B_3) deficiency	Cog	*Pyr*				*NF*		PN					GI		Sk						Alcoholism, malnutrition, increased metabolism are risk factors. Dementia (or acute encephalopathy), diarrhoea, and dermatitis.

NUTRITIONAL DEFICIENCY	Cog	Pyr	BG	Cer	Sen	NF	MR	PN	Aut	CV	Resp	Hep	GI	Ren	Sk	MSk	Hae	End	Infl	Dev	Key points
Pyridoxine (vitamin B_6) deficiency	Cog	*Pyr*	*BG*	*Cer*		*NF*	*MR*	PN		CV			GI		Sk		*Hae*				Risk factors are inflammatory states and some drugs. Can encompass signs of niacin deficiency (q.v.), homocystinaemia (q.v.), ± sideroblastic anaemia.
Cobalamin (vitamin B_{12}) deficiency, and methylmalonic aciduria	Cog	Pyr			Sen			PN	Aut	CV	Resp	Hep	GI				Hae		Infl		Pernicious anaemia, stomach or terminal ileal disorders. Peripheral neuropathy, subacute combined degeneration of the spinal cord, macrocytic anaemia, anorexia, weight loss, fever, optic atrophy (disc pallor).
Folate (vitamin B_9) deficiency	Cog												GI		Sk		Hae		Infl		Dietary deficiency, malabsorption, hypermetabolism, drugs. Glossitis/angular stomatitis, gastrointestinal symptoms, fever, hyperpigmentation, cognitive impairment, macrocytic anaemia.
Zinc deficiency	Cog			Cer	Sen								GI								Anorexia, disruption of taste and smell, dizziness, cerebellar dysfunction.
Starvation	Cog									CV		Hep	GI	*Ren*	Sk	MSk	Hae	End			Hallucinations typically of food, ± effects of nutritional deficiency.

OTHER ACQUIRED METABOLIC DISORDERS	Cog	Pyr	BG	Cer	Sen	NF	MR	PN	Aut	CV	Resp	Hep	GI	Ren	Sk	MSk	Hae	End	Infl	Dev	Key points
Global cerebral hypoxia	Cog	*Pyr*		*Cer*	Sen	NF	*MR*		Aut	CV	Resp										Hypo-oxygenation of blood or hypoperfusion of brain. May be myoclonus after global hypoxia.
Disturbances of pH and hypercapnic encephalopathy	Cog				Sen	NF			Aut	CV	Resp		GI	Ren							Respiratory disease, metabolic alkalosis (ingestion or renal/intestinal disease), metabolic acidosis (typically with compensatory hyperventilation).
Hypoglycaemia	Cog	*Pyr*			Sen	NF			Aut	CV											Commonly insulin/oral hypoglycaemics, alcohol; rarely others (see text). Sympathetic activation (unless autonomic compromise), agitation or decreased consciousness.
Renal failure	Cog		BG		Sen	NF				CV	Resp		GI	Ren	Sk	MSk	Hae	End			Drowsiness, confusion, impaired sleep, headache, visual abnormalities, tremor, muscle twitching/myoclonus.
Hepatic encephalopathy	Cog	*Pyr*		Cer	*Sen*	NF					*Resp*	Hep	GI	*Ren*	Sk		Hae	End			Many causes. Acute liver failure (jaundice, elevated liver enzymes, prolonged PT) or chronic liver failure (peripheral stigmata of chronic liver disease, portal hypertension, coagulopathy, ± jaundice).
Pancreatic encephalopathy	Cog	Pyr				NF							GI					End	Infl		Within the first 2 weeks of severe acute pancreatitis. Markedly raised amylase.

OTHER ACQUIRED METABOLIC DISORDERS	Cog	Pyr	BG	Cer	Sen	NF	MR	PN	Aut	CV	Resp	Hep	GI	Ren	Sk	MSk	Hae	End	Infl	Dev	Key points
Reye's syndrome	Cog					NF						Hep	GI	Ren							Associated with recent viral infection and aspirin use; rare in over-18s. Vomiting, neurological symptoms, hyperammonaemia, hepatic ± renal dysfunction.
Hyponatraemia	Cog	*Pyr*				NF								Ren				End			Many causes (esp. iatrogenic). Nonfocal neurological disturbance when severe.
Hypernatraemia	Cog	*Pyr*				NF								Ren				*End*			Usually due to dehydration. Severe thirst and confusion when severe.
Hypocalcaemia	Cog	Pyr	BG	*Cer*	Sen	NF				CV	Resp		GI	*Ren*		MSk		End			Bronchospasm, arrhythmia, dysphagia, biliary or intestinal colic, bladder dysfunction, muscle spasm and tetany, paraesthesiae and numbness, Chvostek's and Trousseau's signs, irritability, confusion, extrapyramidal movement disorders, seizures.
Hypercalcaemia	Cog	Pyr				NF				CV			GI	Ren		MSk		End			Most commonly from malignancy or primary hyperparathyroidism. "Moans, groans, stones, and bones, with psychic overtones." Depression, abdominal pain, constipation, weakness and joint/muscle pains, polyuria/polydipsia, headaches, hyperreflexia.

OTHER ACQUIRED METABOLIC DISORDERS	Cog	Pyr	BG	Cer	Sen	NF	MR	PN	Aut	CV	Resp	Hep	GI	Ren	Sk	MSk	Hae	End	Infl	Dev	Key points
Hypokalaemia	Cog				Sen					CV			GI	Ren		MSk		End			Palpitations, weakness, muscle cramps, paralysis, paraesthesiae, constipation, nausea, vomiting, abdominal pain, polyuria and polydipsia, delirium. ECG changes.
Hypomagnesaemia				Cer	Sen	NF				CV			GI	Ren		MSk		End			Weakness, tremor, seizures, paraesthesiae, tetany, Chvostek's/Trousseau's signs, nystagmus. ECG changes.
Hypophosphataemia	Cog					NF		PN			Resp		GI			MSk	Hae				Muscle weakness (skeletal, smooth, or cardiac muscle), rhabdomyolysis, neurological dysfunction, haematological impairments.
AUTOIMMUNE RHEUMATIC DISORDERS AND VASCULITIDES	**Cog**	**Pyr**	**BG**	**Cer**	**Sen**	**NF**	**MR**	**PN**	**Aut**	**CV**	**Resp**	**Hep**	**GI**	**Ren**	**Sk**	**MSk**	**Hae**	**End**	**Infl**	**Dev**	**Key points**
Systemic lupus erythematosus	Cog	Pyr	BG	Cer	Sen	NF	MR	PN	Aut	CV	Resp	Hep	GI	Ren	Sk	MSk	Hae	*End*	Infl		Multisystem autoimmune disorder, females>males. Classically raised ESR with normal CRP during flares.
Antiphospholipid syndrome	Cog	Pyr	BG		Sen	NF	*MR*	PN		CV							Hae		Infl		Vascular thrombosis or pregnancy morbidity (see text) with persistent antiphospholipid antibodies (see text).
Sjögren's syndrome		*Pyr*		*Cer*		*NF*	*MR*				Resp	Hep		Ren	Sk	MSk	Hae		Infl		Xerostomia, xerophthalmia, and/or arthritis.

AUTOIMMUNE RHEUMATIC DISORDERS AND VASCULITIDES	Cog	Pyr	BG	Cer	Sen	NF	MR	PN	Aut	CV	Resp	Hep	GI	Ren	Sk	MSk	Hae	End	Infl	Dev	Key points
Systemic sclerosis	*Cog*					*NF*							GI		Sk				Infl		Skin thickening and tethering, smooth muscle atrophy (sometimes with calcinosis, Raynaud's syndrome, oesophageal dysmotility, sclerodactyly, telangiectasia).
Mixed connective tissue disease	Cog	Pyr	BG	Cer	Sen	NF	MR	PN	Aut	CV	Resp	Hep	GI	Ren	Sk	MSk	Hae	*End*	Infl		Features of ≥2 connective tissue disorders.
Giant cell (temporal) arteritis					Sen			PN		CV		Hep		*Ren*		MSk	Hae		Infl		Typically extracranial arteritis (headache, scalp sensitivity, tender thickened arteries, tongue/ jaw claudication, face/ neck pain with nerve damage), ± myalgia, weight loss, malaise, fever, visual disturbance. Raised ESR.
Primary CNS angiitis	Cog	Pyr	BG	Cer	Sen	NF	MR												Infl		Gradual-onset headache, encephalopathy, and (usually) multifocal neurological signs. ESR, CSF, EEG, MRI usually abnormal.
Polyarteritis nodosa	*Cog*	*Pyr*	*BG*	*Cer*	Sen	NF	MR	PN		CV		Hep	GI	Ren	Sk	MSk	Hae		Infl		Multisystem. Systemic features include fever, weight loss, malaise; CNS features include amaurosis fugax. Typically elevated ESR and neutrophilia.
Wegener's granulomatosis		*Pyr*				*NF*		PN			Resp			Ren	Sk	MSk	Hae		Infl		Upper/lower respiratory tract and kidney, ± other systems; ANCA positive.

AUTOIMMUNE RHEUMATIC DISORDERS AND VASCULITIDES	Cog	Pyr	BG	Cer	Sen	NF	MR	PN	Aut	CV	Resp	Hep	GI	Ren	Sk	MSk	Hae	End	Infl	Dev	Key points
Microscopic polyangiitis						NF		PN		CV	Resp		GI	Ren	Sk	MSk	Hae		Infl		Skin, lung, kidney; ANCA positive.
Churg–Strauss syndrome								PN		CV	Resp		GI	Ren	Sk		Hae	End	Infl		Asthma, rhinitis, respiratory infections; then systemic eosinophilia; then systemic vasculitis.
Cogan's syndrome					Sen		MR				Resp	Hep	GI			MSk	Hae		Infl		Eye (interstitial keratitis) and auditory/vestibular symptoms (vertigo, tinnitus, decreased hearing), ± systemic features.
Eales' disease		Pyr			Sen		MR												Infl		Retinal vasculitis (esp. veins) ± vestibuloauditory dysfunction.
Susac's syndrome		*Pyr*		*Cer*	Sen	NF	MR												Infl		Encephalopathy, hearing loss, branch retinal artery occlusions.
Behçet's disease		Pyr					MR	*PN*					GI		Sk	MSk	Hae		Infl		Recurrent oral ulceration, genital ulceration, and eye inflammation, ± arthritis and CNS involvement. Abnormalities on MRI.
Reiter's disease						NF		PN							Sk	MSk	*Hae*		Infl		Seronegative arthropathy, urethritis, conjunctivitis, skin lesions. Autoimmune response (after e.g. gonorrhoea, dysentery).

AUTOIMMUNE RHEUMATIC DISORDERS AND VASCULITIDES	Cog	Pyr	BG	Cer	Sen	NF	MR	PN	Aut	CV	Resp	Hep	GI	Ren	Sk	MSk	Hae	End	Infl	Dev	Key points
Sarcoidosis	Cog	Pyr			Sen	NF	MR	PN		CV	Resp	Hep	*GI*	*Ren*	Sk	MSk		*End*	Infl		Granulomatous disorder with wide racial variation (most common in black races). Systemic features (fever, night sweats, etc.), multisystem involvement, skin disease (including keloid scarring, rashes, lupus pernio). CXR and brain MRI often abnormal.
Scleromyxoedema		*Pyr*				*NF*				CV	Resp		GI		Sk	MSk					Multisystem mucin deposition. Widespread eruption of small, waxy, firm papules on skin.
Thrombotic thrombocytopenic purpura	Cog	Pyr			Sen	NF								Ren	Sk		Hae		Infl		Spontaneous or triggered by drugs or diarrhoeal illness. Microangiopathic haemolytic anaemia, thrombocytopenic purpura, neurological disease, fever, and renal disease.
Polycythaemia	Cog	Pyr	BG		Sen	NF	MR			CV		*Hep*	*GI*				Hae				Thromboses at unusual sites, headaches, visual change, TIAs and strokes, fluctuating cognition.
Cryoglobulinaemia	Cog							PN			Resp		GI	Ren	Sk	MSk	Hae		Infl		Seen in lymphoproliferative disorders and chronic inflammatory disorders. Skin lesions (lesions in dependent areas), livedo reticularis, Raynaud's phenomenon, arthralgia, myalgia, and multisystem disease.

OTHER AUTOIMMUNE ENCEPHALOPATHIES	Cog	Pyr	BG	Cer	Sen	NF	MR	PN	Aut	CV	Resp	Hep	GI	Ren	Sk	MSk	Hae	End	Infl	Dev	Key points
Hashimoto's encephalopathy	Cog	*Pyr*	*BG*	*Cer*		NF						Hep						End	Infl		Otherwise unexplained encephalopathy with either antithyroid antibodies or history of autoimmune thyroiditis.
Autoimmune limbic encephalopathy, including paraneoplastic limbic encephalitis	Cog		BG	Cer		NF	MR	*PN*	Aut		Resp			Ren				*End*	Infl		Subacute onset. Memory/ cognitive impairment, psychiatric symptoms, seizures, hypothalamic dysfunction, brainstem/cerebellar signs. Combination of EEG and MRI rarely both normal. Symptoms vary with antibody (see text). Hyponatraemia in some.
Nonvasculitic autoimmune inflammatory meningoencephalitis	Cog		*BG*			NF													Infl		Acute, subacute, or chronic encephalopathy with fluctuating or increasing confusion and cognitive decline. May overlap with Sjögren's syndrome, hypereosinophilic syndrome, Hashimoto's syndrome, Hashimoto's encephalopathy, and SLE.

POISONING (selected). Therapeutic drug poisoning, recreational drug poisoning, plant poisoning, and poisoning with other organic compounds are not covered here; see Section 1 and poisons databases (e.g. http://www.toxbase.org/; http://www.atsdr.cdc.gov/).	**Cog**	**Pyr**	**BG**	**Cer**	**Sen**	**NF**	**MR**	**PN**	**Aut**	**CV**	**Resp**	**Hep**	**GI**	**Ren**	**Sk**	**MSk**	**Hae**	**End**	**Infl**	**Dev**	**Key points**
Serotonin syndrome	Cog	Pyr	BG			NF			Aut	CV			GI						Infl		Serotonergic drug exposure, mental state changes, autonomic hyperactivity, neuromuscular abnormalities.
Anticholinergic poisoning	Cog	*Pyr*			Sen	NF			Aut	CV			GI		Sk				Infl		Parasympathetic blockade and loss of sweating: "Blind as a bat, mad as a hatter, red as a beet, hot as a hare, and dry as a bone; the bowel and bladder lose their tone, and the heart runs alone." Dilated pupils.
Spider venom	Cog					NF			Aut	CV									Infl		Spider bite, restlessness, hypertension, tachycardia, priapism, facial swelling and trismus.
Amphibian venom																					Ingestion of hallucinogenic toad or frog venom.
Fish poisoning				Cer					Aut				GI								Ingestion of a "dreamfish"; incoordination, malaise, terrifying hallucinations, nightmares, sympathetic arousal.

POISONING (selected). Therapeutic drug poisoning, recreational drug poisoning, plant poisoning, and poisoning with other organic compounds are not covered here; see Section 1 and poisons databases (e.g. http://www.toxbase.org/; http://www.atsdr.cdc.gov/).	**Cog**	**Pyr**	**BG**	**Cer**	**Sen**	**NF**	**MR**	**PN**	**Aut**	**CV**	**Resp**	**Hep**	**GI**	**Ren**	**Sk**	**MSk**	**Hae**	**End**	**Infl**	**Dev**	**Key points**
Ergot poisoning			BG			*NF*			Aut	CV											Ingestion of contaminated cereals. Vasoconstriction ± tremor, convulsions, and hallucinations.
Mercury poisoning	Cog	Pyr		Cer	Sen			PN			Resp	*Hep*	GI		Sk						Chronic poisoning typically industrial. Irritability and nervousness, photophobia, pink discolouration of the hands and feet, polyneuritis, tremor/ataxia, headaches, neuropathy, cognitive impairment.
Arsenic poisoning	Cog					*NF*		PN		CV	Resp		GI		Sk		Hae				Industrial exposure. GI irritation, anaemia, arrhythmias, easy bruising, neuropathy, sore throat, respiratory infection, patches of hyperpigmented skin with interspersed spots of hypopigmentation, and hyperkeratosis on the palms, soles, and torso.

POISONING (selected). Therapeutic drug poisoning, recreational drug poisoning, plant poisoning, and poisoning with other organic compounds are not covered here; see Section 1 and poisons databases (e.g. http://www.toxbase.org/; http://www.atsdr.cdc.gov/).	**Cog**	**Pyr**	**BG**	**Cer**	**Sen**	**NF**	**MR**	**PN**	**Aut**	**CV**	**Resp**	**Hep**	**GI**	**Ren**	**Sk**	**MSk**	**Hae**	**End**	**Infl**	**Dev**	**Key points**
Thallium poisoning	Cog			Cer				PN				*Hep*	GI	*Ren*	Sk						Industrial exposure. Hair loss and dark pigmentation of hair roots, plus GI and CNS effects.
Lead poisoning				*Cer*		*NF*		PN		CV			GI	*Ren*		MSk	Hae				Industrial poisoning, old pipes or paint, children more prone. "Lead colic", constipation/diarrhoea/nausea, joint pains, headache, hypertension, peripheral neuropathy, microcytic anaemia, sometimes a blue-tinged line in the gums.
Manganese poisoning	Cog		BG				MR									MSk					Industrial exposure. Anorexia, malaise, joint pains, muscle cramps; then psychosis; then psychomotor slowing and cognitive decline; then hypersalivation and parkinsonism. "Cock-walk" gait characteristic.
Copper poisoning							MR						GI								Accidental ingestion; mainly GI symptoms.

POISONING (selected). Therapeutic drug poisoning, recreational drug poisoning, plant poisoning, and poisoning with other organic compounds are not covered here; see Section 1 and poisons databases (e.g. http://www.toxbase.org/; http://www.atsdr.cdc.gov/).	**Cog**	**Pyr**	**BG**	**Cer**	**Sen**	**NF**	**MR**	**PN**	**Aut**	**CV**	**Resp**	**Hep**	**GI**	**Ren**	**Sk**	**MSk**	**Hae**	**End**	**Infl**	**Dev**	**Key points**
Aluminium poisoning	Cog					NF								Ren							Haemodialysis using aluminium-containing fluids. Dysarthria, dysphasia, apraxia, personality change, psychosis, myoclonus, seizures, dementia.
Bismuth poisoning	Cog	Pyr		Cer		NF		PN				Hep	GI	Ren	*Sk*	*MSk*	*Hae*				Ingestion, medicinal pastes/ creams. Psychosis usually with chronic exposure. Incoordination, paraesthesiae, cognitive/behavioural change, progressing to overt encephalopathy; ± rashes, renal failure, thrombocytopenia, bone demineralization, paralytic ileus.
Molybdenum poisoning											Resp		GI			MSk		End			Seldom reported.
SLEEP DISORDERS	**Cog**	**Pyr**	**BG**	**Cer**	**Sen**	**NF**	**MR**	**PN**	**Aut**	**CV**	**Resp**	**Hep**	**GI**	**Ren**	**Sk**	**MSk**	**Hae**	**End**	**Infl**	**Dev**	**Key points**
Hypnagogic/hypnopompic hallucinations																					Hallucinations during sleep–wake transitions only.
Night terrors																					Children aged 3–12 waking in terror ~90 minutes after falling asleep and appearing to hallucinate, with amnesia for the event.

SLEEP DISORDERS	Cog	Pyr	BG	Cer	Sen	NF	MR	PN	Aut	CV	Resp	Hep	GI	Ren	Sk	MSk	Hae	End	Infl	Dev	Key points
Sleep deprivation	Cog																				Severe sleep deprivation followed by psychosis.
Sleep apnoea and obesity hypoventilation	Cog					NF				*CV*	Resp										Overweight, snorers. Witnessed apnoea or waking breathless. Daytime somnolence (+ headaches if CO_2 retention).
Narcolepsy						NF															Excessive daytime sleepiness, cataplexy, hypnagogic/hypnopompic hallucinations, sleep paralysis.
Kleine–Levin syndrome	Cog					NF															Adolescents. Recurrent hypersomnia with cognitive changes, overeating, hypersexuality, hallucinations.
Guillain–Barré syndrome					Sen			PN	*Aut*		Resp										REM intrusion disorder seen with psychotic features.
Other parasomnias (q.v.)						*NF*															See text.
SENSORY DEPRIVATION AND IMPAIRMENT	**Cog**	**Pyr**	**BG**	**Cer**	**Sen**	**NF**	**MR**	**PN**	**Aut**	**CV**	**Resp**	**Hep**	**GI**	**Ren**	**Sk**	**MSk**	**Hae**	**End**	**Infl**	**Dev**	**Key points**
Sensory impairment, Charles Bonnet syndrome					Sen																Isolated hallucinations in the impaired sensory modality.
MISCELLANEOUS	**Cog**	**Pyr**	**BG**	**Cer**	**Sen**	**NF**	**MR**	**PN**	**Aut**	**CV**	**Resp**	**Hep**	**GI**	**Ren**	**Sk**	**MSk**	**Hae**	**End**	**Infl**	**Dev**	**Key points**
Coeliac disease				*Cer*		*NF*		*PN*				*Hep*	GI		*Sk*	*MSk*	Hae	*End*			Mainly Caucasians; gluten intolerance. Anaemia, GI upset, mouth ulcers, malabsorption, weight loss, ± dermatitis herpetiformis, "gluten ataxia".
Idiopathic hypereosinophilic syndrome						NF		PN		CV	*Resp*		*GI*	*Ren*	Sk		Hae	*End*			Peripheral eosinophilia, myocarditis, thrombotic phenomena.

SLEEP DISORDERS	Cog	Pyr	BG	Cer	Sen	NF	MR	PN	Aut	CV	Resp	Hep	GI	Ren	Sk	MSk	Hae	End	Infl	Dev	Key points
Idiopathic intracranial pachymeningitis	*Cog*			Cer		NF	MR	PN													Headache, ataxia, cranial neuropathies. Focal pachymeningitis on contrast MRI.
Irradiation (acutely in doses that may be a risk factor for subsequent psychosis)	*Cog*					*NF*							GI	*Ren*	*Sk*		Hae				≥0.3 Sv exposure may be a risk factor for psychosis but is usually asymptomatic acutely. Higher doses disrupt haematological, GI, and CNS function.
Serine- and glycine-evoked psychosis																					Episodic acute polymorphic psychosis; fluctuating emotional state, psychedelic phenomena.
Atrial myxoma	*Cog*	*Pyr*	*BG*		*Sen*	*NF*	*MR*			CV					*Sk*	*MSk*	Hae		Infl		Left/right ventricular failure (sometimes positional); systemic response (fever, weight loss, arthralgia, rash, and Raynaud's phenomenon); tumour "plop"; confusion or psychosis; embolism.
Tinnitus					Sen																Simple auditory hallucinosis; most common causes are otological.
Radio reception (! = beware MRI)							!														Metallic implants, amplitude-modulated radio stations.

CATATONIA	Cog	Pyr	BG	Cer	Sen	NF	MR	PN	Aut	CV	Resp	Hep	GI	Ren	Sk	MSk	Hae	End	Infl	Dev	Key points
Catatonia			*BG*						*Aut*	*CV*											Immobility, mutism, stupor, catalepsy, automatic obedience, posturing, stereotypy, echophenomena, negativism, ambitendency.
Malignant catatonia and neuroleptic malignant syndrome			BG			NF			Aut	CV		Hep		*Ren*		MSk	Hae		Infl		Risk factors include antipsychotic drugs. Autonomic instability (hyperthermia, blood pressure lability, tachycardia, tachpnoea, vasoconstriction, sweating, incontinence); muscle rigidity; dyskinesia; posturing/waxy flexibility/catalepsy; negativism; mutism; dysarthria, dysphagia, sialorrhoea; altered consciousness. Raised CK.
PRIMARY PSYCHIATRIC DISEASE AND NORMAL STATES	**Cog**	**Pyr**	**BG**	**Cer**	**Sen**	**NF**	**MR**	**PN**	**Aut**	**CV**	**Resp**	**Hep**	**GI**	**Ren**	**Sk**	**MSk**	**Hae**	**End**	**Infl**	**Dev**	**Key points**
Schizophrenia	Cog	*Pyr*	*BG*	*Cer*	*Sen*															*Dev*	≥1 month of first-rank symptoms or other bizarre delusions, or two from hallucinations with fleeting delusions or overvalued ideas/thought disorder/catatonia/negative symptoms of schizophrenia; or ≥1 year of negative symptoms and functional decline (ICD-10).

PRIMARY PSYCHIATRIC DISEASE AND NORMAL STATES	Cog	Pyr	BG	Cer	Sen	NF	MR	PN	Aut	CV	Resp	Hep	GI	Ren	Sk	MSk	Hae	End	Infl	Dev	Key points
Manic psychosis																					Mania preceding and with psychotic symptoms.
Depressive psychosis	*Cog*																	*End*			Depression preceding and with psychotic symptoms.
Schizoaffective disorder	Cog																				Simultaneous affective and schizophrenic symptoms fulfilling criteria for neither schizophrenia or an affective disorder.
Schizotypal disorder																					≥2 years of some of: inappropriate affect, odd behaviour or beliefs, magical thinking, social withdrawal, suspiciousness, obsessive ruminations, unusual perceptual experiences, odd thinking patterns without incoherence, transient illusions/hallucinations/delusion-like ideas.
Persistent delusional disorder																					≥3 months (ICD-10) or ≥1 month (DSM-IV equivalent) of a delusion as the main symptom.
Acute and transient psychotic disorders																					<1 month of schizophreniform psychosis, or <3 months of other psychosis.
Induced delusional disorder																					Delusion induced by close links to another person with a psychotic illness, resolving on separation.

PRIMARY PSYCHIATRIC DISEASE AND NORMAL STATES	Cog	Pyr	BG	Cer	Sen	NF	MR	PN	Aut	CV	Resp	Hep	GI	Ren	Sk	MSk	Hae	End	Infl	Dev	Key points
OCD																					Obsessional thoughts and/or compulsive acts. The overlaps with psychosis are obsessions without insight, compulsions evolving into command hallucinations, and others (see text).
Panic attacks with psychotic features									Aut	CV	Resp		GI								Psychotic symptoms purely during panic attacks. Physical features shown as occurring during panic attacks. Sometimes hyperreflexia in anxiety.
Psychosis in the context of eating disorders	Cog									CV		Hep	GI	*Ren*	Sk	MSk	Hae	End			See starvation (above). Physical features shown here as for starvation (above).
Psychosis in the context of personality disorders																					Stress-induced brief psychotic episodes in the context of paranoid, schizoid, or emotionally unstable (borderline type) personality disorders.
Other nonorganic psychotic disorder (inc. chronic hallucinatory psychosis)																					≥3 months of hallucinations, not subsumed under another diagnosis.
Bereavement																					Hallucinations of the deceased, often felt to be helpful.

PRIMARY PSYCHIATRIC DISEASE AND NORMAL STATES	Cog	Pyr	BG	Cer	Sen	NF	MR	PN	Aut	CV	Resp	Hep	GI	Ren	Sk	MSk	Hae	End	Infl	Dev	Key points
Normal experiences																					Transitory developmental psychotic experiences, brief hallucinations without distress.
Prodromal symptoms	Cog																				Attenuated or brief psychotic symptoms, or trait vulnerability plus persistent low general functioning (see text).
Factitious disorder and malingering																					Feigning with (malingering) or without (factitious disorder) clear motivation.

Chapter 27

Further investigations relevant to psychosis

In addition, the tests listed below for rare causes of psychosis should be considered in some circumstances. For psychosis in the context of young-onset dementia, see also [370]. In many cases, these complex investigations will require liaison with and advice from other specialties; this table should be taken only as a guide, and such advice should be sought.

Consider test (*italics* indicate tests to exclude similar disease):	... as part of considering:	... particularly if these features are present:
Genetic ‡		
karyotype	whole-chromosome abnormalities (aneuploidy)	dysmorphism psychosis in childhood features of an identifiable aneuploidy (see text)
22q11 microdeletions	velocardiofacial/DiGeorge syndrome	hypocalcaemia or confirmed hypoparathyroidism congenital structural cardiac abnormalities cleft palate or nasopharyngeal reflux dysmorphic face (see text and [17]) and/or long slender fingers learning disability immunodeficiency or confirmed T cell ($CD4^+$ lymphocyte) deficiency renal abnormalities VCFS in a first-degree relative or family history of congenital structural cardiac abnormality hypernasal speech

Consider test (*italics* indicate tests to exclude similar disease):	... as part of considering:	... particularly if these features are present:
HD CAG repeat expansion *exclude DRPLA*	Huntington's disease	family history movement disorder, dementia, prominent mood or OCD symptoms, anosmia caudate atrophy
FTDP17 (tau mutations)	frontotemporal dementia with parkinsonism	frontotemporal dementia clinically
SCA genes	spinocerebellar ataxia	family history ataxia with pyramidal/extrapyramidal/sensory signs
notch mutations ± skin biopsy for granular osmiophilic material in vascular smooth muscle ± *TREX1 mutations (for HERNS)*	CADASIL ± *HERNS*	white-matter infarcts in the young family history, migraine leukoencephalopathy ± *retinopathy, renal involvement (HERNS)*
DRPLA CAG repeat expansion *exclude HD*	dentatorubropallidoluysian atrophy	clinical features resembling HD MRI: atrophy of the superior cerebellar peduncles, high-intensity T2WI lesions in the pallidum
presenilin-1 mutations ± presenilin-2 mutations ± APP mutations	familial Alzheimer's disease	early-onset dementia, particularly if associated spastic paraparesis, parkinsonism, cerebellar disease, myoclonus, white-matter lesions on MRI, or dilated cardiomyopathy
pantothenate kinase-2 mutations phospholipase A2 G6 mutations serum ferritin	PKAN NBIA2 neuroferritinopathy	movement disorder, dementia, acanthocytosis bilateral T2WI hyperintensity with surrounding hypointensity in the globus pallidus ("eye of the tiger" sign) on MRI
Other neurodegeneration		
formal neuropsychology with specific tests of "lobar" (e.g. frontal lobe) function [33]	dementias	dementia with diagnostic doubt
EEG	distinguishing Alzheimer's disease from frontotemporal dementia	loss of alpha rhythm in Alzheimer's disease, preserved in FTD

Consider test (*italics* indicate tests to exclude similar disease):	... as part of considering:	... particularly if these features are present:
DAT scan (SPECT)	DLB PD PSP	diagnostic ambiguity regarding the presence of DLB or PD (striatal dopamine transporter function is lost in both; the pattern differs); likewise, striatal uptake is also reduced in other parkinsonian syndromes (MSA, PSP, CBGD)
brain SPECT/PET	frontal dementia	sometimes needed if structural imaging normal
Epilepsy		
EEG	epilepsy encephalopathy	focal or generalized seizures, or paroxysmal events suspected of being seizures disturbance of consciousness without obvious cause
24-hour EEG, provocation EEG	epilepsy	strong clinical suspicion of epilepsy despite normal EEG
epilepsy-protocol MRI (high-resolution, thin coronal oblique slices of 1.5–2 mm with no gap using SPGR) ¶	epilepsy	strong clinical suspicion of epilepsy EEG evidence of epilepsy
Malignancy		
CXR	lung cancer	limbic encephalitis young-onset dementia cough, weight loss, haemoptysis, smoking
LP † for cytology (may need large volume) ± brain biopsy	meningeal carcinomatosis potentially malignant CNS lesions	e.g. unexplained meningeal enhancement, doubt as to nature of lesions seen on MRI (such as demyelination versus lymphoma)
hunt for malignancy (according to likely sites and guided by careful clinical examination, e.g. CXR for lung tumours, endoscopy for gastrointestinal tumours, whole-body CT when clinical suspicion very high)	metastatic or paraneoplastic disease from a solid tumour	imaging suggestive of metastatic brain lesions limbic encephalitis (q.v.)
24-hour urinary vanillylmandelic acid, total catecholamines, and metanephrines ± plasma metanephrines	phaeochromocytoma	paroxysmal headache, sweating, palpitations, hypertension; suspicion of multiple endocrine neoplasia (e.g. parathyroid adenoma)

Consider test (*italics* indicate tests to exclude similar disease):	... as part of considering:	... particularly if these features are present:
24-hour urinary 5-hydroxyindoleacetic acid	carcinoid syndrome	diarrhoea, flushing, fatigue, wheeze and dyspnoea, palpitations, hypotension liver metastases
Infection		
LP † for culture/serology/PCR	viral/bacterial meningitis, encephalitis, meningoencephalitis, subacute encephalitis	meningism; fever; new seizures (LP only after imaging if any clinical suspicion of raised intracranial pressure) imaging suggestive of meningitis/encephalitis subacute encephalitis/ SSPE: personality change/ intellectual decline 7–12 years after measles infection (faster in the immunosuppressed); multiple lesions on MRI PML: immunosuppression; focal neurological deficits, seizures, memory impairment, psychomotor retardation, inattentiveness
Lyme disease (*Borrelia*) serum serology LP including CSF Lyme serology *investigations for Whipple's disease and cerebrotendinous xanthomatosis (q.v.)*	Lyme disease (borreliosis)	travel to endemic area erythema migrans intermittent inflammatory arthritis; cranial nerve palsies; meningoradiculitis; chronic fatigue
Bartonella serology	bacillary angiomatosis	lice/tick/cat-scratch contact; immunosuppressed patient, multi-organ involvement including skin nodules
CXR	tuberculosis	high-risk groups (endemic areas, immunosuppressed) pulmonary symptoms of TB (e.g. cough, weight loss, night sweats) young-onset dementia
brucella serology LP† blood ± tissue special cultures	neurobrucellosis	occupational history of potential exposure (unvaccinated livestock) fever, systemic illness, organo-megaly, rashes, BG calcification

Consider test (*italics* indicate tests to exclude similar disease):	... as part of considering:	... particularly if these features are present:
tissue biopsy (jejunal, ± other affected tissue e.g. synovium/synovial fluid, lymph nodes, CSF ± brain, aqueous humour, cardiac valve, intervertebral disk) (for electron microscopy, immunohistochemistry, and/or PCR) *investigations for Lyme disease and cerebrotendinous xanthomatosis (q.v.)*	CNS Whipple's disease	diarrhoea, weight loss, abdominal pain, and arthralgia with CNS disease oculomasticatory myorhythmia or oculo-facial-skeletal myorhythmia
HIV 1+2 serology (or if known HIV infection, $CD4^+$ T-lymphocyte count and viral load by PCR)	HIV encephalopathy	risk factors for HIV infection evidence of immunodeficiency markedly raised ESR with normal CRP unexplained encephalopathy
Toxoplasma gondii serology	toxoplasmosis	brain cysts latent infection is implicated in psychosis, but good evidence as to its role and what to do about it is lacking
LP † with India ink stain/ cryptococcal antigen testing	cryptococcosis	typically immunosuppressed patients; fever, malaise, headache, and altered cognition, behaviour, and/or level of consciousness; dilated Virchow–Robin spaces or miliary enhancing lesions on MRI
LP †, serology	neurocysticercosis	infected pork; epilepsy, headaches, intracranial hypertension, eosinophilic meningitis, stroke
EEG LP † for 14–3-3 protein and tau protein MRI¶ including DWI and FLAIR (occasionally, tonsil biopsy and/or brain biopsy) *blood or urine bismuth levels* *antithyroid antibodies* *paraneoplastic autoantibodies*ǁ	CJD	rapidly progressive cognitive impairment, cerebellar signs, myoclonus; sensory impairment (variant CJD) characteristic periodic sharp waves/spikes on EEG bilateral increased MRI signal intensity in the globus pallidus, putamen, caudate (CJD), or pulvinar and mediodorsal thalamus (vCJD)

Consider test (*italics* indicate tests to exclude similar disease):	... as part of considering:	... particularly if these features are present:
investigations covered in main text	leptospirosis typhus typhoid Rocky Mountain spotted fever atypical pneumonia with meningoencephalitis rabies malaria trypanosomiasis	features covered in text; all are acute and systemic disease is generally obvious
Endocrine		
urinary 24-h free cortisol ± low-dose dexamethasone suppression test	Cushing's syndrome	myopathy, weight gain, depression, obesity, plethora, moon face, hypertension, diabetes, infections, bruising, gastric ulceration
short Synacthen® test	adrenal insufficiency	weakness, abdominal pain, pigmented mucous membranes, vitiligo postural hypotension low Na, high K, hypoglycaemia
pituitary MRI ¶	pituitary insufficiency	combination of pituitary-dependent hormone deficiencies
PTH	hypoparathyroidism hyperparathyroidism	hypocalcaemia hypercalcaemia
Inborn errors of metabolism		
ammonia *	urea cycle disorders hepatic encephalopathy (if doubt)	intermittent encephalopathy hepatic failure low urea
acutely, urinary porphyrins (PBG and ALA) in remission, consider porphobilinogen deaminase assay, faecal porphyrins, fluorescence emission spectroscopy of plasma *Note photosensitivity of specimens; discuss with lab.* *Consider also lead, arsenic, thallium poisoning, tyrosinaemia.*	porphyria	neurovisceral attacks: abdominal pain (or other GI, urinary, or cardiovascular disturbance), neuropathy, psychiatric symptoms; hyponatraemia history of recurrence, exploratory laparotomy

Consider test (*italics* indicate tests to exclude similar disease):	... as part of considering:	... particularly if these features are present:
urinary/plasma amino acids (all standard amino acids are screened)	Hartnup's disease	clinical features of pellagra (q.v.) or cerebellar ataxia
urinary/plasma homocysteine (may be done separately)	intermittent maple syrup urine disease mitochondrial disease hyperhomocysteinaemia/ homocystinuria	ataxia, lethargy, seizures ± coma triggered by catabolic stress evidence of mitochondrial disease thromboembolism
slit-lamp examination serum caeruloplasmin serum copper ± 24h urinary copper	Wilson's disease	movement disorder, including clumsiness hepatic dysfunction/abnormal LFTs Kayser–Fleischer rings dementia if patient aged <40 characteristic MRI findings (atrophy, T1WI BG hypointensities, T2WI hyperintensities in BG/white matter/thalamus, or "face of the giant panda" sign)
ophthalmological examination (slit-lamp, retina) abdominal ultrasound	suspected storage disorder	chronic progressive disorder with neurological and multi-organ involvement where diagnosis unclear [115]
urinary sediment dolichols biopsy of muscle/rectum/ skin for lipofuscin ± palmitoyl-protein thioesterase assay	neuronal ceroid lipofuscinoses	seizures, myoclonus, dementia, extrapyramidal/cerebellar signs
assay of cholesterol processing in skin fibroblasts ± bone marrow aspirate and biopsy for sea-blue histiocytes	Niemann–Pick disease, type C	subtle vertical supranuclear ophthalmoplegia in 80%, movement disorder, dementia, splenomegaly, hepatomegaly high index of suspicion (often neurologically normal with psychosis)
plasma/leukocyte lysosomal enzyme screen ("white cell enzymes"), which includes the following (preceded by "..."):		metabolic disorder dementia in patient aged <40

Consider test (*italics* indicate tests to exclude similar disease):	**... as part of considering:**	**... particularly if these features are present:**
... chitotriosidase (non-specific marker, elevated in lysosomal lipid storage disorders and others)	lysosomal lipid storage disorders; see below	
... hexosaminidase B	Sandhoff's disease	lower motor neuron disease, cerebellar ataxia, dystonia; cherry-red macular spots
... hexosaminidase A	Tay–Sachs disease	lower motor neuron disease, cerebellar ataxia, dystonia; cherry-red macular spots
... α-mannosidase (also: urine oligosaccharides)	α-mannosidosis	mental retardation, sensorineural hearing loss, immunodeficiency, dysmorphism, hepatosplenomegaly, visual impairment, cerebellar ataxia, pyramidal signs
... aspartylglucosaminidase (glycoasparaginase) (also: urinary oligosaccharides)	aspartylglucosaminuria	mental retardation, facial/cranial/skeletal abnormalities, periodic hyperactivity, recurrent infections, vacuolated lymphocytes
... α-galactosidase (also: glycolipid in urine or plasma)	Fabry's disease	lancinating pain in the extremities; angiokeratomas; diarrhoea after eating; febrile attacks with abdominal pain; other features of autonomic neuropathy
... leucocyte β-glucosidase (glucosylceramidase)	Gaucher's disease	CNS involvement, bone disease, visceral disease, cytopenia, skin changes
... leucocyte galactocerebrosidase	Krabbe leucodystrophy	pes cavus, optic disc pallor, progressive spastic tetraparesis, sensorimotor demyelinating neuropathy, demyelination on MRI
leukocyte arylsulfatase A level ± urine sulfatide levels, functional cell assay, genetic testing	metachromatic leukodystrophy	cognitive impairment, motor involvement, MRI white matter abnormalities high index of suspicion (often neurologically normal with psychosis)

Consider test (*italics* indicate tests to exclude similar disease):	... as part of considering:	... particularly if these features are present:
serum VLCFA	X-linked adrenoleukodystrophy	suspicion of adrenal, gonadal, or neurological involvement demyelination on MRI metabolic disorder dementia in patient aged <40
sterols (for cholestanol) *investigations for Lyme disease and Whipple's disease (q.v.)*	cerebrotendinous xanthomatosis	cerebellar ataxia, pseudobulbar palsy, other neurological features, low-normal serum cholesterol
MRS[¶]	vanishing white matter leukodystrophy	predominantly cerebellar ataxia and spasticity diffuse cystic degeneration of white matter on MRI
serum lactate[*] ± LP[†] with CSF lactate[*] ± genetic tests[‡] for common mitochondrial mutations ± skeletal muscle biopsy	mitochondrial encephalopathy	unexplained encephalopathy diabetes, deafness, short stature, cardiac involvement, renal involvement, sideroblastic anaemia, dementia, ataxia, myoclonus, seizures, stroke-like episodes, myopathy, peripheral neuropathy if mitochondrial disease is strongly suspected, hunt for other evidence of respiratory chain disease (see text: ECG, echocardiography, oral glucose tolerance test, thyroid function, alkP, fasting calcium, PTH, urinary organic and amino acids)
blood film looking for acanthocytes	neuroacanthocytosis	movement disorder, raised CK, caudate atrophy or "eye of the tiger" on MRI
urinary organic acids (multiple compounds are screened by gas chromatography and mass spectrometry; screens for multiple metabolic disorders)	organic acidaemias mitochondrial disease succinic semialdehyde dehydrogenase deficiency (needs volatile organic acid assay) xylene and toluene toxicity	hyperammonaemia evidence of mitochondrial disease developmental delay, abnormal eye movements, hyporeflexia/ hypotonia, seizures, EEG abnormalities, hallucinations appropriate poisoning history
screen for haemolysis (as above)	G6PD deficiency[∫]	haemolysis triggered by infections, oxidative drugs, broad beans

Consider test (*italics* indicate tests to exclude similar disease):	... as part of considering:	... particularly if these features are present:
plasma serine taurine/(serine × methionine) ratio oral serine provocation test	serine-sensitive polymorphic psychosis	acute polymorphic psychosis with sensory perceptual disturbances
Nutritional		
methylmalonic acid (blood/urine) homocysteine (blood/urine)	vitamin B_{12} deficiency methylmalonic aciduria	doubt about presence of vitamin B_{12} deficiency after serum measurement clinical picture of B_{12} deficiency with normal/high serum B_{12}
anti-gastric parietal cell antibodies anti-intrinsic factor	pernicious anaemia	vitamin B_{12} deficiency
trial of thiamine	thiamine deficiency	alcoholism, malnutrition, malabsorption, hypermetabolic states; tachycardia, weakness, decreased deep tendon reflexes, peripheral neuropathy; Wernicke's encephalopathy: mental state changes, ± eye signs, ataxia
trial of niacin (± serum/urinary niacin/metabolites)	niacin deficiency	alcoholism, malnutrition, increased metabolism; dementia (or acute encephalopathy), diarrhoea, dermatitis
serum pyridoxal 5′-phosphate	pyridoxine deficiency	inflammatory states/drugs (e.g. isoniazid); signs of niacin deficiency (q.v.), homocystinaemia (q.v.), ± sideroblastic anaemia
Other acquired metabolic disorders		
venous bicarbonate, venous pH, or arterial pH	screening test for metabolic acidosis	hyperventilation (Kussmaul breathing) drowsiness suspected poisoning renal failure suspected mitochondrial diseases suspected MC/NMS
amylase and/or lipase	pancreatic encephalopathy	abdominal pain, nausea, vomiting, unwell, abdominal bruising, hypocalcaemia

Consider test (*italics* indicate tests to exclude similar disease):	… as part of considering:	… particularly if these features are present:
Autoimmune		
LP †	CNS inflammation, autoimmunity	any unexplained diffuse or focal CNS lesions [see 28]
antistreptococcal antibodies (ASO titre, ± anti-DNAse, antihyaluronidase) anti-basal ganglia antibodies	autoimmune neuropsychiatric disorders associated with recent streptococcal infection	recent sore throat evidence of rheumatic fever (arthritis, carditis, chorea, erythema marginatum, and/or skin nodules) children, pregnant women with movement disorder
ANA urine dip and microscopy complement C3 and C4 levels	systemic lupus erythematosus	known positive ANA or strong clinical suspicion of SLE
antiphospholipid antibodies (lupus anticoagulant, anticardiolipin IgG and IgM, anti-β_2 glycoprotein-1 antibody)	antiphospholipid syndrome Behçet's disease	known autoimmune disease (e.g. SLE) history of miscarriage, or arterial or venous thrombosis, particularly if young-onset multiple hyperintense lesions on MRI, especially if aged <40 young-onset dementia recurrent oral ulceration, genital ulceration, eye inflammation, arthritis, CNS involvement, abnormalities on MRI
ANA RhF salivary gland biopsy	Sjögren's syndrome	xerostomia, xerophthalmia, arthritis
ANA anti-Scl-70 antibodies anti-smooth muscle antibodies ± skin biopsy	systemic sclerosis scleromyxoedema	skin thickening and tethering, calcinosis, Raynaud's syndrome, oesophageal dysmotility, sclerodactyly, telangiectasia widespread eruption of small, waxy, firm papules on skin
temporal artery biopsy	GCA	features of extracranial arteritis (headache, scalp sensitivity, tender thickened arteries, tongue/jaw claudication, face/neck pain with nerve damage), myalgia, weight loss, malaise, fever, visual disturbance; raised ESR

Consider test (*italics* indicate tests to exclude similar disease):	... as part of considering:	... particularly if these features are present:
echocardiography (?endocarditis [transthoracic echo, plus transoesophageal if strong suspicion]; ?right-to-left defect) HIV, hepatitis B, hepatitis C serology malignancy screen (if strong suspicion, whole-body CT ± PET) consider mitochondrial DNA testing cryoglobulins *screen for causes of multiple strokes*	mimics of CNS vasculitis	suspicion of CNS vasculitis (q.v.)
magnetic resonance angiography ¶	cerebral vasculitis moyamoya disease	suspected cerebral vasculitis (q.v.) intracranial haemorrhage
retinal photography ?CNS angiography ± labelled leukocyte imaging, SPECT ± brain biopsy *CRP, complement, cryoglobulins, immune complexes, ANA, ANCA, anti-Ro, anti-La, RhF, ACE, anticardiolipin, protein electrophoresis* LP † *including for cytology*	CNS vasculitis/PACNS	gradual-onset headache, encephalopathy, multifocal neurological signs systemic and/or CSF inflammatory response inflammatory changes on MRI systemic vasculitis or (for PACNS) exclusion of other causes
mesenteric angiography hepatitis B serology	polyarteritis nodosa	multisystem (see text); CNS features inc. amaurosis fugax; raised ESR/neutrophila
ANCA	ANCA-associated vasculitis	respiratory tract and renal involvement (WG) skin, lung, and renal involvement (MPA) multisystem; CNS features inc. amaurosis fugax (PAN) other suspected systemic or CNS vasculitis young-onset dementia

Consider test (*italics* indicate tests to exclude similar disease):	... as part of considering:	... particularly if these features are present:
RhF ANA HLA typing hunt for infectious triggers (inc. *Chlamydia*, *Neisseria gonorrhoeae*, diarrhoeal illnesses)	Reiter's syndrome	seronegative arthropathy, urethritis, conjunctivitis, skin lesions
CXR, MRI, serum ACE, RhF, immunoglobulins, serum lysozyme, urinary calcium ± LP [†] with CSF ACE (± CT, bronchoscopy with lavage, gallium scan, biopsy)	sarcoid	racial predilection; systemic features (fever, night sweats, etc.), multisystem involvement, skin disease (keloid scarring, rashes, lupus pernio) young-onset dementia
screen for haemolysis (FBC, blood film, reticulocyte count, LDH, haptoglobin, LFTs, ± direct Coomb's/ antiglobulin test) clotting, D-dimer, fibrinogen	TTP	spontaneous/drugs/diarrhoeal illness; microangiopathic haemolytic anaemia, thrombocytopenic purpura, neurological disease, fever, renal disease
antithyroid antibodies (anti-thyroid peroxidase ± antithyroglobulin)	autoimmune thyroiditis Hashimoto's encephalopathy	raised TSH encephalopathy of unknown cause young-onset dementia suspected CJD
cryoglobulins	cryoglobulinaemia	lymphoproliferative disorders, chronic inflammatory disorders (e.g. hepatitis C) skin lesions in dependent areas, livedo reticularis, Raynaud's phenomenon, arthralgia, myalgia, multisystem disease
serum electrophoresis immunoglobulin levels	monoclonal gammopathy, inc. scleromyxoedema paraproteinaemia causing hyperviscosity (many other inflammatory disorders may also affect these tests)	small, waxy, firm papules oronasal bleeding, retinal haemorrhages, and variable neurological symptoms unexplained TIAs/CVAs young-onset dementia suspected paraneoplastic disease
trial of steroids (± other immunosuppressive regimes, plasma exchange)	Hashimoto's encephalopathy limbic encephalitis other autoimmune inflammatory encephalopathies	evidence of autoimmune encephalopathy and no other cause identified after a thorough hunt

Consider test (*italics* indicate tests to exclude similar disease):	**... as part of considering:**	**... particularly if these features are present:**
antineuronal antibodies[II]	limbic encephalitis	subacute onset; mnemonic impairment; seizures EEG/MRI evidence of encephalitis unexplained hyponatraemia (anti-VGKC antibodies) autonomic instability (anti-$NMDA_R$) peripheral neuropathy (anti-Hu) known cancer young-onset dementia suspected CJD
coeliac serology (anti-endomysial = anti-tissue transglutaminase antibodies, with simultaneous total IgA level) ± endoscopy and duodenal biopsy	coeliac disease[J]	anaemia due to iron, folate, or B_{12} deficiency weight loss or growth retardation gastrointestinal disturbance (discomfort, bloating, flatulence, altered bowel habit, steatorrhoea, overt malabsorption) mouth ulcers dermatitis herpetiformis
Poisoning (discuss also with a national poisons service if any doubt)		
blood manganese level	manganese poisoning	industrial exposure; anorexia, malaise, joint pains, muscle cramps; psychomotor slowing, cognitive decline, hypersalivation, parkinsonism; "cock-walk" gait increased T1WI signal in the basal ganglia on MRI
blood film iron studies urate blood lead level hunt for source (inc. swallowed) if confirmed	lead poisoning	history suggestive of lead exposure (industrial, old pipes/paint) "lead colic", joint pains, headache, hypertension, peripheral neuropathy, microcytic anaemia, blue-tinged gum line

Consider test (*italics* indicate tests to exclude similar disease):	... as part of considering:	... particularly if these features are present:
CK LDH	NMS/MC	antipsychotic drug use; autonomic instability (hyperthermia, blood pressure lability, tachycardia, tachpnoea, vasoconstriction, sweating, incontinence); muscle rigidity; dyskinesia; posturing/waxy flexibility/ catalepsy; negativism; mutism; dysarthria, dysphagia, sialorrhoea; altered consciousness
biopsy of skin lesions	(*multiple*)	psychotic disorders with rash or other skin lesions of uncertain cause
reassess and repeat investigations later	—	any psychosis of unknown biological aetiology, if clinical features evolve

Notes:

† LP is an invasive procedure, so best done only once. Ensure there is no contraindication (in particular, obtain urgent imaging first if there is a possibility of raised intracranial pressure, and beware bleeding tendencies). Measure the opening pressure. Consider sending CSF for [472, 852] some subset of:

- ***biochemistry***: protein§, glucose§ (the lab may require a separate CSF sample in a fluoride tube), electrophoresis for oligoclonal bands§ (as evidence for intrathecal IgG synthesis), 14-3-3 protein ± tau protein (if CJD is suspected), ACE (if neurosarcoidosis suspected)
- ***microbiology***: microscopy for cell counts and organisms§, special stains (e.g. acid-fast bacilli), cultures (bacterial§, viral, fungal), PCR (viral e.g. enterovirus [RNA], HSV, VZV, HHV-6, adenovirus, influenza [RNA], HIV [RNA], West Nile virus [RNA], JC virus; bacterial e.g. *Bartonella* species, *Tropheryma whipplei*, *Borrelia*, *Mycoplasma*, *Chlamydophila pneumoniae* and *Chlamydophila psittaci*), serology (for e.g. syphilis, *Brucella*, *Mycoplasma pneumoniae*, other encephalitis viruses such as arboviruses, measles), antigen detection (e.g. cryptococcal antigen)
- ***cytology***

Minimal standard tests are indicated by §. Send a simultaneous venous glucose.

* Ammonia (typically EDTA) and lactate (typically fluoride) samples need to be placed on ice rapidly for transportation to the laboratory.

¶ MRI scans can be time-consuming and are usually in high demand, so it is worthwhile choosing the protocol in advance so that only one session is required. Discuss with a radiologist, including any potential need for intravenous contrast (and any contraindications to it).

‡ Genetic testing often carries potential implications for family members, and this must be discussed if possible. Sample requirements for cytogenetic testing (karyotype or fluorescent *in situ* hybridization for chromosomal abnormalities; typically a lithium–heparin sample transported on ice) are different from those used for mutation analysis by PCR (typically an EDTA sample).

‖ Antibodies associated with limbic encephalitis include anti-Hu (50% of patients with PLE and lung cancer), anti-Ri (less common in PLE; most typically opsoclonus and cerebellar ataxia in women with breast cancer), anti-CV2 (some patients with PLE and lung cancer), PCA-2, ANNA-3, anti-Ma2 (majority of patients with PLE and testicular cancer), anti-VGKC (45% of patient with limbic encephalitis and neuronal surface antigens in one study), anti-$NMDA_R$ (17% of patient with limbic encephalitis and neuronal surface antigens in one study), anti-GAD, and anti-amphiphysin (some patients with PLE and lung cancer) [860, 1295, 1296].

Several other autoantibodies have been described in PLE: for a more complete list, see Chapter 14.2.3▶ and Chapter 14.2.4▶. There are also antineuronal and anti-brain antibodies whose antigen has not yet been characterized (Chapter 14.2▶); identification of these requires direct immunohistochemistry, which is not always available in clinical settings, but which allows determination of the presence of antineuronal antibodies without the need to specify in advance which type they might be.

Some antibody testing requires separate samples to be sent to a reference laboratory (in the UK in 2009, anti-VGKC and anti-$NMDA_R$ antibodies are via the Neuroimmunology Laboratory, John Radcliffe Hospital, Oxford).

∫ For these diseases, there is some evidence for a population association with psychosis, rather than psychosis associated with an acute flare of disease (see text).

Chapter 28

Classificatory approach for psychosis of unknown aetiology

The approach shown in Chapter 28.1 ▶ is based on our reading of the ICD-10 and the review presented here, and is intended as a rough and approximate clinical guide to ICD-10 classification of psychosis [4]. All tentative diagnoses reached using this approach should be rechecked against formal diagnostic criteria [4, 10]. A DSM-IV version is given in Chapter 28.5 ▶, adapted and extended from DSM-IV-TR Appendix A; likewise, diagnoses should be rechecked against formal criteria [5]. Computerized classification can give accurate diagnoses across a range of classificatory systems simultaneously (e.g. OPCRIT [1297]; http://sgdp.iop.kcl.ac.uk/opcrit/).

Checklists are provided on the pages that follow Figures 28.1 and 28.2, showing ICD-10 and DSM-IV criteria for mood episodes (depressive, manic, hypomanic, mixed; Chapter 28.2 ▶/Chapter 28.6 ▶), schizophrenia (Chapter 28.3 ▶/Chapter 28.7 ▶), and personality disorders that can present with brief psychotic symptoms (Chapter 28.4 ▶/ Chapter 28.8 ▶), together with one examination technique and set of criteria for catatonia (Chapter 28.9 ▶/Chapter 28.10 ▶).

ICD-10 criteria shown in this book are reproduced with permission of the World Health organization. DSM-IV criteria are reprinted, with permission, from the *Diagnostic and Statistical Manual of Mental Disorders*, Fourth Edition, Text Revision (copyright ©2000, American Psychiatric Association).

28.1 Classificatory approach to psychosis of unknown aetiology, based on ICD-10

Figure 28.1 Classificatory approach to psychosis of unknown aetiology, based on ICD-10. This tree is based on our reading of ICD-10 definitions of primary psychiatric disorders in which psychosis can be a feature. Part 1 of 3.

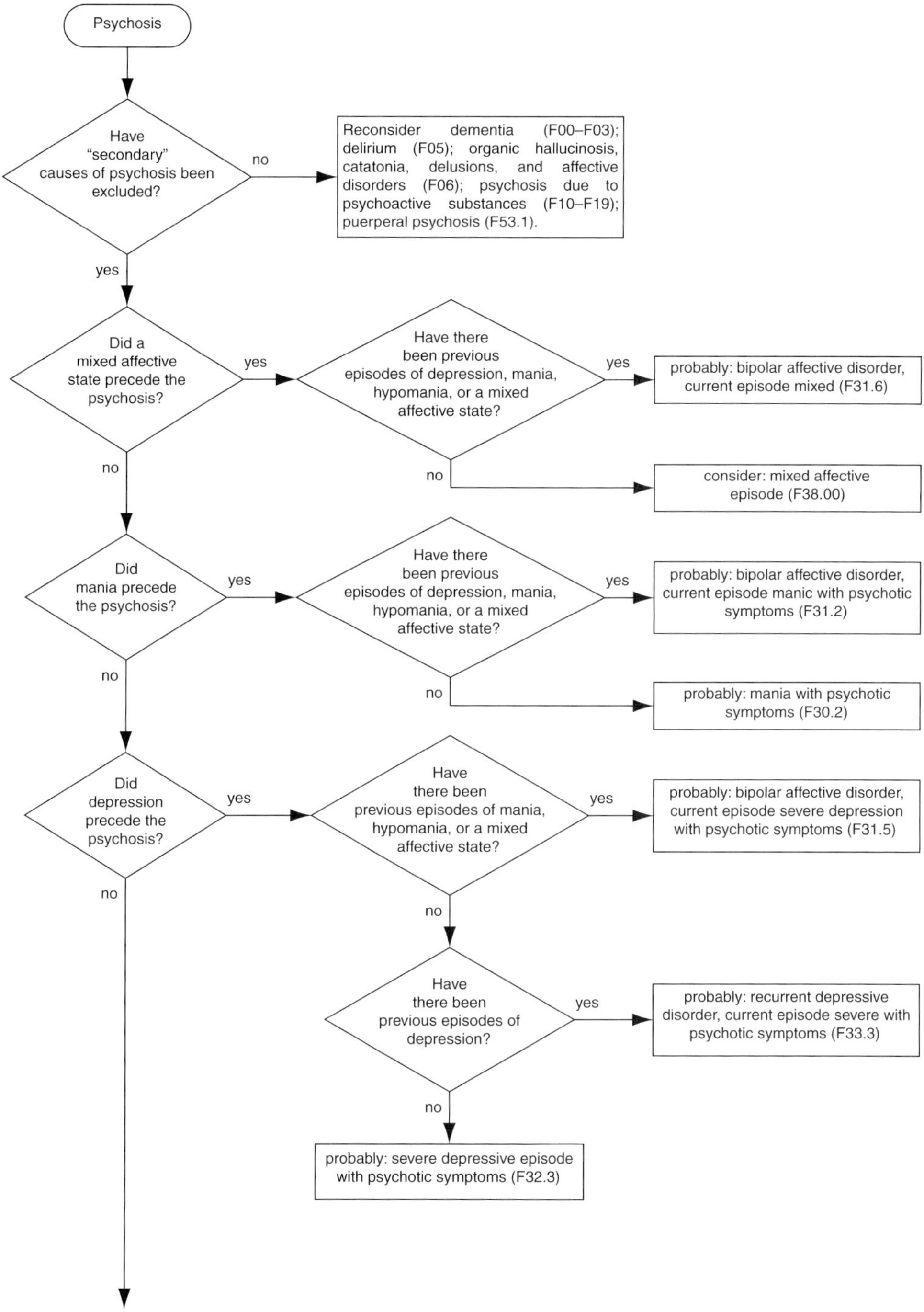

Figure 28.1 Part 2 of 3.

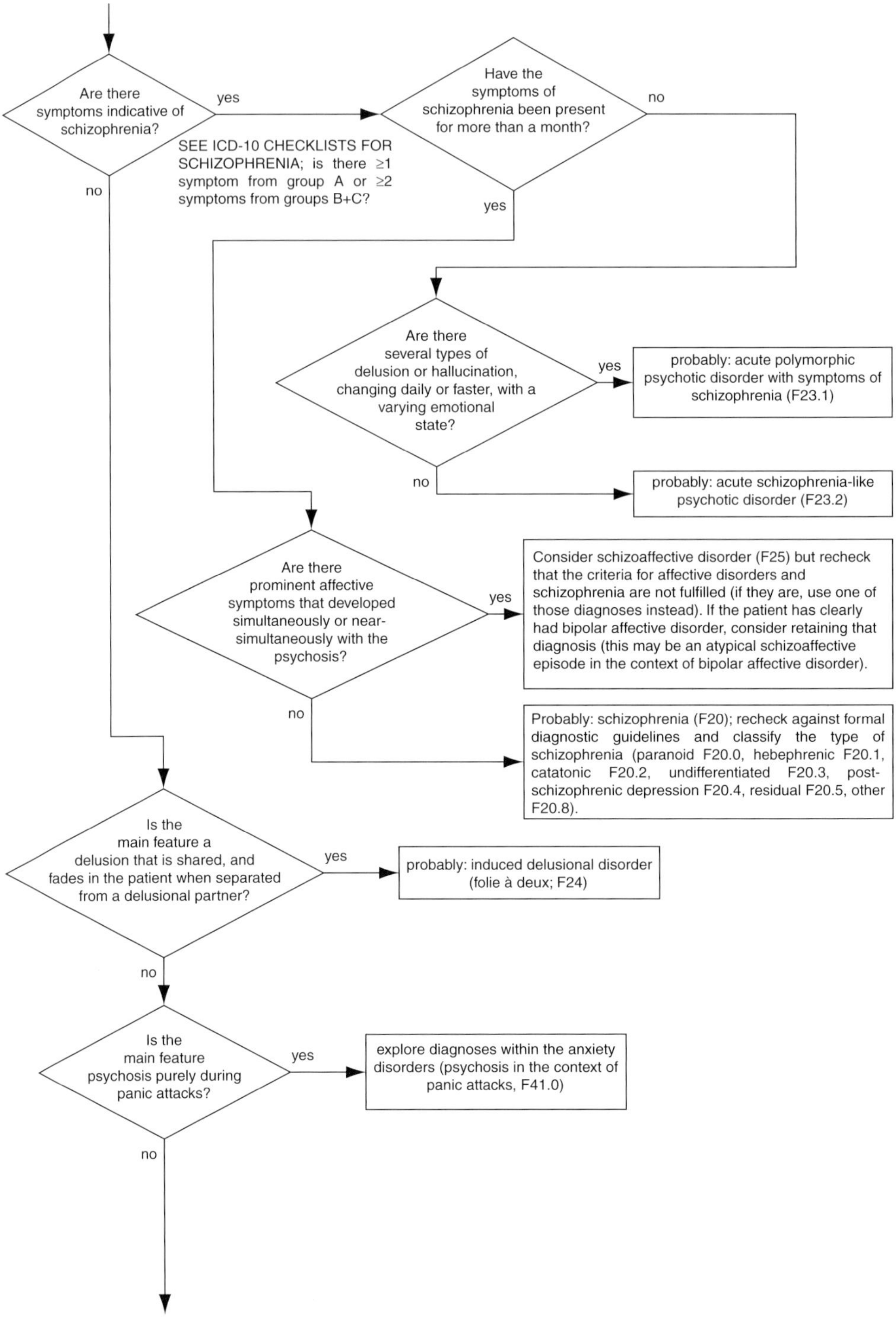

Figure 28.1 Part 3 of 3.

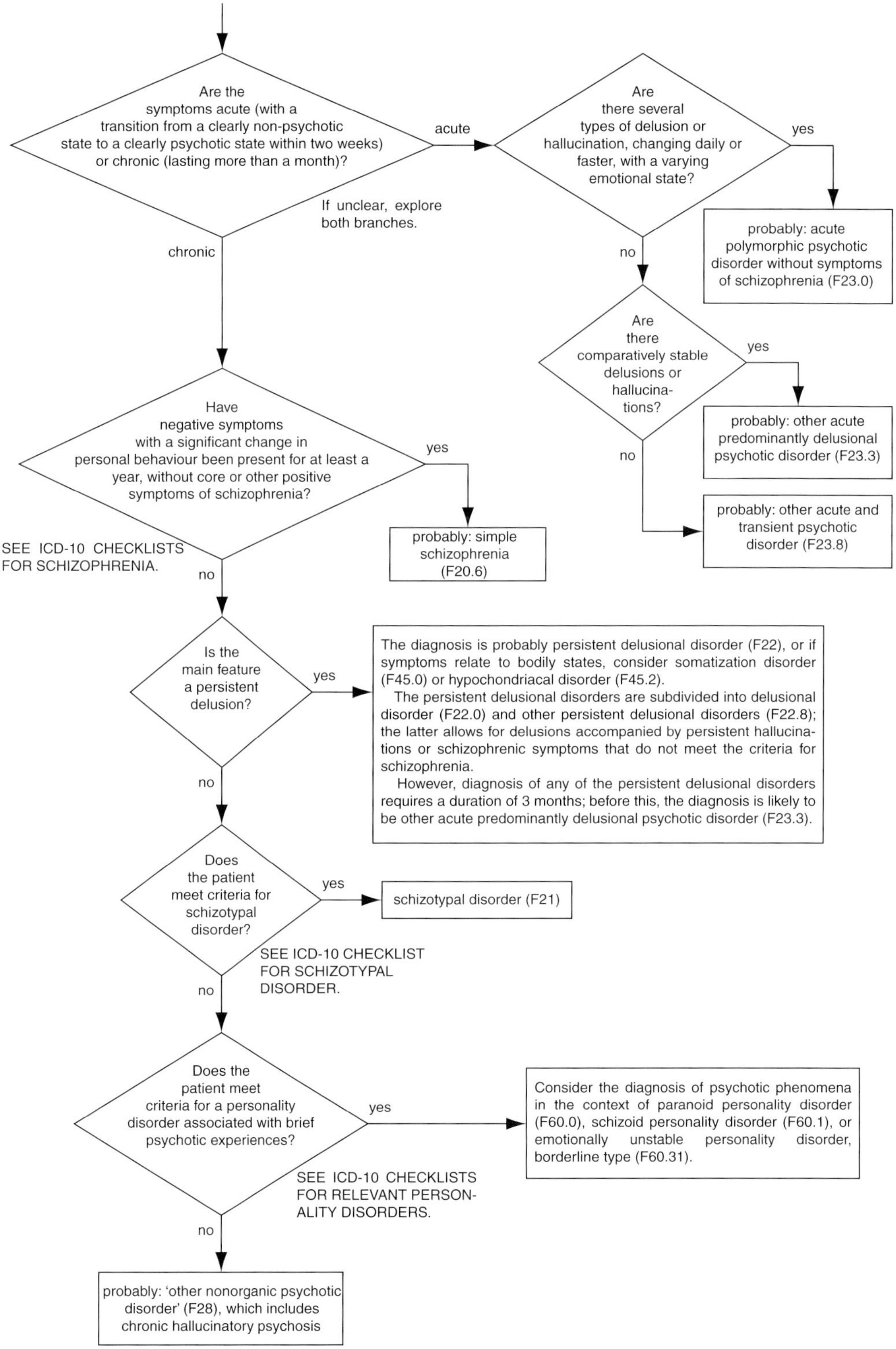

28.2 ICD-10 criteria for mood disorders

Date: ____________ Assessor: ____________	Patient details

DEPRESSION. ICD-10 criteria for depressive episodes. Headings in bold are written so as to approach an acronym; plain text and other diagnostic criteria are taken from ICD-10 [10].

A. Core symptom (= part of somatic syndrome)*	*Absent*	*Present*
Mood: depressed mood to a degree that is definitely abnormal for the individual, present for most of the day and almost every day, largely uninfluenced by circumstances, and sustained for at least 2 weeks.		
Anhedonia (*): loss of interest or pleasure in activities that are normally pleasurable.		
Energy: decreased energy or increased fatigability.		
Total symptoms in category A:		
B. Other key diagnostic symptoms (= part of somatic syndrome)*	*Absent*	*Present*
Sleep: sleep disturbance of any type.		
Worth: loss of confidence and self-esteem.		
Appetite (*): change in appetite (decrease or increase) with corresponding weight change.		
Guilt: unreasonable feelings of self-reproach or excessive and inappropriate guilt.		
Concentration: complaints or evidence of diminished ability to think or concentrate, such as indecisiveness or vacillation.		
Activity (*): change in psychomotor activity, with agitation or retardation (either subjective or objective).		
Death: recurrent thoughts of death or suicide, or any suicidal behaviour.		
Total symptoms in category B:		
Total symptoms in categories A + B:		
C. Somatic syndrome of depression	*Absent*	*Present*
Anhedonia (as above): marked loss of interest or pleasure in activities that are normally pleasurable.		
Psychomotor agitation/retardation ("activity" as above): objective evidence of marked psychomotor retardation or agitation (remarked on or reported by other people).		
Appetite (as above): marked loss of appetite.		
Weight (as above): weight loss (5% or more of body weight in the past month).		
Morning mood: depression worse in the morning.		

Unresponsive emotionally: lack of emotional reactions to events or activities that normally produce an emotional response.		
Libido: marked loss of libido.		
Early morning waking: waking in the morning 2 hours or more before the usual time.		
Total symptoms in category C:		
General criteria for a depressive episode (F32)	*False*	*True*
The depressive episode should last for at least 2 weeks. (*Diagnosis after a shorter period may still be reasonable if symptoms are unusually severe and of rapid onset.*)		
There have been no hypomanic or manic episodes in the individual's lifetime. (*If false, the diagnosis simply changes from a depressive episode to an episode of bipolar depression.*)		
The episode is not attributable to psychoactive substance use or organic mental disorder.		

- A ***mild depressive episode*** requires 2 symptoms from group A and a total of ≥4 symptoms from across groups A & B.
- A ***moderate depressive episode*** requires 2 symptoms from group A and ≥6 symptoms from across groups A & B.
- A ***severe depressive episode*** requires all 3 symptoms from group A and ≥8 symptoms from across groups A & B, or a clinical impression of "severe" in a patient with marked agitation or retardation who is unwilling or unable to describe their symptoms in detail.
    - For *severe depressive episode without psychotic symptoms*, there must be no hallucinations, delusions, or depressive stupor.
    - For *severe depressive episode with psychotic symptoms*, there may be any of these, other than "typically schizophrenic" symptoms.† ICD-10 is silent on what to call what appear to be depressive episodes with psychotic features of that kind; note that such symptoms can occur in severe depression with psychosis [1164]. The depressive psychotic symptoms may be specified as *mood-congruent* or *mood-incongruent*.
- The ***somatic syndrome*** of depression requires 4 symptoms in category C.

ICD-10 criteria for mood disorders, continued.

Date: ________________ Assessor: ________________	Patient details

MANIA AND HYPOMANIA. ICD-10 criteria for hypomanic and manic episodes. Layout as before. Some criteria are phrased almost identically for hypomania and mania, and have been combined below with the actual text shown [10].

A. Core symptom of hypomania and mania	*Absent*	*Present*
Mood: The mood is "elevated or irritable" [hypomania] or "predominantly elevated, expansive or irritable" [mania] to a degree that is definitely abnormal for the individual concerned.		
B. Other symptoms of hypomania and mania	*Absent*	*Present*
Distractible: difficulty in concentration or distractibility [from the criteria for hypomania]; distractibility or constant changes in activity or plans [from the criteria for mania].		
Activity: increased activity or physical restlessness.		
Sleep: decreased need for sleep.		
Talkative: increased talkativeness (pressure of speech).		
Recklessness: mild spending sprees, or other types of reckless or irresponsible behaviour [hypomania]; behaviour which is foolhardy or reckless and whose risks the subject does not recognize e.g. spending sprees, foolish enterprises, reckless driving [mania].		
Disinhibition socially: increased sociability or over-familiarity [hypomania]; loss of normal social inhibitions resulting in behaviour which is inappropriate to the circumstances [mania].		
Sexual energy: increased sexual energy [hypomania]; marked sexual energy or sexual indiscretions [mania].		
Total symptoms in category B:		
C. Other symptoms of mania	*Absent*	*Present*
Grandiosity: Inflated self-esteem or grandiosity.		
Flight of ideas: Flight of ideas or the subjective experience of thoughts racing.		
Total symptoms in category C:		
Total symptoms in category B + C:		

- ***Hypomania*** requires mood symptom A for at least 4 days, at least 3 symptoms from group B, and some interference with personal functioning in daily living.
- ***Mania*** requires mood symptom A for at least 7 days (unless it is severe enough to require hospital admission), plus at least 3 symptoms from across groups B and C (or at least 4 symptoms from those groups if the mood is merely irritable), plus severe interference with personal functioning in daily living.
  - *Mania without psychotic symptoms* may include perceptual changes (e.g. hyperacusis, visual hyperaesthesia) but not hallucinations or delusions.
  - *Mania with psychotic symptoms* requires delusions or hallucinations, other than those that are "typically schizophrenic".†
- Exclusion criteria apply (including psychoactive substance use, organic mental disorder, schizophrenia, and schizoaffective disorder).

MIXED AFFECTIVE STATE. ICD-10 criteria for mixed affective episode [10].

Criteria for mixed affective episode (F38.00)	*False*	*True*
A. Mixed state: There is either a mixture or a rapid alternation (within a few hours) of hypomanic, manic, and depressive symptoms		
B. Duration/severity: Both manic and depressive symptoms must be prominent most of the time during a period of at least two weeks.		

† "Typically schizophrenic" symptoms that are excluded are (a) delusions of control, influence, or passivity, clearly referred to body or limb movements or specific thoughts, actions, or sensations, and delusional perception; (b) hallucinatory voices giving a running commentary on the patient's behaviour, or discussing him between themselves, or other types of hallucinatory voices coming from some part of the body; (c) persistent delusions of other kinds that are culturally inappropriate and completely impossible. Note, however, that Schneiderian first-rank symptoms can occur in manic psychosis [1157].

28.3 ICD-10 criteria for schizophrenia

Date: ________________ Assessor: ________________	Patient details

SCHIZOPHRENIA. ICD-10 criteria for schizophrenia [10]. Layout as before. Further explanation of individual symptoms is given in italics.

*A. Core symptoms of schizophrenia**	*Absent*	*Present*
Passivity: delusions of control, influence, or passivity, clearly referred to body or limb movements...		
... or to specific thoughts, actions, or sensations.		
Third-person auditory hallucinations: hallucinatory voices giving a running commentary on the patient's behaviour		
... or discussing the patient among themselves		
... or other types of hallucinatory voices coming from some part of the body.		
Delusions: persistent delusions of other kinds that are culturally inappropriate and completely impossible, such as religious or political identity, or superhuman powers and abilities (e.g. being able to control the weather, or being in communication with aliens from another world).		
Delusional perception *(a normal perception, delusionally interpreted* [1298]).		
Thought **e**cho *(hearing one's own thoughts aloud, just before, just after, or simultaneously with the thought* [1298])		
... thought **w**ithdrawal (*the feeling that one's thoughts have been removed by an outside agency* [1298])		
... thought **i**nsertion *(the feeling that one's thoughts have been placed there from outside* [1298])		
... or thought **b**roadcasting (*the feeling that one's thoughts leave oneself and are diffused widely* [1298], *or are audible to others, or that others think the same thoughts in unison* [1299]).		
B. Other positive symptoms of schizophrenia	*Absent*	*Present*
Hallucinations: persistent hallucinations in any modality, when accompanied either by fleeting or half-formed delusions without clear affective content, or by persistent over-valued ideas, or when occurring every day for weeks or months on end.		
Thought disorder: breaks or interpolations in the train of thought, resulting in incoherence or irrelevant speech, or neologisms.		
Catatonia: catatonic behaviour, such as excitement, posturing, or waxy flexibility, negativism, mutism, and stupor (*see template for catatonia*).		

C. Negative symptoms of schizophrenia	*Absent*	*Present*
Negative symptoms: "negative" symptoms such as marked apathy, paucity of speech, and blunting or incongruity of emotional responses, usually resulting in social withdrawal and lowering of social performance; it must be clear that these are not due to depression or to neuroleptic medication.		
D. Additional criteria used in the diagnosis of simple schizophrenia	*Absent*	*Present*
A significant and consistent change in the overall quality of some aspects of personal behaviour, manifest as loss of interest, aimlessness, idleness, a self-absorbed attitude, and social withdrawal.		
Marked decline in social, scholastic, or occupational performance.		

- ***Schizophrenia*** requires at least 1 of group A, or at least 2 of groups B+C, present for most of the time for a month.
- Other diagnoses are used if these symptoms are present for less than a month (see Figure 28.1).
- Exclusion criteria apply:
  - If the patient also meets criteria for a manic episode or depressive episode, the criteria for schizophrenia must have been met before the disturbance of mood developed.
  - The disorder is not attributable to organic brain disease or to alcohol or drug intoxication, dependence, or withdrawal.
- Subtypes of schizophrenia are shown on the next page.

* These core symptoms of schizophrenia are essentially Schneider's first-rank symptoms of schizophrenia [18], with the addition of persistent delusions not relating to passivity. The first-rank symptoms are audible thoughts, voices arguing or discussing, voices commenting on the patient's action, delusional perception, somatic passivity, made thoughts, made impulses, made volitional acts, made feelings, thought insertion, thought withdrawal, and thought broadcasting [1298, 1300].

ICD-10 schizophrenia, continued.

Date: ______________ Assessor: ______________	Patient details

E. Subtypes of schizophrenia	*Absent*	*Present*
Paranoid: dominated by delusions or hallucinations.		
Hebephrenic: dominated by affective changes (shallow, flat, incongruous, or inappropriate affect), and either pronounced thought disorder or aimless, disjointed behaviour is present.		
Catatonic: psychomotor disturbances dominate (such as stupor, mutism, excitement, posturing, negativism, rigidity, waxy flexibility, command automatisms, or verbal perseveration).		
Undifferentiated: schizophrenia with active psychosis fitting none or more than one of the above three types.		
Post-schizophrenic depression: in which a depressive episode has developed for at least 2 weeks following a schizophrenic episode within the last 12 months and in which schizophrenic symptoms persist but are not as prominent as the depression.		
Residual: in which previous psychotic episodes of schizophrenia have given way to a chronic condition with "negative" symptoms of schizophrenia for at least 1 year.		
Simple schizophrenia, in which "negative" symptoms (C) with a change in personal behaviour (D) develop for at least one year without any psychotic episodes (no symptoms from groups A or B), and with a marked decline in social, scholastic, or occupational performance.		
Cenesthopathic: body image aberration (e.g. desomatization, loss of bodily boundaries, feelings of body size change) or abnormal bodily sensations (e.g. numbness, stiffness, feeling strange, depersonalization, or sensations of pain, temperature, electricity, heaviness, lightness, or discomfort when touched) dominate		

Formal criteria for these subtypes are given in [10].

28.4 ICD-10 criteria for schizotypal disorder and personality disorders associated with psychotic symptoms

Date: ______________ Assessor: ______________	Patient details

SCHIZOTYPAL DISORDER. ICD-10 criteria [10]. Layout as before.

Symptoms of schizotypal disorder	*Absent*	*Present*
Suspicious: Suspiciousness or paranoid ideas.		
Thought abnormalities: Vague, circumstantial, metaphorical, over-elaborate, or stereotyped thinking, manifested by odd speech or in other ways, without gross incoherence.		
Obsessions: Obsessive ruminations without inner resistance, often with dysmorphophobic, sexual or aggressive contents.		
Magical thinking: Odd beliefs or magical thinking, influencing behaviour and inconsistent with subcultural norms.		
Psychosis: occasional transient quasi-psychotic episodes with intense illusions, auditory or other hallucinations, and delusion-like ideas, usually occurring without external provocation.		
Social difficulties: Poor rapport with others and a tendency to social withdrawal.		
Odd: Behaviour or appearance that is odd, eccentric, or peculiar.		
Aloof: Inappropriate or constricted affect (the individual appears cold and aloof).		
Perceptual abnormalities: Unusual perceptual experiences including somatosensory (bodily) or other illusions, depersonalization or derealization.		

- ***Schizotypal disorder*** requires at least 4 of these, manifested (either continuously or repeatedly) over at least 2 years.
- The patient must never have met the criteria for schizophrenia.

Date: ____________ Assessor: ____________	Patient details

PERSONALITY DISORDERS ASSOCIATED WITH PSYCHOTIC SYMPTOMS:

GENERAL CRITERIA FOR PERSONALITY DISORDER. ICD-10 criteria [10].

A. General definition of a personality disorder: ALL criteria must be met.	*False*	*True*
Pathological (1): The individual's enduring patterns of inner experience and behaviour deviate markedly from the cultural norm, manifest in more than one of cognition, affect, impulse control, and interpersonal relationships.		
Pathological (2): It causes personal distress or adverse social consequences.		
Pervasive: The deviation is pervasive, not situation-specific.		
Persistent: It is stable and long-lasting, having its onset in late childhood or adolescence.		
Primary (1): It is not a consequence of other adult mental disorders.		
Primary (2): Organic brain disease is excluded as a cause.		

PARANOID PERSONALITY DISORDER. ICD-10 criteria [10].

Need all general criteria for personality disorder plus 4 of:	*Absent*	*Present*
Conspiratorial: Preoccupation with unsubstantiated conspiratorial explanations of events around the subject or in the world at large.		
Aggrieved: A combative and tenacious sense of personal rights out of keeping with the actual situation.		
Touchy: Excessive sensitivity to setbacks and rebuffs.		
Suspicious: Suspiciousness and a pervasive tendency to distort experience by misconstruing the neutral or friendly actions of others as hostile or contemptuous.		
Jealous: Recurrent suspicions, without justification, regarding sexual fidelity of spouse or sexual partner.		
Important: Persistent self-referential attitude, associated particularly with excessive self-importance.		
Grudges: A tendency to bear grudges persistently.		

ICD-10 criteria for personality disorders associated with psychotic symptoms, continued.

Date: ________________ Assessor: ________________	Patient details

SCHIZOID PERSONALITY DISORDER. ICD-10 criteria [10]. Layout as before.

Need all general criteria for personality disorder plus 3 of:	*Absent*	*Present*
Fantasy: Excessive preoccupation with fantasy and introspection.		
Indifferent: Appears indifferent to either praise or criticism of others.		
Solitary: Almost always chooses solitary activities.		
Cold: A limited capacity to express warm, tender feelings for others as well as anger.		
Anhedonia: Few, if any, activities provide pleasure.		
Loner: Neither desires, nor has, any close friends or confiding relationships, or has only one.		
Asexual: Little interest in having sexual experiences with another person, taking into account age.		
Insensitive: Marked insensitivity to prevailing social norms and conventions, with breach of them being unintentional.		
Detached: Emotional coldness, detachment, or flattened affectivity.		

EMOTIONALLY UNSTABLE PERSONALITY DISORDER, BORDERLINE TYPE. ICD-10 criteria [10]. Layout as before.

Need all general criteria for personality disorder plus 3 of:	*Absent*	*Present*
Quarrelsome: A marked tendency to quarrelsome behaviour and to conflicts with others, especially when impulsive acts are thwarted or criticised.		
Unstable and capricious mood.		
Outcomes must be immediate: Difficulty in maintaining any course of action that offers no immediate reward.		
Impulsive: A marked tendency to act unexpectedly and without consideration of the consequences.		
Temper: Liability to outbursts of anger or violence, with inability to control the resulting behavioural explosions.		
... and 2 of:	*Absent*	*Present*
Avoid abandonment: Excessive efforts to avoid abandonment.		
Self-image uncertain: Disturbances in and uncertainty about self-image, aims and internal, including sexual, preferences.		
Intense/unstable relationships: Liability to become involved in intense and unstable relationships, often leading to emotional crises.		
Deliberate self-harm: Recurrent threats or acts of self-harm.		
Emptiness: Chronic feelings of emptiness.		

28.5 Classifactory approach to psychosis of unknown aetiology, based on DSM-IV-TR

Figure 28.2 Classificatory approach to psychosis of unknown aetiology, based on DSM-IV-TR. DSM-IV-TR provides its own decision trees for some psychotic conditions.

PRELIMINARY TREE: conditions not considered primary causes of psychosis by DSM-IV-TR, but which can have psychotic features, or omitted from its psychosis tree

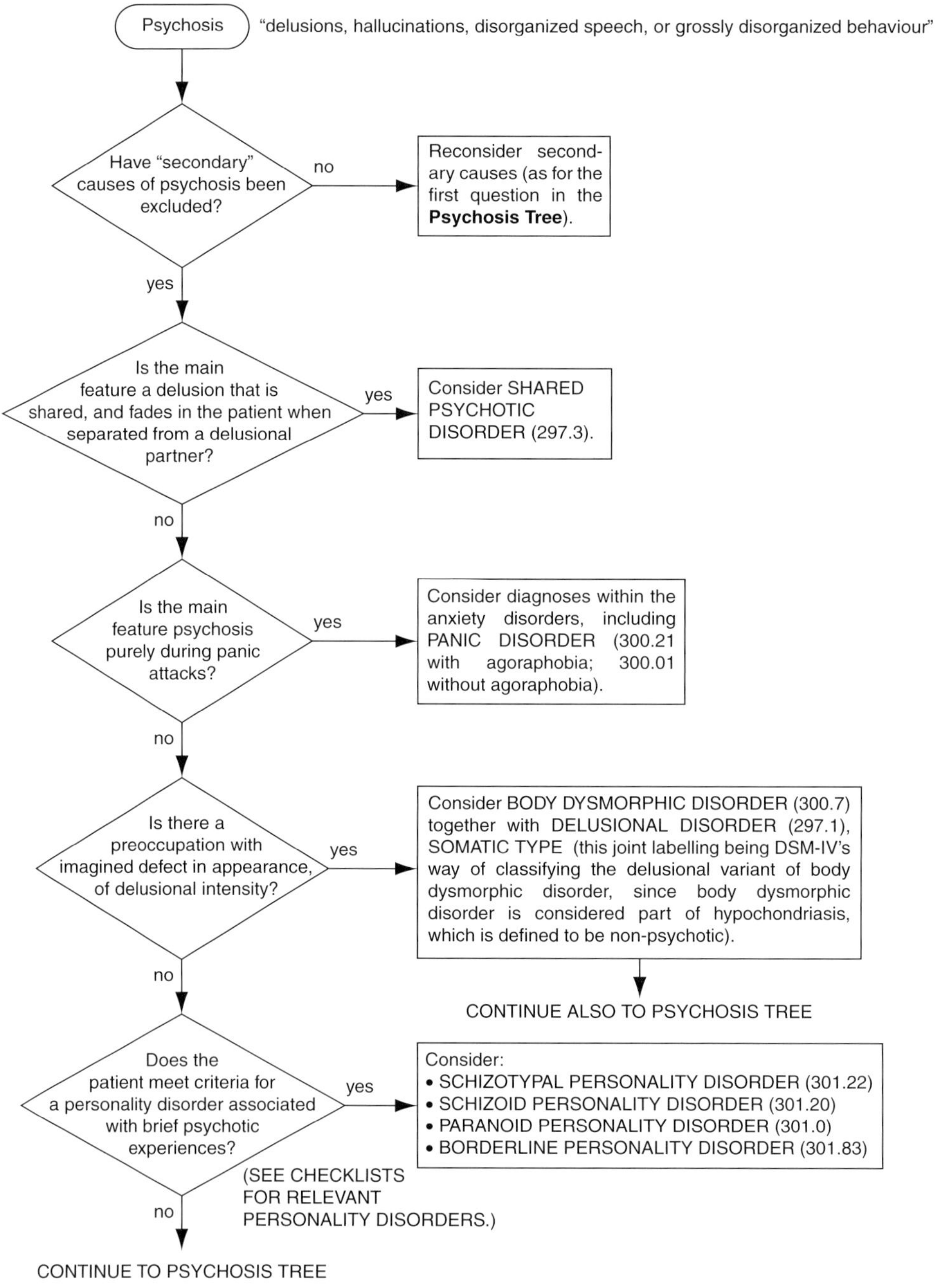

PSYCHOSIS TREE, adapted from DSM-IV-TR

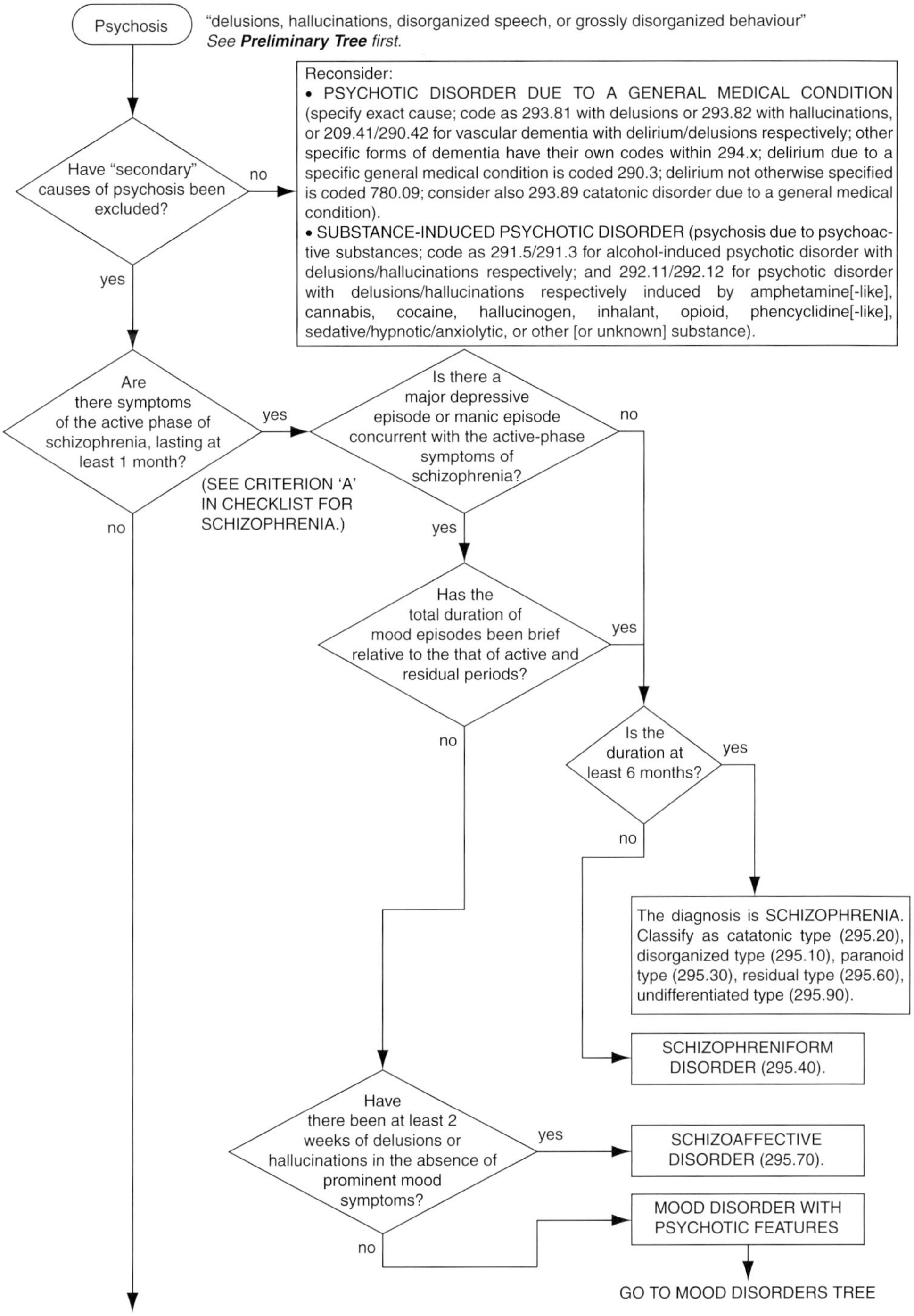

PSYCHOSIS TREE, adapted from DSM-IV-TR (continued)

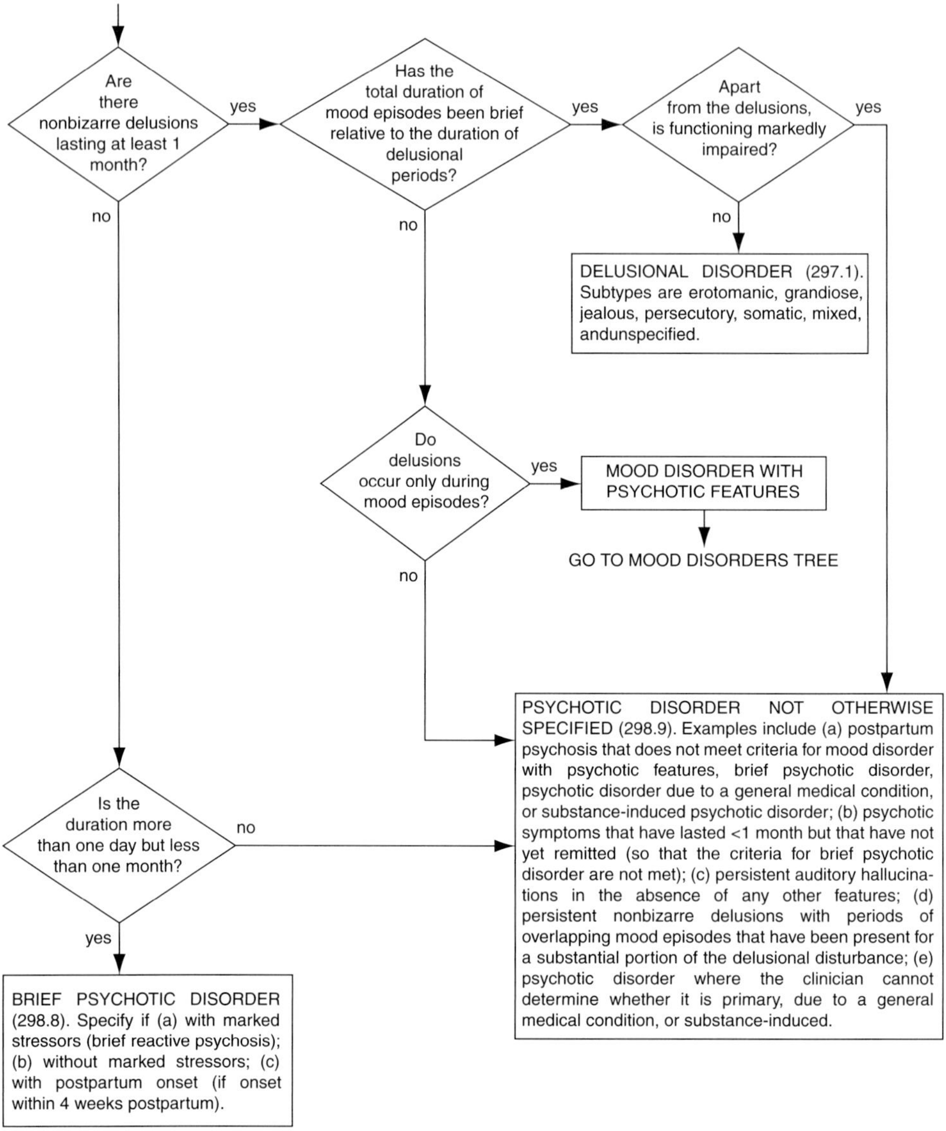

MOOD DISORDERS TREE, adapted from DSM-IV-TR, for mood disorders with psychosis

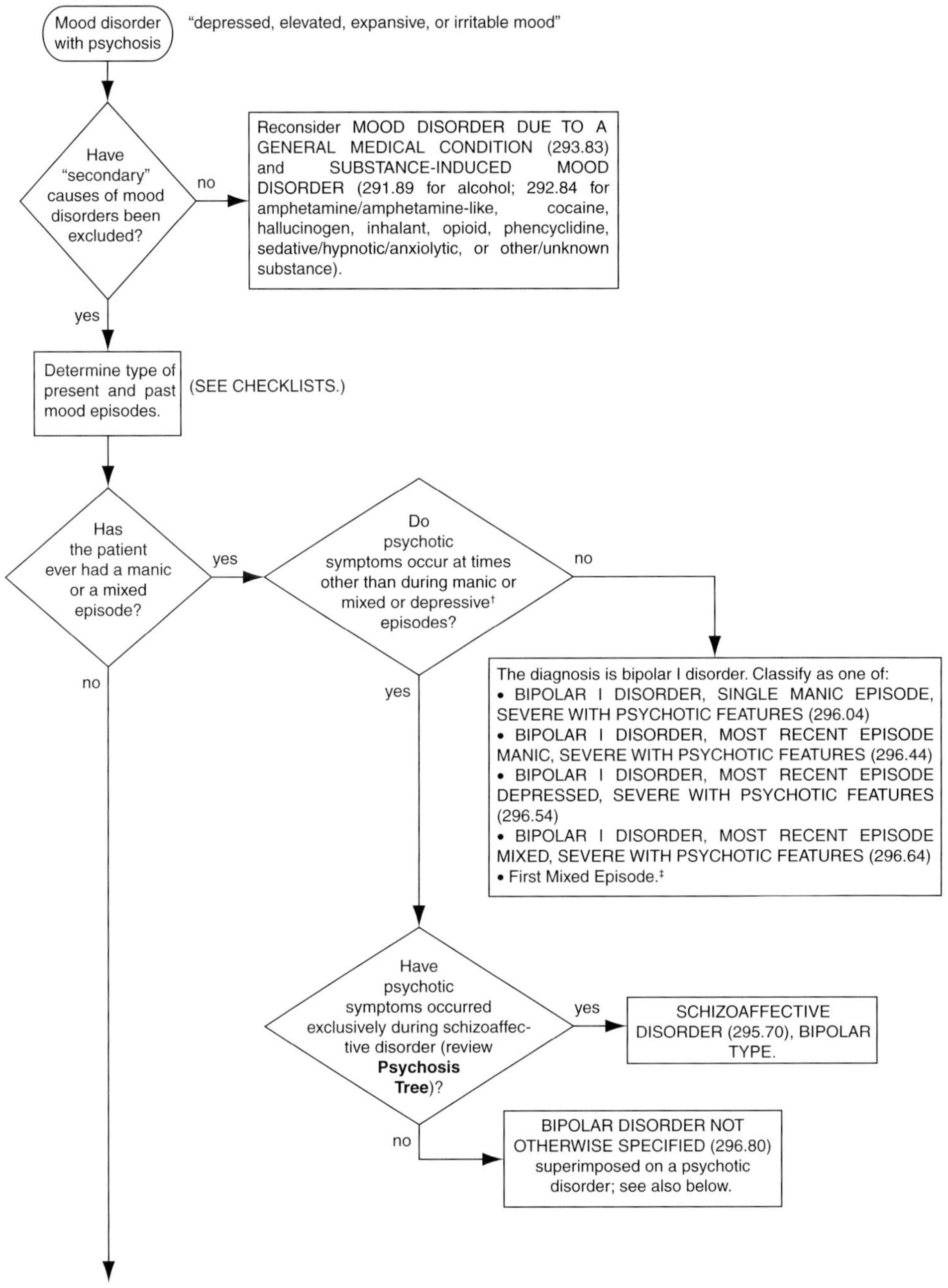

† We have added "or depressive", since we think that otherwise, a diagnosis of bipolar I disorder with psychotic depression (but never psychotic mania) would be misclassified as bipolar disorder not otherwise specified, superimposed on a psychotic disorder.

‡ This is not in the DSM-IV-TR decision tree; note that DSM-IV criteria for bipolar I disorder are not fulfilled by a first mixed episode, without a previous depressive or mixed or manic episode, and there is no numerical code for a first mixed episode.

MOOD DISORDERS TREE, adapted from DSM-IV-TR, for mood disorders with psychosis (continued)

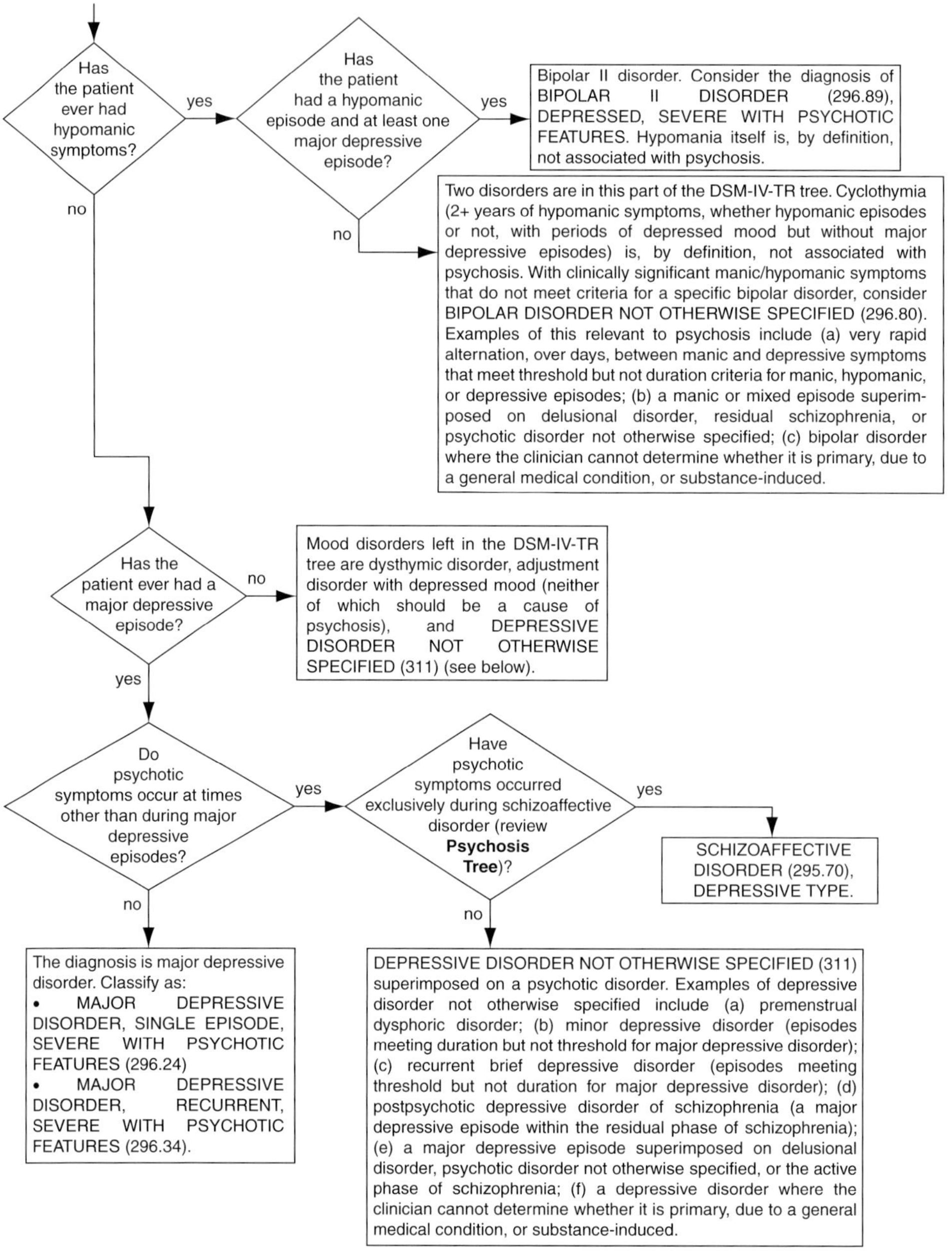

28.6 DSM-IV criteria for mood disorders

Date: ________________ Assessor: ________________	Patient details

DEPRESSION. DSM-IV-TR criteria for Major Depressive Episode [5].

A. Core symptoms	*Absent*	*Present*
Mood: depressed mood most of the day, nearly every day, as indicated by either subjective report (e.g. feels sad or empty) or observation made by others (e.g. appears tearful). *In children and adolescents, can be irritable mood.*		
Anhedonia: markedly diminished interest or pleasure in all, or almost all, activities most of the day, nearly every day (as indicated by either subjective account or observation made by others)		
Total symptoms in category A:		
B. Other key diagnostic symptoms (do NOT include symptoms that are clearly due to a general medical condition, or mood-incongruent delusions or hallucinations)	*Absent*	*Present*
Energy: fatigue or loss of energy nearly every day		
Sleep: insomnia or hypersomnia nearly every day		
Worth/Guilt: feelings of worthless or excessive or inappropriate guilt (which may be delusional) nearly every day (not merely self-reproach or guilt about being sick)		
Appetite: significant weight loss when not dieting or weight gain (e.g. a change of >5% of body weight in a month), or decrease or increase in appetite nearly every day. *In children and adolescents, consider failure to make expected weight gains.*		
Concentration: diminished ability to think or concentrate, or indecisiveness, nearly every day (either by subjective account or as observed by others)		
Activity: psychomotor agitation or retardation nearly every day (observable by others, not merely subjective feelings of restlessness or being slowed down)		
Death: recurrent thoughts of death (not just fear of dying), recurrent suicidal ideation without a specific plan, or a suicide attempt or a specific plan for committing suicide.		
Total symptoms in category B:		
Total symptoms in categories A + B:		

DSM-IV criteria for mood disorders, continued.

Date: _______________ Assessor: _______________	Patient details

Criteria: Number of symptoms and duration (all must be true)	*False*	*True*
At least one symptom from group A and a total of ≥5 symptoms from across groups A and B…		
Criteria: Number of symptoms and duration (all must be true)	*False*	*True*
… present during the same 2-week period and representing a change from previous functioning.		
Exclusion criteria (all must be true)	*False*	*True*
The symptoms do not meet criteria for a Mixed Episode.		
The symptoms cause clinically significant distress or impairment in social, occupational, or other important areas of functioning.		
Not due to a substance or to a general medical condition.		
Symptoms not better accounted for by Bereavement (i.e. after the loss of a loved one, the symptoms persist for >2 months or are characterized by marked functional impairment, morbid preoccupation with worthlessness, suicidal ideation, psychotic symptoms, or psychomotor retardation).		

DSM-IV criteria for mood disorders, continued.

Date: ____________ Assessor: ____________	Patient details

MANIA AND HYPOMANIA. DSM-IV-TR criteria for hypomanic and manic episodes [5].

A. Core symptom of hypomania and mania	*Absent*	*Present*
Mood: A distinct period of abnormally and persistently elevated, expansive, or irritable mood.		
B. Other symptoms of hypomania and mania	*Absent*	*Present*
Distractible: attention too easily drawn to unimportant or irrelevant external stimuli		
Activity: increase in goal-directed activity (either socially, at work or school, or sexually) or psychomotor agitation		
Sleep: decreased need for sleep (e.g., feels rested after only 3 hours of sleep).		
Talkative: more talkative than usual or pressure to keep talking.		
Recklessness: excessive involvement in pleasurable activities that have a high potential for painful consequences (e.g. engaging in unrestrained buying sprees, sexual indiscretions, or foolish business investments)		
Grandiosity: Inflated self-esteem or grandiosity.		
Flight of ideas: Flight of ideas or the subjective experience that thoughts are racing.		
Total symptoms in category B:		
C. Criteria for diagnosis of MANIC EPISODE (all must be true)	*False*	*True*
Mood symptom A for at least 7 days (or it is severe enough to require hospital admission), plus at least 3 symptoms from group B (or at least 4 symptoms if the mood is merely irritable) present to a significant degree.		
C. Criteria for diagnosis of MANIC EPISODE (all must be true)	*False*	*True*
Symptoms do not meet criteria for a Mixed Episode.		
Marked impairment in occupational functioning, or in usual social activities or relationships with others, or such as to necessitate hospitalization to prevent harm to self/others, or there are psychotic features.		
Not due to a substance or to a general medical condition.		

DSM-IV criteria for mood disorders, continued.

Date: ________________ Assessor: ________________	Patient details

D. Criteria for diagnosis of HYPOMANIC EPISODE (all must be true)	*False*	*True*
Mood symptom A for at least 4 days (clearly different from the usual nondepressed mood), and at least 3 symptoms from group B (4 if the mood is merely irritable) present to a significant degree.		
Episode associated with an unequivocal change in functioning that is uncharacteristic of the person when not symptomatic.		
Mood disturbance and change in functioning are observable by others.		
The episode is not severe enough to cause marked impairment in social or occupational functioning, or to necessitate hospitalization, and there are no psychotic features.		
Not due to a substance or to a general medical condition.		

MIXED AFFECTIVE STATE. DSM-IV-TR criteria for mixed episode [5].

Criteria for Mixed Episode (all must be true)	*False*	*True*
The criteria are met both for a Manic Episode and for a Major Depressive Episode (except for duration) nearly every day during at least a 1-week period.		
Marked impairment in occupational functioning, or in usual social activities or relationships with others, or such as to necessitate hospitalization to prevent harm to self/others, or there are psychotic features.		
Not due to a substance or to a general medical condition.		

28.7 DSM-IV criteria for schizophrenia

Date: ______________ Assessor: ______________	Patient details

SCHIZOPHRENIA. DSM-IV-TR criteria for schizophrenia [5]. Layout modified.

A1. Core symptoms of schizophrenia	*Absent*	*Present*
Bizarre delusions		
Hallucinatory voice keeping up a running commentary on the person's behaviour or thoughts		
Two or more voices conversing with each other		
A2. Other symptoms of schizophrenia	*Absent*	*Present*
Delusions		
Hallucinations		
Disorganized speech (e.g. frequent derailment or incoherence)		
Grossly disorganized or catatonic behaviour		
Negative symptoms, i.e. affective flattening, alogia, or avolition		
Criterion A. Symptom criterion for schizophrenia (must be true)	*False*	*True*
One symptom from group A1, or ≥2 symptoms from group A2, each present for a significant portion of time during a 1-month period (or less if successfully treated)		
B–F. Other criteria (all must be true)	*False*	*True*
Functioning. For a significant portion of the time since the onset of the disturbance, one or more major areas of functioning such as work, interpersonal relations, or self-care are markedly below the level achieved prior to the onset (or when the onset is in childhood or adolescence, failure to achieve expected level of interpersonal, academic, or occupational achievement).		
Duration. Continuous signs of the disturbance persist for at least 6 months (which period must include at least one month of active-phase symptoms, i.e. criterion A, but which may include periods of prodromal or residual symptoms, manifested by only negative symptoms, or ≥2 group A symptoms in attenuated form, such as odd beliefs and unusual perceptual experiences).		
Schizoaffective disorder and mood disorder with psychotic features have been excluded, because either (1) no major depressive, manic, or mixed episodes have occurred concurrently with the active-phase symptoms, or (2) if mood episodes have occurred during active-phase symptoms, their total duration has been brief relative to the duration of the active and residual periods.		
Not due to a substance or general medical condition.		
Either no history of autistic disorder or another pervasive developmental disorder, or if there is such a history, prominent delusions or hallucinations have also been present for at least a month (or less if successfully treated).		

DSM-IV criteria for schizophrenia, continued.

Date: ____________ Assessor: ____________	Patient details

TYPES OF SCHIZOPHRENIA. From DSM-IV-TR [5].

PARANOID SCHIZOPHRENIA (295.30): need schizophrenia criteria and all of:	*False*	*True*
Preoccupation with one or more delusions or frequent auditory hallucinations.		
None of the following is prominent: disorganized speech, disorganized or catatonic behaviour, or flat or inappropriate affect.		
DISORGANIZED SCHIZOPHRENIA (295.10): need schizophrenia criteria and all of:	*False*	*True*
Prominent disorganized speech.		
Prominent disorganized behaviour.		
Prominent flat or inappropriate affect.		
The criteria are not met for Catatonia type.		
CATATONIC SCHIZOPHRENIA (295.20): need schizophrenia criteria and the clinical picture dominated by ≥2 of:	*False*	*True*
Motoric immobility as evidenced by catalepsy (including waxy flexibility) or stupor.		
Excessive motor activity (that is apparently purposeless and not influenced by external stimuli).		
Extreme negativism (an apparently motiveless resistance to all instructions or maintenance of a rigid posture against attempts to be moved) or mutism.		
Peculiarities of voluntary movement as evidenced by posturing (voluntary assumption of inappropriate or bizarre postures), stereotyped movements, prominent mannerisms, or prominent grimacing.		
Echolalia or echopraxia		
UNDIFFERENTIATED SCHIZOPHRENIA (295.90): need schizophrenia criteria and all of:	*False*	*True*
Criteria are not met for the paranoid, disorganized, or catatonic types.		
RESIDUAL SCHIZOPHRENIA (295.60): need at least one episode of schizophrenia and all of:	*False*	*True*
Absence of prominent delusions, hallucinations, disorganized speech, and grossly disorganized or catatonic behaviour.		
There is continuing evidence of the disturbance, as indicated by the presence of negative symptoms or two or more symptoms listed in Criterion A for Schizophrenia, present in an attenuated form (e.g. odd beliefs, unusual perceptual experiences).		

28.8 DSM-IV criteria for personality disorders associated with psychotic symptoms

Date: ______________ Assessor: ______________	Patient details

PARANOID PERSONALITY DISORDER (CLUSTER A). DSM-IV-TR criteria [5].

A. Symptoms	*Absent*	*Present*
Doubting: Is preoccupied with unjustified doubts about the loyalty or trustworthiness of friends or associates.		
Overinterpretive: Reads hidden demeaning or threatening meanings into benign remarks or events.		
Grudges: Persistently bears grudges, i.e. is unforgiving of insults, injuries, or slights.		
Suspicious: Suspects, without sufficient basis, that others are exploiting, harming, or deceiving him or her.		
Jealous: Has recurrent suspicions, without justification, regarding sexual fidelity of spouse or sexual partner.		
Unconfiding: Is reluctant to confide in others because of unwarranted fear that the information will be used maliciously against him or her.		
Touchy: Perceives attacks on his or her character or reputation that are not apparent to others and is quick to react angrily or to counterattack.		
Total symptoms:		
B. Criteria (all must be met)	*False*	*True*
Symptoms: A pervasive distrust and suspiciousness of others such that their motives are interpreted as malevolent, as indicated by **≥4** symptoms from those listed above.		
Pervasive: The characteristics are present in a variety of contexts.		
Persistent: It begins by early adulthood.		
Primary (1): Does not occur exclusively during the course of schizophrenia, a mood disorder with psychotic features, or another psychotic disorder.		
Primary (2): Not due to a general medical condition.		

DSM-IV personality disorders associated with psychotic symptoms, continued.

Date: ________________ Assessor: ________________	Patient details

SCHIZOID PERSONALITY DISORDER (CLUSTER A). DSM-IV-TR criteria [5]. Layout as before.

A. Symptoms	*Absent*	*Present*
Loner (1): Neither desires nor enjoys close confiding relationships, including being part of a family.		
Anhedonia: Takes pleasure in few, if any, activities.		
Detached: Emotional coldness, detachment, or flattened affectivity.		
Solitary: Almost always chooses solitary activities.		
Asexual: Has little, if any, interest in having sexual experiences with another person.		
Indifferent: Appears indifferent to either praise or criticism of others.		
Loner (2): Lacks close friends or confidants other than first-degree relatives.		
Total symptoms:		
B. Criteria (all must be met)	*False*	*True*
Symptoms: A pervasive pattern of detachment from social relationships and a restricted range of expression in emotions in interpersonal settings, as indicated by **≥4** symptoms from those listed above.		
Pervasive: The characteristics are present in a variety of contexts.		
Persistent: It begins by early adulthood.		
Primary (1): Does not occur exclusively during the course of schizophrenia, a mood disorder with psychotic features, another psychotic disorder, or a pervasive developmental disorder.		
Primary (2): Not due to a general medical condition.		

DSM-IV personality disorders associated with psychotic symptoms, continued.

Date: ____________ Assessor: ____________	Patient details

SCHIZOTYPAL PERSONALITY DISORDER (CLUSTER A). DSM-IV-TR criteria [5]. Layout as before.

A. Symptoms	*Absent*	*Present*
Magical thinking: Odd beliefs or magical thinking that influences behaviour and inconsistent with subcultural norms (e.g. superstitiousness, belief in clairvoyance, telepathy, or "sixth sense"; in children and adolescents, bizarre fantasies or preoccupations).		
Affect: Inappropriate or constricted affect.		
Ideas of reference: ideas of reference (excluding delusions of reference).		
Loner: lack of close friends or confidants other than first-degree relatives.		
Suspicious: Suspiciousness or paranoid ideation.		
Thought abnormalities: Odd thinking and speech (e.g. vague, circumstantial, metaphorical, over-elaborate, or stereotyped).		
Odd: Behaviour or appearance that is odd, eccentric, or peculiar.		
Perceptual abnormalities: Unusual perceptual experiences, including bodily illusions.		
Social anxiety: Excessive social anxiety that does not diminish with familiarity and tends to be associated with paranoid fears rather than negative judgements about self.		
Total symptoms:		
B. Criteria (all must be met)	*False*	*True*
Symptoms: A pervasive pattern of social and interpersonal deficits marked by acute discomfort with, and reduced capacity for, close relationships as well as by cognitive or perceptual distortions and eccentricities of behaviour, as indicated by **≥5** symptoms from those above.		
Pervasive: The characteristics are present in a variety of contexts.		
Persistent: It begins by early adulthood.		
Primary: Does not occur exclusively during the course of schizophrenia, a mood disorder with psychotic features, another psychotic disorder, or a pervasive developmental disorder.		

DSM-IV personality disorders associated with psychotic symptoms, continued.

Date: ______________ Assessor: ______________	Patient details

BORDERLINE PERSONALITY DISORDER (CLUSTER B). DSM-IV-TR criteria [5]. Layout as before.

A. Symptoms	*Absent*	*Present*
Impulsive: Impulsivity in at least two areas that are potentially self-damaging (e.g. spending, sex, substance abuse, reckless driving, binge eating). *Do not include suicidal or self-mutilating behaviour covered in "deliberate self-harm".*		
Paranoia/dissociation: Transient, stress-related paranoid ideation or severe dissociative symptoms.		
Unstable mood: Affective instability due to a marked reactivity of mood (e.g. intense episodic dysphoria, irritability, or anxiety usually lasting a few hours and only rarely more than a few days).		
Temper: Inappropriate, intense anger or difficulty controlling anger (e.g. frequent displays of temper, constant anger, recurrent physical fights).		
Avoid abandoment: Frantic efforts to avoid real or imagined abandonment. *Do not include suicidal or self-mutilating behaviour covered in "deliberate self-harm".*		
Self-image uncertain: Identity disturbance: markedly and persistently unstable self-image or sense of self.		
Intense/unstable relationships: A pattern of unstable and intense interpersonal relationships characterized by alternating between extremes of idealization and devaluation.		
Deliberate self-harm: Recurrent suicidal behaviour, gestures, or threats, or self-mutilating behaviour.		
Emptiness: Chronic feelings of emptiness.		
	Total symptoms:	
B. Criteria (all must be met)	*False*	*True*
Symptoms: A pervasive pattern of instability of interpersonal relationships, self-image, and affects, and marked impulsivity, as indicated by **≥5** symptoms from those listed above.		
Pervasive: The characteristics are present in a variety of contexts.		
Persistent: It begins by early adulthood.		

28.9 Examination for catatonia

Date: ______________ Assessor: ______________	Patient details

From [31, 1130].

Procedure:	Examines:
1. Observe patient while trying to engage in a conversation.	Activity level, abnormal movements, abnormal speech.
2. Examiner scratches head in exaggerated manner.	Echopraxia
3. Examine arm for cogwheeling. Attempt to reposition, instructing patient to "keep your arm loose". Move arm with alternating lighter and heavier force.	Rigidity, negativism, waxy flexibility
4. Ask patient to extend arm. Place one finger beneath hand and try to raise slowly after stating, "DO NOT let me raise your arm."	Passive obedience
5. Extend hand stating, "DO NOT shake my hand."	Ambitendence
6. Reach into your pocket and state, "Stick out your tongue, I want to stick a pin in it."	Automatic obedience
7. Examine for the grasp reflex.	Grasp reflex
8. Examine the patient's chart for oral intake, vital signs, and unusual incidents.	
9. Observe the patient indirectly for a brief period each day.	

28.10 Fink & Taylor criteria for catatonia

Date: ____________ Assessor: ____________	Patient details

Criteria for catatonia [31, 1132].

Symptom group A	*Absent*		*Present*
Stupor lasting ≥1 hour (conscious but unresponsive with hypoactivity and reduced or altered arousal; fails to respond to queries ± to pain).			
Immobility lasting ≥1 hour.			
Mutism lasting ≥1 hour.			
Symptom group B	*Absent*	*1 occasion*	*≥2 occasions*
Catalepsy (postural perseveration, waxy flexibility).			
Automatic obedience (permits an examiner's light touch to move patient's limbs into a new posture, despite instructions to the contrary).			
Posturing (maintains abnormal posture of limbs/body/face for long periods).			
Symptom group C	*Absent*	*1 occasion*	*≥2 occasions*
Stereotypy (repetitive, awkward, or stiff, apparently senseless, movements).			
Ambitendency (the state of becoming "stuck" between two alternative actions, such as when given conflicting verbal and non-verbal instructions).			
Negativism (includes resisting of examiner's manipulations with force equal to that applied, or refusing or performing the opposite of any request).			
Echophenomena (echolalia, echopraxia, utilization behaviour, speech-promptness).			

These criteria for catatonia [31, 1132] require either of:

- one symptom from group A, associated with at least one symptom from group B seen or elicited on ≥2 occasions;
- two symptoms from across groups B and C seen or elicited on ≥2 occasions.

Chapter 29

Conclusion

Psychosis is a common response to a wide variety of neurological insults, but also a common syndrome occurring in primary psychiatric disease. Correct diagnosis may allow treatment of specific causes, where such causes can be identified, in addition to symptom-based treatments, such as with antipsychotic drugs.

Overall, how common are primary and secondary psychoses? One recent DSM-IV-based Finnish study suggested that the lifetime prevalence of psychotic disorders is 3.06% (3.48% including survey nonresponders), with lifetime prevalences of 0.87% for schizophrenia, 0.45% for psychotic disorder not otherwise specified, 0.42% for substance-induced psychotic disorders, 0.35% for major depressive disorder with psychotic features, 0.32% for schizoaffective disorder, 0.21% for psychotic disorders due to a general medical condition, 0.18% for delusional disorder, 0.12% for bipolar I disorder with psychotic features, 0.07% for schizophreniform disorder, and 0.05% for brief psychotic disorder [1162]. Past studies have found that 12% of patients admitted to a psychiatric hospital had a physical illness that was an important causative factor in their mental disorder, and that 13% of patients admitted to old-age psychiatric wards had an acute (and 30% had an acute-on-chronic) physical cause for their symptoms [25]. One large series surveying patients within psychiatric care, both inpatient and outpatient, concluded that physical illness caused the mental disorder in 6% and exacerbated a mental disorder in 9% [1301]. Relevant organic disease was found in 6% of patients with first-episode psychosis in another study [824]. Of course, as primary psychoses are diagnoses of exclusion, there is always potential for the discovery of new causes of secondary psychosis.

What is the relative importance of psychopathology in the diagnosis of primary and secondary psychosis? We have emphasized the non-psychiatric phenotype in the diagnosis of secondary psychosis, and psychopathology in the diagnosis of primary psychosis (not forgetting, of course, that psychopathology may be key to symptomatic treatment, regardless of the cause). Further refinement by considering the psychopathology of secondary psychoses may be useful. However, as described in Chapter 1, there is considerable overlap with the psychopathology of primary psychoses, and at present there is no evidence that exclusion of secondary psychosis can be made reliably based on the mental state alone, though certain "red flag" symptoms may strongly suggest secondary psychosis. We refer the reader to other works for detailed descriptions of psychopathology in secondary psychosis [5, 14–17, 20, 22, 33].

Does our review of the causes of psychosis add significantly to our understanding of the neurobiological mechanisms of psychosis? No. However, a number of contemporary

Inborn errors of metabolism. Abetalipoproteinemia (MIM 200100, though see neuroacanthocytosis [Chapter 5.10 ▶]); Batten's disease (CLN 3, MIM 204200); Canavan's disease (aspartoacylase deficiency, MIM 271900); creatine deficiency (MIM 300352) [1317]; cystinosis (OMIM 219800, 219750); Farber's disease (ceramidase deficiency, disseminated lipogranulomatosis, MIM 228000); Forbes' disease (Cori's disease, glycogen storage disease III, MIM 232400); fucosidosis (MIM 230000); galactosaemia (MIM 230400); GM1 and GM3 gangliosidosis (MIM 230500, 230600, 230650); glycine encephalopathy (non-ketotic hyperglycinemia, MIM 605899); haemochromatosis (MIM 235200); hyperasparaginemia (see above); β-mannosidosis (MIM 248510); Menke's disease (kinky hair disease; X-linked copper deficiency, MIM 300011, 309400); neuraminidase deficiency (sialidosis, MIM 256550); polyglucosan body disease, adult form (MIM 263570); Pompe's disease (glycogen storage disease II, acid maltase deficiency, MIM 232300); Refsum's disease (MIM 266500); Sanfilippo syndrome (mucopolysaccharidosis type IIIA, MIM 252900) [1318]; Schindler's disease (α-N-acetylgalactosaminidase deficiency, MIM 609241, 609242); Sly's syndrome (mucopolysaccharidosis type VII, MIM 253220); Tangier disease (MIM 205400); von Gierke's disease (glycogen storage disease I, MIM 232200); Wolman's disease (lysosomal acid lipase deficiency, MIM 278000).

Infections. Anaplasmosis; babesiosis; BK virus; Borna virus (though there is a suggestion of an association and this is one to watch [22, 1319–1321]); dengue; diphtheria; Hendra virus; HSV causing postencephalitic as opposed to acute psychosis [20, 1322]; leprosy (as discussed above); postencephalitic psychosis in general, excepting postencephalitic parkinsonism (see encephalitis lethargica, Chapter 8.7.2 ▶); viral meningitis (without encephalitis).

Miscellaneous. Anemia (in isolation); disseminated intravascular coagulation (in isolation); hepatitis (in isolation); Fanconi's syndrome (this can refer to Prader–Labhart–Willi–Fanconi syndrome, better known as Prader–Willi syndrome [Chapter 4.5 ▶], but much more commonly to renal tubular acidosis); idiopathic intracranial hypertension (benign intracranial hypertension, pseudotumor cerebri); malignant hyperthermia (anaesthetic-induced); Morgagni's syndrome (hyperostosis frontalis interna).

Neoplastic. Bronchogenic carcinoma (aside from mechanisms discussed in the text); Castleman's disease (a disorder of B cell hyperproliferation; case [1323] has a range of possible other causes); pancreatic carcinoma (as above).

Neurodegenerative. familial encephalopathy with neuroserpin inclusion bodies (FENIB, MIM 604218); Marchiafava–Bignami syndrome (corpus callosum degeneration in the context of alcoholism; some reports suggest psychosis has occurred [1324], but see Chapter 4.4 ▶); neurofibromatosis (type 1 MIM 162200, type 2 MIM 101000; potentially associated with "childhood psychosis" but using a definition of psychosis principally that of autism [1325]); sudanophilic cerebral sclerosis (but see also diffuse sclerosis [Chapter 10.5.14 ▶] and note some naming confusion; MIM 272100; some cases such as [1326] are hard to distinguish from e.g. diffuse myelinoclastic sclerosis); Zellweger's syndrome (cerebrohepatorenal syndrome; MIM 214100).

Nutritional. Biotin deficiency; vitamin E deficiency.

Other genetic and congenital conditions. Alexander's disease (MIM 203450) [17, 94]; Alpers' syndrome (Alpers' diffuse degeneration of cerebral gray matter with hepatic cirrhosis; MIM 203700); chromosome 18q deletion (MIM 601808) [1327]; Cockayne's syndrome (MIM 216400, 133540); congenital myotonia (myotonia congenita) [33]; juvenile myoclonic epilepsy (in isolation [1329]; MIM 245570; see also Landau–Kleffner syndrome [Chapter 4.8 ▶]); Kartagener's syndrome (primary ciliary dyskinesia I, MIM 244400; scant evidence [1330]); Leber's hereditary optic atrophy (MIM 535000); Miller–Dieker lissencephaly syndrome (chromosome 17p13.3 deletion, MIM 247200).

Other metabolic. Acromegaly [33]; Paget's disease of bone (no evidence; [1331]).

Psychological. Severe pain (though see also Chapter 21.20.3 ▶).

Rheumatological. Polymyositis.

Toxic. Antimony; aspartame (though perhaps mania with high-dose aspartame [1332]) carbidopa (in isolation); formaldehyde; ketoconazole (somewhat unconvincing [1333, 1334]); lathyrism; mannitol (though conceivably but not convincingly mania [1335]); methyldopa withdrawal (though mania [1336]); oxygen toxicity (hyperoxia); tiagabine withdrawal [1337]; vinyl chloride; vitamin D toxicity (except with hypercalcaemia).

Vascular (other). Autosomal dominant vascular retinopathy, migraine and Raynaud's syndrome (MIM 192315); Ehlers–Danlos syndrome (MIM 130000); fibromuscular dysplasia (MIM 135580); hereditary cerebral hemorrhage with amyloidosis, Dutch type (MIM 605714); Köhlmeier–Degos disease (papulosis atrophicans maligna, MIM 602248); pseudoxanthoma elasticum (single case report only; see Chapter 13.2.5 ▶).

Appendix B: Relevant changes proposed in DSM-V

DSM-IV-TR is currently undergoing revision to DSM-V, due for publication in 2013. Classificatory issues are under discussion, but a number of proposals have relevance to the current work [24]. The major proposed changes relating to psychosis, described in more detail below, are:

- the proposal of a new psychosis risk syndrome or attenuated psychotic symptoms syndrome;
- some changes to the criteria for schizophrenia (including de-emphasizing bizarre delusions and Schneiderian first-rank symptoms), with corresponding changes to the criteria for schizophreniform disorder;
- the removal of all subtypes of schizophrenia;
- greater clarity in the criteria for schizoaffective disorder;
- removal of shared psychotic disorder;
- minor changes to the definition of manic, hypomanic and depressive episodes, with "mixed features" becoming a specifier applied to other episodes (rather than distinct "mixed episodes");
- with regard to depressive episodes and depressive disorder, removal of the exclusion relating to bereavement, removal of the exclusion of mood-incongruent psychotic symptoms, and recognition that psychotic depression is not always severe depression;
- representation of insight as a continuum (with delusions at one end of it) in body dysmorphic disorder, obsessive–compulsive disorder, and a new condition, olfactory reference syndrome;
- reworking of personality disorders into a predominantly dimensional approach, though with the retention of five personality disorders (including schizotypal and borderline personality disorders, but not paranoid or schizoid personality disorder).

In more detail, the relevant changes proposed at the time of writing are as follows.

General

There is a proposal to **collapse Axes I, II, and III**, to a single axis encompassing all medical and psychiatric diagnoses.

Neurodegenerative disorders

There is a proposal to **re-label "dementia" as "major neurocognitive disorder"**, within a group of neurocognitive disorders (viz. delirium, major neurocognitive disorder, and minor neurocognitive disorder) and to categorize e.g. psychosis and depression within them.

Catatonia

Catatonia may be changed from a disorder ("catatonic disorder due to…") to a catatonia specifier ("… with catatonia"), applicable to any diagnosis within the schizophrenic, mood, and medical disorders. Catatonia would be defined as ≥3 of catalepsy, waxy flexibility, stupor, agitation, mutism, negativism, posturing, mannerisms, stereotypies, grimacing, echolalia, or echopraxia.

Schizophrenia and related disorders

Psychosis risk syndrome or **attenuated psychotic symptoms syndrome** may be added, characterized by at least one of delusions, hallucinations, or disorganized speech, in attenuated form with intact reality testing, but severe and/or frequent enough that it is not ignored. These symptons must have occured at least weekly in the past month, begun or progressed in the past year, led the patient or their carer to seek help, and not be explained better by another diagnosis; criteria for a psychotic disorder should never have been met.

Schizophrenia criteria (Chapter 21.1, 28.7 ►) may be modified. The principal proposed changes are to criterion A (characteristic symptoms). "Disorganized behavior" is removed, "negative symptoms" are clarified, the privileged status of bizarre delusions and Schneiderian first-rank hallucinations is removed, and a requirement for psychotic symptoms is added. The required symptoms therefore become ≥2 from delusions, hallucinations, disorganized speech, catatonia, and negative symptoms ("restricted affect or avolition/asociality"), with at least one symptom from the first three of these. The required duration does not change, and neither do the rest of criteria B–F (social/occupational dysfunction, duration, exclusion of schizoaffective/mood/substance-induced/general medical disorders, and the relationship to pervasive developmental disorders).

Subtypes of schizophrenia may be removed from DSM-V, with a move towards a dimensional system.

Shared psychotic disorder may be removed from DSM-V.

The criteria for **schizophreniform disorder** (the DSM's category for a disorder meeting the criteria for schizophrenia apart from its duration) will change to reflect the new proposed criteria for schizophrenia (as above).

The criteria for **schizoaffective disorder** may become more precise. Any changes to the definition of schizophrenia or mood disorders will be reflected. The criterion of delusions or hallucinations for ≥2 weeks in the absence of "prominent mood symptoms" may be strengthened (to the absence of a major mood episode), or removed. A requirement may be introduced that the patient meets criteria for a major mood episode for >30–50% of the lifetime duration of the illness.

The criteria for the **somatic type of delusional disorder** are changed in a minor way, by specifying that the delusion must be of having some general medical condition (to distinguish this disorder more clearly from body dysmorphic disorder of deluional intensity).

The criteria for **brief psychotic disorder** may undergo minor revision to separate the description of disorganized speech and psychomotor symptoms.

Mood disorders

The diagnostic criteria for **mania** and **hypomania** may be changed slightly. The main mood criterion for mania may be amended so that the abnormal mood must be present for "most of the day, nearly every day" (for a week, unless hospitalized, as before). A requirement for persistently increased activity or energy may be added. Clarification is added that the other symptoms should represent a change from usual behaviour, and "pleasurable" is removed from "excessive involvement in pleasurable activities that have a high potential for painful consequences". A note is also added to the effect that a full (but only a full) manic episode emerging during, and persisting beyond, antidepressant therapy should be classed as such. Similar changes are likely to be made to the definition of a hypomanic episode.

The category of **bipolar I disorder, most recent episode mixed** may be removed and be replaced by a **mixed** [affective state] **specifier** ("... with mixed features"), applicable to depressive, hypomanic, and manic episodes, with concomitant changes to the definitions of other affective disorders. If the episode is predominantly manic/hypomanic, then full criteria for a manic/hypomanic episode must be met, plus ≥3 persistent depressive symptoms (dysphoria/depressed mood; anhedonia; psychomotor retardation; fatigue; worthlessness/guilt; thoughts of death). If the episode is predominantly depressive, then full criteria for a depressive episode must be met, plus ≥3 persistent manic symptoms (elevated/expensive mood; grandiosity/increased self-esteem; talkativeness; flight of ideas/racing thoughts; increased energy/activity; risky activities; decreased need for sleep). If full criteria for manic and depressed episodes are met, the episode is classified as manic with mixed features (mania "trumps" depression).

There may also be changes to **bipolar disorder not otherwise specified**, perhaps with a new category encompassing those with short-duration symptoms, symptoms of subthreshold intensity, or hypomania only.

The criteria for **major depressive episode** are likely to change in the following ways:

- The text requiring a certain "number of symptoms" becomes "number of criteria" to reduce confusion.
- The exclusion of mood-incongruent psychotic symptoms is removed.
- The exclusion of symptoms caused by bereavement is removed, as there is no evidence that depression in this context is any different [1338].

With regard to **major depressive disorder**, the following significant changes are likely to be made:

- DSM-V is likely to recognize that depression with psychotic features is not always severe depression [1163].
- Where mood-incongruent and mood-congruent psychotic features exist, precedence may be given in a hierarchy to mood-incongruent psychotic features.
- The duration of the "postpartum" period for postpartum depression is extended to 6 months [1339].

Insight as a continuum

For **body dysmorphic disorder**, the "psychotic or not" dichotomy is likely to be replaced by more of a continuum, in which the body dysmorphic disorder beliefs are held with good/fair insight (the patient recognizes that they are definitely/probably not true, or that they may or may not be true), poor insight (thinks they are probably true), or no insight (completely convinced, i.e. delusional beliefs). The same approach is also proposed for **obsessive–compulsive disorder**, and a new condition, **olfactory reference syndrome** (likely to be included in an appendix as a condition for further research, and characterized by preoccupation with the belief that one emits a foul or offensive body odour, which is not perceived by others).

Personality disorders and personality traits

There is a proposal to rework the classification system for personality disorders entirely in DSM-V, to a dimensional system. In essence, the proposal is to rate individuals on 6 broad personality *trait domains*, each composed of more specific *trait facets*. The draft proposed trait domains and facets [24] are:

- **Negative emotionality**: The subject experiences a wide range of negative emotions (e.g., anxiety, depression, guilt, shame, worry), and their behavioural and interpersonal consequences. The trait facets are: emotional lability, anxiousness, submissiveness, separation insecurity, pessimism, low self-esteem, guilt/shame, self-harm, depressivity, and suspiciousness.
- **Introversion**: Withdrawal from other people, and restricted affective experience and expression. The trait facets are: social withdrawal, social detachment, restricted affectivity, anhedonia, and intimacy avoidance.
- **Antagonism**: Antipathy toward others and exaggerated self-importance. The trait facets are: callousness, manipulativeness, narcissism, histrionism, hostility, aggression, oppositionality, and deceitfulness.
- **Disinhibition**: Being oriented to the present, so that behaviour is driven by current internal and external stimuli, rather than by past learning and future consequences. The trait facets are: impulsivity, distractibility, recklessness, and irresponsibility.
- **Compulsivity**: The tendency to think and act according to a narrow and unchanging ideal, and the expectation that this ideal should be adhered to by everyone. The trait facets are: perfectionism, perseveration, rigidity, orderliness, and risk aversion.
- **Schizotypy**: Odd or unusual behaviours and cognitions, including abnormalities of perceptions and beliefs. The trait facets are: unusual perceptions, unusual beliefs, eccentricity, cognitive dysregulation, and dissociation proneness.

Trait levels are assessed on a four-point scale based on how descriptive they are of the patient.

Five personality disorders are retained as categorical entities in the proposal: schizotypal, antisocial/psychopathic, borderline, avoidant, and obsessive–compulsive personality disorders. Prominent personality traits are listed for these and for the other DSM-IV personality disorders.

General criteria for personality disorder are proposed. Personality disorders are defined as a failure to develop a sense of self-identity and capacity for interpersonal functioning that is culturally adaptive. An impaired sense of self-identity may manifest as a limited sense of personal unity and continuity, a changing definition of the self or changing self-states, poorly delineated interpersonal boundaries, and a sense of inner emptiness or difficulty describing self-attributes. Impaired interpersonal functioning may be manifest as poor empathy, impaired capacity for intimate relationships, poor social cooperativeness, and less complex and poorly integrated representations of other people. The adaptive failure is associated with extreme levels of one or more personality traits, is stable across time and situations, has an onset in adolescence or earlier, and is not solely the consequence of another mental disorder, a psychoactive drug, or a general medical disorder.

21. Asher, R. (1949). Myxoedematous madness. *British Medical Journal* **2**: 555–562. PMID 18148089.
22. Sadock, B. J. & Sadock, V. A., Eds. (2005). *Kaplan & Sadock's Comprehensive Textbook of Psychiatry*. Eighth edition. Philadelphia, PA: Lippincott Williams & Wilkins.
23. Bayes, T. (1763). An essay towards solving a problem in the doctrine of chances. *Philosophical Transactions of the Royal Society of London* **53**: 370–418.
24. American Psychiatric Association (2010). DSM-5 Development. URL: http://www.dsm5.org/. Accessed 30 March 2010 and 5 Januaury 2011.
25. Lishman, W. A. (1997). *Organic Psychiatry: The psychological consequences of cerebral disorder*. Third edition. Oxford: Blackwell.
26. Warrell, D. A., Cox, T. M., Firth, J. D. & Benz, E. J., Eds. (2003). *Oxford Textbook of Medicine*. Fourth edition. Oxford: Oxford University Press.
27. British Medical Association & Royal Pharmaceutical Society of Great Britain (2007). *British National Formulary (BNF) 54 [September 2007]*. London: BMJ Publishing Group Ltd & RPS Publishing.
28. Goetz, C. G., Ed. (2007). *Textbook of Clinical Neurology*. Philadelphia, PA: Saunders Elsevier.
29. Stein, G. & Wilkinson, G., Eds. (2007). *Seminars in General Adult Psychiatry*. Second edition. London: Gaskell (Royal College of Psychiatrists).
30. Johnstone, E. C., Cunningham Owens, D. G., Lawrie, S. M., Sharpe, M. & Freeman, C. P. L., Eds. (2004). *Companion to Psychiatric Studies*. Seventh edition. Edinburgh: Churchill Livingstone.
31. Fink, M. & Taylor, M. A. (2003). *Catatonia: A clinician's guide to diagnosis and treatment*. Cambridge: Cambridge University Press.
32. Lloyd, G. G. & Guthrie, E., Eds. (2007). *Handbook of Liaison Psychiatry*. Cambridge: Cambridge University Press.
33. David, A. S., Fleminger, S., Kopelman, M. D., Lovestone, S. & Mellers, J. D. C., Eds. (2009). *Lishman's Organic Psychiatry: A textbook of neuropsychiatry*. Fourth edition. Chichester: Wiley-Blackwell.
34. Leucht, S., Burkard, T., Henderson, J. H., Maj, M. & Sartorius, N. (2007). *Physical Illness and Schizophrenia: A review of the evidence*. Cambridge: Cambridge University Press.
35. Propping, P. (1983). Genetic disorders presenting as "schizophrenia". Karl Bonhoeffer's early view of the psychoses in the light of medical genetics. *Human Genetics* **65**: 1–10. PMID 6357993.
36. Cummings, J. L. (1985). Organic delusions: phenomenology, anatomical correlations, and review. *British Journal of Psychiatry* **146**: 184–197. PMID 3156653.
37. OMIM (2008). Online Mendelian Inheritance in Man. Johns Hopkins University, Baltimore, MD. URL: http://www.ncbi.nlm.nih.gov/omim/. Accessed 8 June 2008.
38. RxList (2008). RxList: the Internet drug index. WebMD, San Clemente, California. URL: http://www.rxlist.com/. Accessed 26 October 2008.
39. Porter, N., Ed. (1913). *Webster's Revised Unabridged Dictionary*. Springfield, MA: C. & G. Merriam Co.
40. Alagiakrishnan, K. & Blanchette, P. (2007). Delirium. eMedicine. URL: http://www.emedicine.com/med/topic3006.htm. Accessed 4 April 2008.
41. Levkoff, S. E., Safran, C., Cleary, P. D., Gallop, J. & Phillips, R. S. (1988). Identification of factors associated with the diagnosis of delirium in elderly hospitalized patients. *Journal of the American Geriatrics Society* **36**: 1099–1104. PMID 3192888.
42. Alexander, J. J., Jacob, A., Cunningham, P., Hensley, L. & Quigg, R. J. (2008). TNF is a key mediator of septic encephalopathy acting through its receptor, TNF receptor-1. *Neurochemistry International* **52**: 447–456. PMID 17884256.
43. Papadopoulos, M. C., Davies, D. C., Moss, R. F., Tighe, D. & Bennett, E. D. (2000). Pathophysiology of septic encephalopathy: a review. *Critical Care Medicine* **28**: 3019–3024. PMID 10966289.
44. Guttmann, O. (1952). Psychic disturbances in typhus fever. *Psychiatric Quarterly* **26**: 478–491.
45. Arom, K. V., Nicoloff, D. M., Lindsay, W. G., Northrup, W. F. & Kersten, T. E. (1984). Should valve replacement and related procedures be performed in elderly

patients? *Annals of Thoracic Surgery* **38**: 466–472. PMID 6333851.

46. Giltay, E. J., Huijskes, R. V., Kho, K. H., Blansjaar, B. A. & Rosseel, P. M. (2006). Psychotic symptoms in patients undergoing coronary artery bypass grafting and heart valve operation. *European Journal of Cardio-Thoracic Surgery* **30**: 140–147. PMID 16723244.
47. Grossman, R. I. & Yousem, D. M. (2003). *Neuroradiology: The requisites*. Second edition. Philadelphia, PA: Mosby/Elsevier.
48. Simon, H. B. (1993). Hyperthermia. *New England Journal of Medicine* **329**: 483–487. PMID 8332154.
49. O'Driscoll, B. R., Howard, L. S. & Davison, A. G. (2008). BTS guideline for emergency oxygen use in adult patients. *Thorax* **63 Suppl 6**: vi1–68. PMID 18838559.
50. Bisognano, J. D. & Orsini, A. N. (2006). Hypertension, malignant. eMedicine. URL: http://www.emedicine.com/med/topic1107.htm. Accessed 18 April 2008.
51. Sund-Levander, M., Forsberg, C. & Wahren, L. K. (2002). Normal oral, rectal, tympanic and axillary body temperature in adult men and women: a systematic literature review. *Scandinavian Journal of Caring Sciences* **16**: 122–128. PMID 12000664.
52. Karayiorgou, M., Morris, M. A., Morrow, B., Shprintzen, R. J., Goldberg, R., Borrow, J., Gos, A., Nestadt, G., Wolyniec, P. S., Lasseter, V. K., Eisen, H., Childs, B. Kazazian, H. H., Kucherlapati, R., Antonarakis, S. E., Pulver, A. E. & Housman, D. E. (1995). Schizophrenia susceptibility associated with interstitial deletions of chromosome 22q11. *Proceedings of the National Academy of Sciences of the United States of America* **92**: 7612–7616. PMID 7644464.
53. Gothelf, D. & Lombroso, P. J. (2001). Genetics of childhood disorders: XXV. Velocardiofacial syndrome. *Journal of the American Academy of Child and Adolescent Psychiatry* **40**: 489–491. PMID 11314577.
54. Papolos, D. F., Faedda, G. L., Veit, S., Goldberg, R., Morrow, B., Kucherlapati, R. & Shprintzen, R. J. (1996). Bipolar spectrum disorders in patients diagnosed with velo-cardio-facial syndrome: does a hemizygous deletion of chromosome 22q11 result in bipolar affective disorder? *American Journal of Psychiatry* **153**: 1541–1547. PMID 8942449.
55. Ardinger, H. H. & Ardinger, R. H. (2002). Historical perspectives of velo-cardio-facial syndrome. *Progress in Pediatric Cardiology* **15**: 89–92.
56. Robin, N. H. & Shprintzen, R. J. (2005). Defining the clinical spectrum of deletion 22q11.2. *Journal of Pediatrics* **147**: 90–96. PMID 16027702.
57. Tonelli, A. R., Kosuri, K., Wei, S. & Chick, D. (2007). Seizures as the first manifestation of chromosome 22q11.2 deletion syndrome in a 40-year old man: a case report. *Journal of Medical Case Reports* **1**: 167. PMID 18053182.
58. Botto, L. D., May, K., Fernhoff, P. M., Correa, A., Coleman, K., Rasmussen, S. A., Merritt, R. K., O'Leary, L. A., Wong, L. Y., Elixson, E. M., Mahle, W. T. & Campbell, R. M. (2003). A population-based study of the 22q11.2 deletion: phenotype, incidence, and contribution to major birth defects in the population. *Pediatrics* **112**: 101–107. PMID 12837874.
59. Murphy, K. C., Jones, L. A. & Owen, M. J. (1999). High rates of schizophrenia in adults with velo-cardio-facial syndrome. *Archives of General Psychiatry* **56**: 940–945. PMID 10530637.
60. Sugama, S., Namihira, T., Matsuoka, R., Taira, N., Eto, Y. & Maekawa, K. (1999). Psychiatric inpatients and chromosome deletions within 22q11.2. *Journal of Neurology, Neurosurgery and Psychiatry* **67**: 803–806. PMID 10567504.
61. Arinami, T., Ohtsuki, T., Takase, K., Shimizu, H., Yoshikawa, T., Horigome, H., Nakayama, J. & Toru, M. (2001). Screening for 22q11 deletions in a schizophrenia population. *Schizophrenia Research* **52**: 167–170. PMID 11705710.
62. Bassett, A. S., Hodgkinson, K., Chow, E. W., Correia, S., Scutt, L. E. & Weksberg, R. (1998). 22q11 deletion syndrome in adults with schizophrenia. *American Journal of Medical Genetics* **81**: 328–337. PMID 9674980.
63. Usiskin, S. I., Nicolson, R., Krasnewich, D. M., Yan, W., Lenane, M., Wudarsky, M., Hamburger, S. D. & Rapoport, J. L. (1999). Velocardiofacial syndrome in childhood-onset schizophrenia. *Journal of the American Academy of Child and*

Adolescent Psychiatry **38**: 1536–1543. PMID 10596254.

64. Karayiorgou, M., Gogos, J. A., Galke, B. L., Wolyniec, P. S., Nestadt, G., Antonarakis, S. E., Kazazian, H. H., Housman, D. E. & Pulver, A. E. (1998). Identification of sequence variants and analysis of the role of the catechol-O-methyl-transferase gene in schizophrenia susceptibility. *Biological Psychiatry* **43**: 425–431. PMID 9532347.
65. Handoko, H. Y., Nyholt, D. R., Hayward, N. K., Nertney, D. A., Hannah, D. E., Windus, L. C., McCormack, C. M., Smith, H. J., Filippich, C., James, M. R. & Mowry, B. J. (2005). Separate and interacting effects within the catechol-O-methyltransferase (COMT) are associated with schizophrenia. *Molecular Psychiatry* **10**: 589–597. PMID 15505638.
66. Shifman, S., Bronstein, M., Sternfeld, M., Pisante-Shalom, A., Lev-Lehman, E., Weizman, A., Reznik, I., Spivak, B., Grisaru, N., Karp, L., Schiffer, R., Kotler, M., Strous, R. D., Swartz-Vanetik, M., Knobler, H. Y., Shinar, E., Beckmann, J. S., Yakir, B., Risch, N., Zak, N. B. & Darvasi, A. (2002). A highly significant association between a COMT haplotype and schizophrenia. *American Journal of Human Genetics* **71**: 1296–1302. PMID 12402217.
67. Caspi, A., Moffitt, T. E., Cannon, M., McClay, J., Murray, R., Harrington, H., Taylor, A., Arseneault, L., Williams, B., Braithwaite, A., Poulton, R. & Craig, I. W. (2005). Moderation of the effect of adolescent-onset cannabis use on adult psychosis by a functional polymorphism in the catechol-O-methyltransferase gene: longitudinal evidence of a gene X environment interaction. *Biological Psychiatry* **57**: 1117–1127. PMID 15866551.
68. Zammit, S., Spurlock, G., Williams, H., Norton, N., Williams, N., O'Donovan, M. C. & Owen, M. J. (2007). Genotype effects of CHRNA7, CNR1 and COMT in schizophrenia: interactions with tobacco and cannabis use. *British Journal of Psychiatry* **191**: 402–407. PMID 17978319.
69. Gothelf, D., Feinstein, C., Thompson, T., Gu, E., Penniman, L., Van Stone, E., Kwon, H., Eliez, S. & Reiss, A. L. (2007). Risk factors for the emergence of psychotic disorders in adolescents with 22q11.2 deletion syndrome. *American Journal of Psychiatry* **164**: 663–669. PMID 17403981.
70. Gothelf, D., Eliez, S., Thompson, T., Hinard, C., Penniman, L., Feinstein, C., Kwon, H., Jin, S., Jo, B., Antonarakis, S. E., Morris, M. A. & Reiss, A. L. (2005). COMT genotype predicts longitudinal cognitive decline and psychosis in 22q11.2 deletion syndrome. *Nature Neuroscience* **8**: 1500–1502. PMID 16234808.
71. Mimmack, M. L., Ryan, M., Baba, H., Navarro-Ruiz, J., Iritani, S., Faull, R. L., McKenna, P. J., Jones, P. B., Arai, H., Starkey, M., Emson, P. C. & Bahn, S. (2002). Gene expression analysis in schizophrenia: reproducible up-regulation of several members of the apolipoprotein L family located in a high-susceptibility locus for schizophrenia on chromosome 22. *Proceedings of the National Academy of Sciences of the United States of America* **99**: 4680–4685. PMID 11930015.
72. Ardinger, H. H. & Ardinger, R. H. (2002). Clinical presentation of velo-cardio-facial syndrome. *Progress in Pediatric Cardiology* **15**: 93–97.
73. Chen, H. (2007). Down syndrome. eMedicine. URL: http://www.emedicine.com/ped/topic615.htm. Accessed 18 April 2008.
74. Blackwood, D. H., Fordyce, A., Walker, M. T., St Clair, D. M., Porteous, D. J. & Muir, W. J. (2001). Schizophrenia and affective disorders – cosegregation with a translocation at chromosome 1q42 that directly disrupts brain-expressed genes: clinical and P300 findings in a family. *American Journal of Human Genetics* **69**: 428–433. PMID 11443544.
75. Millar, J. K., Wilson-Annan, J. C., Anderson, S., Christie, S., Taylor, M. S., Semple, C. A., Devon, R. S., St Clair, D. M., Muir, W. J., Blackwood, D. H. & Porteous, D. J. (2000). Disruption of two novel genes by a translocation co-segregating with schizophrenia. *Human Molecular Genetics* **9**: 1415–1423. PMID 10814723.
76. Owen, M. J., Craddock, N. & Jablensky, A. (2007). The genetic deconstruction of psychosis. *Schizophrenia Bulletin* **33**: 905–911. PMID 17551090.
77. van Rijn, S., Aleman, A., Swaab, H. & Kahn, R. (2006). Klinefelter's syndrome (karyotype 47, XXY) and schizophrenia-spectrum

pathology. *British Journal of Psychiatry* **189**: 459–460. PMID 17077438.

78. DeLisi, L. E., Maurizio, A. M., Svetina, C., Ardekani, B., Szulc, K., Nierenberg, J., Leonard, J. & Harvey, P. D. (2005). Klinefelter's syndrome (XXY) as a genetic model for psychotic disorders. *American Journal of Medical Genetics. Part B, Neuropsychiatric Genetics* **135**: 15–23. PMID 15729733.
79. Kumra, S., Wiggs, E., Krasnewich, D., Meck, J., Smith, A. C., Bedwell, J., Fernandez, T., Jacobsen, L. K., Lenane, M. & Rapoport, J. L. (1998). Brief report: association of sex chromosome anomalies with childhood-onset psychotic disorders. *Journal of the American Academy of Child and Adolescent Psychiatry* **37**: 292–296. PMID 9519634.
80. Otter, M. (2007). X-chromosome abnormality and schizophrenia. *British Journal of Psychiatry* **190**: 450; author reply 450. PMID 17470966.
81. Lee, J. W. (1996). An XXYY male with schizophrenia. *Australian and New Zealand Journal of Psychiatry* **30**: 553–556. PMID 8887709.
82. Sperber, M. A. (1975). Schizophrenia and organic brain syndrome with trisomy 8 (group-C trisomy 8 [47, XX, 8+]). *Biological Psychiatry* **10**: 27–43. PMID 1120174.
83. DeLisi, L. E., Friedrich, U., Wahlstrom, J., Boccio-Smith, A., Forsman, A., Eklund, K. & Crow, T. J. (1994). Schizophrenia and sex chromosome anomalies. *Schizophrenia Bulletin* **20**: 495–505. PMID 7973466.
84. Chen, H. (2007). Klinefelter syndrome. eMedicine. URL: http://www.emedicine.com/ped/topic1252.htm. Accessed 18 April 2008.
85. Visootsak, J. & Graham, J. M., Jr. (2006). Klinefelter syndrome and other sex chromosomal aneuploidies. *Orphanet Journal of Rare Diseases* **1**: 42. PMID 17062147.
86. Flatt, A. E. (2005). The troubles with pinkies. *Proceedings (Baylor University Medical Center)* **18**: 341–344. PMID 16252026.
87. Tartaglia, N. R., Howell, S., Sutherland, A., Wilson, R. & Wilson, L. (2010). A review of trisomy X (47, XXX). *Orphanet Journal of Rare Diseases* **5**: 8. PMID 20459843.
88. Wisniewska, M. & Mazurek, M. (2002). Trisomy 8 mosaicism syndrome. *Journal of Applied Genetics* **43**: 115–118. PMID 12084977.
89. Reiss, A. L., Feinstein, C., Toomey, K. E., Goldsmith, B., Rosenbaum, K. & Caruso, M. A. (1986). Psychiatric disability associated with the fragile X chromosome. *American Journal of Medical Genetics* **23**: 393–401. PMID 3953657.
90. Vantalon, V., Briard-Luginbuhl, V. & Mouren, M. C. (2005). [Fragile X syndrome and very early onset schizophrenia: a female case study]. *Archives de Pediatrie* **12**: 176–179. PMID 15694544.
91. Reiss, A. L., Hagerman, R. J., Vinogradov, S., Abrams, M. & King, R. J. (1988). Psychiatric disability in female carriers of the fragile X chromosome. *Archives of General Psychiatry* **45**: 25–30. PMID 3337608.
92. Prior, T. I., Chue, P. S. & Tibbo, P. (2000). Investigation of Turner syndrome in schizophrenia. *American Journal of Medical Genetics* **96**: 373–378. PMID 10898917.
93. Sybert, V. P. & McCauley, E. (2004). Turner's syndrome. *New England Journal of Medicine* **351**: 1227–1238. PMID 15371580.
94. Walterfang, M., Wood, S. J., Velakoulis, D., Copolov, D. & Pantelis, C. (2005). Diseases of white matter and schizophrenia-like psychosis. *Australian and New Zealand Journal of Psychiatry* **39**: 746–756. PMID 16168032.
95. Berman, S. A., Hardjasurarma, M. & Dinnerstein, E. (2007). Marchiafava-Bignami disease. eMedicine. URL: http://emedicine.medscape.com/article/1146086-overview. Accessed 26 August 2009.
96. Meyer, J., Scherer, S. J., Mössner, R. & Lesch, K. P. (2002). Reply concerning KIAA0027 (WKL1, MLC1) and psychosis: white matters. *Molecular Psychiatry* 7: 1037–1038.
97. Filteau, M. J., Pourcher, E., Bouchard, R. H., Baruch, P., Mathieu, J., Bedard, F., Simard, N. & Vincent, P. (1991). Corpus callosum agenesis and psychosis in Andermann syndrome. *Archives of Neurology* **48**: 1275–1280. PMID 1668979.
98. Gupta, S. & Popli, A. (1995). Psychosis in Apert's syndrome with partial agenesis of

the corpus callosum. *Journal of Psychiatry and Neuroscience* **20**: 307–309. PMID 7647085.
99. Soni, S., Whittington, J., Holland, A. J., Webb, T., Maina, E., Boer, H. & Clarke, D. (2007). The course and outcome of psychiatric illness in people with Prader-Willi syndrome: implications for management and treatment. *Journal of Intellectual Disability Research* **51**: 32–42. PMID 17181601.
100. Soni, S., Whittington, J., Holland, A. J., Webb, T., Maina, E. N., Boer, H. & Clarke, D. (2008). The phenomenology and diagnosis of psychiatric illness in people with Prader-Willi syndrome. *Psychological Medicine* **38**: 1505–1514. PMID 18177526.
101. Verhoeven, W. M., Tuinier, S. & Curfs, L. M. (2003). Prader-Willi syndrome: the psychopathological phenotype in uniparental disomy. *Journal of Medical Genetics* **40**: e112. PMID 14569135.
102. McBean, M. S. & Stephenson, J. B. (1968). Treatment of classical phenylketonuria. *Archives of Disease in Childhood* **43**: 1–7. PMID 4868338.
103. Lindsay, S., Splitt, M., Edney, S., Berney, T. P., Knight, S. J., Davies, K. E., O'Brien, O., Gale, M. & Burn, J. (1996). PPM-X: a new X-linked mental retardation syndrome with psychosis, pyramidal signs, and macroorchidism maps to Xq28. *American Journal of Human Genetics* **58**: 1120–1126. PMID 8651288.
104. Purandare, K. N. & Markar, T. N. (2005). Psychiatric symptomatology of Lujan-Fryns syndrome: an X-linked syndrome displaying Marfanoid symptoms with autistic features, hyperactivity, shyness and schizophreniform symptoms. *Psychiatric Genetics* **15**: 229–231. PMID 16094260.
105. Weiss, M., Meshulam, B. & Wijsenbeek, H. (1981). The possible relationship between Laurence–Moon–Biedl–Bardet syndrome and a schizophrenic-like psychosis. *Journal of Nervous and Mental Disease* **169**: 259–260. PMID 7217934.
106. Todd, J. (1955). A case of the Laurence–Moon–Biedl syndrome with paranoid psychosis. *American Journal of Mental Deficiency* **60**: 331–334. PMID 13258608.
107. Swift, R. G., Sadler, D. B. & Swift, M. (1990). Psychiatric findings in Wolfram syndrome homozygotes. *Lancet* **336**: 667–669. PMID 1975860.
108. d'Annunzio, G., Minuto, N., D'Amato, E., de Toni, T., Lombardo, F., Pasquali, L. & Lorini, R. (2008). Wolfram syndrome (diabetes insipidus, diabetes, optic atrophy, and deafness): clinical and genetic study. *Diabetes Care* **31**: 1743–1745. PMID 18566338.
109. Raybarman, C. (2002). Landau–Kleffner syndrome: a case report. *Neurology India* **50**: 212–213. PMID 12134193.
110. Clarke, D. J. & Buckley, M. E. (1989). Familial association of albinism and schizophrenia. *British Journal of Psychiatry* **155**: 551–553. PMID 2611578.
111. Baron, M. (1976). Albinism and schizophreniform psychosis: a pedigree study. *American Journal of Psychiatry* **133**: 1070–1073. PMID 961931.
112. Zalewska, A. & Schwartz, R. A. (2009). Sjögren–Larsson syndrome. eMedicine. URL: http://emedicine.medscape.com/article/1114823-overview. Accessed 8 November 2009.
113. Donnet, A. & Samuelian, J. C. (1988). [Congenital neuroichthyosis and psychiatric involvement. Apropos of a case]. *Encephale* **14**: 427–429. PMID 3068048.
114. Mochizuki, H., Tobo, M. & Itoi, K. (1980). A case of ichthyosis vulgalis associated with schizophrenia-like psychosis and spike-wave stupor. *Folia Psychiatrica et Neurologica Japonica* **34**: 392–393. PMID 7216063.
115. Sedel, F., Baumann, N., Turpin, J. C., Lyon-Caen, O., Saudubray, J. M. & Cohen, D. (2007). Psychiatric manifestations revealing inborn errors of metabolism in adolescents and adults. *Journal of Inherited Metabolic Disease* **30**: 631–641. PMID 17694356.
116. Gibson, K. M., Gupta, M., Pearl, P. L., Tuchman, M., Vezina, L. G., Snead, O. C., 3rd, Smit, L. M. & Jakobs, C. (2003). Significant behavioral disturbances in succinic semialdehyde dehydrogenase (SSADH) deficiency (gamma-hydroxybutyric aciduria). *Biological Psychiatry* **54**: 763–768. PMID 14512218.

117. Thomas, C. S., Toone, B. K. & Rose, P. E. (1988). Neurocutaneous melanosis and psychosis. *American Journal of Psychiatry* **145**: 649–650. PMID 3358470.
118. Azzoni, A., Argentieri, R. & Raja, M. (2001). Neurocutaneous melanosis and psychosis: a case report. *Psychiatry and Clinical Neurosciences* **55**: 93–95. PMID 11285085.
119. Holroyd, S. & Laurie, S. (1999). Correlates of psychotic symptoms among elderly outpatients. *International Journal of Geriatric Psychiatry* **14**: 379–384. PMID 10389042.
120. Kujlis, R. O. (2007). Alzheimer disease. eMedicine. URL: http://www.emedicine.com/neuro/topic13.htm. Accessed 19 March 2008.
121. Ropacki, S. A. & Jeste, D. V. (2005). Epidemiology of and risk factors for psychosis of Alzheimer's disease: a review of 55 studies published from 1990 to 2003. *American Journal of Psychiatry* **162**: 2022–2030. PMID 16263838.
122. Borroni, B., Grassi, M., Agosti, C., Archetti, S., Costanzi, C., Cornali, C., Caltagirone, C., Caimi, L., Di Luca, M. & Padovani, A. (2006). Cumulative effect of COMT and 5-HTTLPR polymorphisms and their interaction with disease severity and comorbidities on the risk of psychosis in Alzheimer disease. *American Journal of Geriatric Psychiatry* **14**: 343–351. PMID 16582043.
123. Borroni, B., Grassi, M., Costanzi, C., Zanetti, M., Archetti, S., Franzoni, S., Caimi, L. & Padovani, A. (2007). Haplotypes in cathechol-O-methyltransferase gene confer increased risk for psychosis in Alzheimer disease. *Neurobiology of Aging* **28**: 1231–1238. PMID 16837108.
124. Hirono, N., Mori, E., Yasuda, M., Ikejiri, Y., Imamura, T., Shimomura, T., Ikeda, M., Hashimoto, M. & Yamashita, H. (1998). Factors associated with psychotic symptoms in Alzheimer's disease. *Journal of Neurology, Neurosurgery and Psychiatry* **64**: 648–652. PMID 9598682.
125. McKhann, G., Drachman, D., Folstein, M., Katzman, R., Price, D. & Stadlan, E. M. (1984). Clinical diagnosis of Alzheimer's disease: report of the NINCDS-ADRDA Work Group under the auspices of Department of Health and Human Services Task Force on Alzheimer's Disease. *Neurology* **34**: 939–944. PMID 6610841.
126. Hauser, R. A., Pahwa, R., Lyons, K. E. & McClain, T. A. (2007). Parkinson disease. eMedicine. URL: http://www.emedicine.com/neuro/topic304.htm. Accessed 4 March 2008.
127. Papapetropoulos, S. & Mash, D. C. (2005). Psychotic symptoms in Parkinson's disease. From description to etiology. *Journal of Neurology* **252**: 753–764. PMID 15999234.
128. Ferreri, F., Agbokou, C. & Gauthier, S. (2006). Recognition and management of neuropsychiatric complications in Parkinson's disease. *Canadian Medical Association Journal* **175**: 1545–1552. PMID 17146092.
129. Fenelon, G., Mahieux, F., Huon, R. & Ziegler, M. (2000). Hallucinations in Parkinson's disease: prevalence, phenomenology and risk factors. *Brain* **123**: 733–745. PMID 10734005.
130. Holroyd, S., Currie, L. & Wooten, G. F. (2001). Prospective study of hallucinations and delusions in Parkinson's disease. *Journal of Neurology, Neurosurgery and Psychiatry* **70**: 734–738. PMID 11385005.
131. Goetz, C. G., Wuu, J., Curgian, L. M. & Leurgans, S. (2005). Hallucinations and sleep disorders in PD: six-year prospective longitudinal study. *Neurology* **64**: 81–86. PMID 15642908.
132. Weintraub, D., Morales, K. H., Duda, J. E., Moberg, P. J. & Stern, M. B. (2006). Frequency and correlates of co-morbid psychosis and depression in Parkinson's disease. *Parkinsonism and Related Disorders* **12**: 427–431. PMID 16797214.
133. Dalvi, A. & Bloomfield, S. M. (2005). Parkinson-plus syndromes. eMedicine. URL: http://www.emedicine.com/neuro/topic596.htm. Accessed 4 March 2008.
134. Diedrich, A. & Robertson, D. (2007). Multiple system atrophy. eMedicine. URL: http://www.emedicine.com/neuro/topic671.htm. Accessed 18 April 2008.
135. Eggenberger, E. R. & Vanek, Z. F. (2007). Progressive supranuclear palsy.

eMedicine. URL: http://www.emedicine.com/neuro/topic328.htm. Accessed 18 April 2008.

136. Janati, A. & Appel, A. R. (1984). Psychiatric aspects of progressive supranuclear palsy. *Journal of Nervous and Mental Disease* **172**: 85–89. PMID 6693866.

137. McKeith, I. G., Galasko, D., Kosaka, K., Perry, E. K., Dickson, D. W., Hansen, L. A., Salmon, D. P., Lowe, J., Mirra, S. S., Byrne, E. J., Lennox, G., Quinn, N. P., Edwardson, J. A., Ince, P. G., Bergeron, C., Burns, A., Miller, B. L., Lovestone, S., Collerton, D., Jansen, E. N., Ballard, C., de Vos, R. A., Wilcock, G. K., Jellinger, K. A. & Perry, R. H. (1996). Consensus guidelines for the clinical and pathologic diagnosis of dementia with Lewy bodies (DLB): report of the consortium on DLB international workshop. *Neurology* **47**: 1113–1124. PMID 8909416.

138. McKeith, I., Mintzer, J., Aarsland, D., Burn, D., Chiu, H., Cohen-Mansfield, J., Dickson, D., Dubois, B., Duda, J. E., Feldman, H., Gauthier, S., Halliday, G., Lawlor, B., Lippa, C., Lopez, O. L., Carlos Machado, J., O'Brien, J., Playfer, J. & Reid, W. (2004). Dementia with Lewy bodies. *Lancet Neurology* **3**: 19–28. PMID 14693108.

139. Neary, D., Snowden, J. S., Gustafson, L., Passant, U., Stuss, D., Black, S., Freedman, M., Kertesz, A., Robert, P. H., Albert, M., Boone, K., Miller, B. L., Cummings, J. & Benson, D. F. (1998). Frontotemporal lobar degeneration: a consensus on clinical diagnostic criteria. *Neurology* **51**: 1546–1554. PMID 9855500.

140. Waddington, J. L., Youssef, H. A., Farrell, M. A. & Toland, J. (1995). Initial 'schizophrenia-like' psychosis in Pick's disease: case study with neuroimaging and neuropathology, and implications for frontotemporal dysfunction in schizophrenia. *Schizophrenia Research* **18**: 79–82. PMID 8929764.

141. Mendez, M. F., Shapira, J. S., Woods, R. J., Licht, E. A. & Saul, R. E. (2008). Psychotic symptoms in frontotemporal dementia: prevalence and review. *Dementia and Geriatric Cognitive Disorders* **25**: 206–211. PMID 18204254.

142. Loy, C. T., Kril, J. J., Trollor, J. N., Kiernan, M. C., Kwok, J. B., Vucic, S., Halliday, G. M. & Hodges, J. R. (2010). The case of a 48 year-old woman with bizarre and complex delusions. *Nature Reviews Neurology* **6**: 175–179. PMID 20212429.

143. Velakoulis, D., Walterfang, M., Mocellin, R., Pantelis, C. & McLean, C. (2009). Frontotemporal dementia presenting as schizophrenia-like psychosis in young people: clinicopathological series and review of cases. *British Journal of Psychiatry* **194**: 298–305. PMID 19336778.

144. Skoglund, L., Viitanen, M., Kalimo, H., Lannfelt, L., Jonhagen, M. E., Ingelsson, M., Glaser, A. & Herva, R. (2008). The tau S305S mutation causes frontotemporal dementia with parkinsonism. *European Journal of Neurology* **15**: 156–161. PMID 18093153.

145. Bird, T. D., Wijsman, E. M., Nochlin, D., Leehey, M., Sumi, S. M., Payami, H., Poorkaj, P., Nemens, E., Rafkind, M. & Schellenberg, G. D. (1997). Chromosome 17 and hereditary dementia: linkage studies in three non-Alzheimer families and kindreds with late-onset FAD. *Neurology* **48**: 949–954. PMID 9109883.

146. Burnstein, M. H. (1981). Familial amyotrophic lateral sclerosis, dementia, and psychosis. *Psychosomatics* **22**: 151, 155–157. PMID 7208781.

147. Goodman, A. B. (1994). A family history study of schizophrenia spectrum disorders suggests new candidate genes in schizophrenia and autism. *Psychiatric Quarterly* **65**: 287–297. PMID 7831415.

148. Federico, A., Palmeri, S., Malandrini, A., Fabrizi, G., Mondelli, M. & Guazzi, G. C. (1991). The clinical aspects of adult hexosaminidase deficiencies. *Developmental Neuroscience* **13**: 280–287. PMID 1840098.

149. Nakamura, K., Chen, C. K., Sekine, Y., Iwata, Y., Anitha, A., Loh el, W., Takei, N., Suzuki, A., Kawai, M., Takebayashi, K., Suzuki, K., Minabe, Y., Tsuchiya, K., Yamada, K., Iyo, M., Ozaki, N., Inada, T., Iwata, N., Harano, M., Komiyama, T., Yamada, M., Sora, I., Ujike, H., Ball, D. M., Yoshikawa, T.,

Lin, S. K. & Mori, N. (2006). Association analysis of SOD2 variants with methamphetamine psychosis in Japanese and Taiwanese populations. *Human Genetics* **120**: 243–252. PMID 16807759.

150. Akyol, O., Yanik, M., Elyas, H., Namli, M., Canatan, H., Akin, H., Yuce, H., Yilmaz, H. R., Tutkun, H., Sogut, S., Herken, H., Ozyurt, H., Savas, H. A. & Zoroglu, S. S. (2005). Association between Ala-9Val polymorphism of Mn-SOD gene and schizophrenia. *Progress in Neuro-Psychopharmacology and Biological Psychiatry* **29**: 123–131. PMID 15610954.

151. Michel, T. M., Thome, J., Martin, D., Nara, K., Zwerina, S., Tatschner, T., Weijers, H. G. & Koutsilieri, E. (2004). Cu, Zn- and Mn-superoxide dismutase levels in brains of patients with schizophrenic psychosis. *Journal of Neural Transmission* **111**: 1191–1201. PMID 15338334.

152. Mukherjee, S., Mahadik, S. P., Scheffer, R., Correnti, E. E. & Kelkar, H. (1996). Impaired antioxidant defense at the onset of psychosis. *Schizophrenia Research* **19**: 19–26. PMID 9147492.

153. Lauterbach, E. C., Cummings, J. L., Duffy, J., Coffey, C. E., Kaufer, D., Lovell, M., Malloy, P., Reeve, A., Royall, D. R., Rummans, T. A. & Salloway, S. P. (1998). Neuropsychiatric correlates and treatment of lenticulostriatal diseases: a review of the literature and overview of research opportunities in Huntington's, Wilson's, and Fahr's diseases. A report of the ANPA Committee on Research. American Neuropsychiatric Association. *Journal of Neuropsychiatry and Clinical Neurosciences* **10**: 249–266. PMID 9706533.

154. Huff, J. S. (2007). Huntington disease. eMedicine. URL: http://www.emedicine.com/emerg/topic254.htm. Accessed 4 March 2008.

155. Rawlins, M. (2010). Huntington's disease out of the closet? *Lancet*. PMID 20594589.

156. van Duijn, E., Kingma, E. M. & van der Mast, R. C. (2007). Psychopathology in verified Huntington's disease gene carriers. *Journal of Neuropsychiatry and Clinical Neurosciences* **19**: 441–448. PMID 18070848.

157. Correa, B. B., Xavier, M. & Guimaraes, J. (2006). Association of Huntington's disease and schizophrenia-like psychosis in a Huntington's disease pedigree. *Clinical Practice and Epidemiology in Mental Health* **2**: 1. PMID 16480508.

158. Mendez, M. F. (1994). Huntington's disease: update and review of neuropsychiatric aspects. *International Journal of Psychiatry in Medicine* **24**: 189–208. PMID 7890478.

159. Rosenblatt, A. & Leroi, I. (2000). Neuropsychiatry of Huntington's disease and other basal ganglia disorders. *Psychosomatics* **41**: 24–30. PMID 10665265.

160. Lovestone, S., Hodgson, S., Sham, P., Differ, A. M. & Levy, R. (1996). Familial psychiatric presentation of Huntington's disease. *Journal of Medical Genetics* **33**: 128–131. PMID 8929949.

161. Madhusoodanan, S., Brenner, R., Moise, D., Sindagi, J. & Brafman, I. (1998). Psychiatric and neuropsychological abnormalities in Huntington's disease: a case study. *Annals of Clinical Psychiatry* **10**: 117–120. PMID 9781475.

162. Weigell-Weber, M., Schmid, W. & Spiegel, R. (1996). Psychiatric symptoms and CAG expansion in Huntington's disease. *American Journal of Medical Genetics* **67**: 53–57. PMID 8678115.

163. Tsuang, D., Almqvist, E. W., Lipe, H., Strgar, F., DiGiacomo, L., Hoff, D., Eugenio, C., Hayden, M. R. & Bird, T. D. (2000). Familial aggregation of psychotic symptoms in Huntington's disease. *American Journal of Psychiatry* **157**: 1955–1959. PMID 11097960.

164. Pirogovsky, E., Gilbert, P. E., Jacobson, M., Peavy, G., Wetter, S., Goldstein, J., Corey-Bloom, J. & Murphy, C. (2007). Impairments in source memory for olfactory and visual stimuli in preclinical and clinical stages of Huntington's disease. *Journal of Clinical and Experimental Neuropsychology* **29**: 395–404. PMID 17497563.

165. Moberg, P. J. & Doty, R. L. (1997). Olfactory function in Huntington's disease patients and at-risk offspring.

International Journal of Neuroscience **89**: 133–139. PMID 9134451.
166. Bylsma, F. W., Moberg, P. J., Doty, R. L. & Brandt, J. (1997). Odor identification in Huntington's disease patients and asymptomatic gene carriers. *Journal of Neuropsychiatry and Clinical Neurosciences* **9**: 598–600. PMID 9447504.
167. Warner, T. T., Williams, L. D., Walker, R. W., Flinter, F., Robb, S. A., Bundey, S. E., Honavar, M. & Harding, A. E. (1995). A clinical and molecular genetic study of dentatorubropallidoluysian atrophy in four European families. *Annals of Neurology* **37**: 452–459. PMID 7717681.
168. Adachi, N., Arima, K., Asada, T., Kato, M., Minami, N., Goto, Y., Onuma, T., Ikeuchi, T., Tsuji, S., Hayashi, M. & Fukutani, Y. (2001). Dentatorubral-pallidoluysian atrophy (DRPLA) presenting with psychosis. *Journal of Neuropsychiatry and Clinical Neurosciences* **13**: 258–260. PMID 11449034.
169. Lee, I. H., Soong, B. W., Lu, Y. C. & Chang, Y. C. (2001). Dentatorubropallidoluysian atrophy in Chinese. *Archives of Neurology* **58**: 1905–1908. PMID 11709002.
170. Burke, J. R., Wingfield, M. S., Lewis, K. E., Roses, A. D., Lee, J. E., Hulette, C., Pericak-Vance, M. A. & Vance, J. M. (1994). The Haw River syndrome: dentatorubropallidoluysian atrophy (DRPLA) in an African-American family. *Nature Genetics* **7**: 521–524. PMID 7951323.
171. Pearce, J. M. (2001). The subthalamic nucleus and Jules Bernard Luys (1828–97). *Journal of Neurology, Neurosurgery and Psychiatry* **71**: 783. PMID 11723202.
172. Shulman, L. M., Lang, A. E., Jankovic, J., David, N. J. & Weiner, W. J. (1995). Case 1, 1995: psychosis, dementia, chorea, ataxia, and supranuclear gaze dysfunction. *Movement Disorders* **10**: 257–262. PMID 7651440.
173. Prasad, A., Prasad, C. & Greenberg, C. R. (2007). Ataxia with identified genetic and biochemical defects. eMedicine. URL: http://www.emedicine.com/neuro/topic556.htm. Accessed 4 March 2008.
174. Vincent, J. B., Yuan, Q. P., Schalling, M., Adolfsson, R., Azevedo, M. H., Macedo, A., Bauer, A., DallaTorre, C., Medeiros, H. M., Pato, M. T., Pato, C. N., Bowen, T., Guy, C. A., Owen, M. J., O'Donovan, M. C., Paterson, A. D., Petronis, A. & Kennedy, J. L. (2000). Long repeat tracts at SCA8 in major psychosis. *American Journal of Medical Genetics* **96**: 873–876. PMID 11121201.
175. Vincent, J. B., Paterson, A. D., Strong, E., Petronis, A. & Kennedy, J. L. (2000). The unstable trinucleotide repeat story of major psychosis. *American Journal of Medical Genetics* **97**: 77–97. PMID 10813808.
176. Salbenblatt, M. J., Buzan, R. D. & Dubovsky, S. L. (2000). Risperidone treatment for psychosis in end-stage Friedreich's ataxia. *American Journal of Psychiatry* **157**: 303. PMID 10671420.
177. Dinnerstein, E., Berman, S. A. & Arroyo-Muñiz, M. (2006). Neuroacanthocytosis. eMedicine. URL: http://www.emedicine.com/neuro/topic246.htm. Accessed 4 March 2008.
178. Gross, K. B. & Lorenzo, N. Y. (2007). Neuroacanthocytosis syndromes. eMedicine. URL: http://www.emedicine.com/neuro/topic502.htm. Accessed 4 March 2008.
179. Habermeyer, B., Fuhr, P., Hiss, B., Alber, C. & Muller-Spahn, F. (2006). Obsessive-compulsive disorder due to neuroacanthocytosis treated with citalopram. A case report. *Pharmacopsychiatry* **39**: 193–194. PMID 16944412.
180. Bruneau, M. A., Lesperance, P. & Chouinard, S. (2003). Schizophrenia-like presentation of neuroacanthocytosis. *Journal of Neuropsychiatry and Clinical Neurosciences* **15**: 378–380. PMID 12928518.
181. Miranda, M., Castiglioni, C., Frey, B. M., Hergersberg, M., Danek, A. & Jung, H. H. (2007). Phenotypic variability of a distinct deletion in McLeod syndrome. *Movement Disorders* **22**: 1358–1361. PMID 17469188.
182. Hewer, E., Danek, A., Schoser, B. G., Miranda, M., Reichard, R., Castiglioni, C., Oechsner, M., Goebel, H. H.,

Heppner, F. L. & Jung, H. H. (2007). McLeod myopathy revisited: more neurogenic and less benign. *Brain* **130**: 3285–3296. PMID 18055495.

183. Walker, R. H., Jung, H. H., Dobson-Stone, C., Rampoldi, L., Sano, A., Tison, F. & Danek, A. (2007). Neurologic phenotypes associated with acanthocytosis. *Neurology* **68**: 92–98. PMID 17210889.
184. Danek, A., Jung, H. H., Melone, M. A., Rampoldi, L., Broccoli, V. & Walker, R. H. (2005). Neuroacanthocytosis: new developments in a neglected group of dementing disorders. *Journal of the Neurological Sciences* **229–230**: 171–186. PMID 15760637.
185. Danek, A. & Walker, R. H. (2005). Neuroacanthocytosis. *Current Opinion in Neurology* **18**: 386–392. PMID 16003113.
186. Jung, H. H., Danek, A. & Walker, R. H. (2009). Neuroacanthocytosis. *Advances in Clinical Neuroscience and Rehabilitation* **9**: 16–20.
187. Rauschkolb, P. K. & Berman, S. A. (2010). Neuroacanthocytosis. eMedicine. URL: http://emedicine.medscape.com/article/1150817-overview. Accessed 9 March 2010.
188. Lopez-Villegas, D., Kulisevsky, J., Deus, J., Junque, C., Pujol, J., Guardia, E. & Grau, J. M. (1996). Neuropsychological alterations in patients with computed tomography-detected basal ganglia calcification. *Archives of Neurology* **53**: 251–256. PMID 8651878.
189. Cummings, J. L., Gosenfeld, L. F., Houlihan, J. P. & McCaffrey, T. (1983). Neuropsychiatric disturbances associated with idiopathic calcification of the basal ganglia. *Biological Psychiatry* **18**: 591–601. PMID 6860732.
190. Ostling, S., Andreasson, L. A. & Skoog, I. (2003). Basal ganglia calcification and psychotic symptoms in the very old. *International Journal of Geriatric Psychiatry* **18**: 983–987. PMID 14618548.
191. Abraham, M. R. & Khardori, R. (2007). Pseudohypoparathyroidism. eMedicine. URL: http://www.emedicine.com/med/topic1940.htm. Accessed 4 March 2008.
192. Rastogi, R., Beauchamp, N. J. & Ladenson, P. W. (2003). Calcification of the basal ganglia in chronic hypoparathyroidism. *Journal of Clinical Endocrinology and Metabolism* **88**: 1476–1477. PMID 12679425.
193. Mousa, A. M., Muhtaseb, S. A., Reddy, R. R., Senthilselvan, A., Al-Mudallal, D. S. & Marafie, A. A. (1987). The high rate of prevalence of CT-detected basal ganglia calcification in neuropsychiatric (CNS) brucellosis. *Acta Neurologica Scandinavica* **76**: 448–456. PMID 3434203.
194. Swaiman, K. F. (2001). Hallervorden–Spatz syndrome. *Pediatric Neurology* **25**: 102–108. PMID 11551740.
195. Sachin, S., Goyal, V., Singh, S., Shukla, G., Sharma, M. C., Gaikwed, S. & Behari, M. (2009). Clinical spectrum of Hallervorden–Spatz syndrome in India. *Journal of Clinical Neuroscience* **16**: 253–258. PMID 19056277.
196. Hayflick, S. J., Westaway, S. K., Levinson, B., Zhou, B., Johnson, M. A., Ching, K. H. & Gitschier, J. (2003). Genetic, clinical, and radiographic delineation of Hallervorden–Spatz syndrome. *New England Journal of Medicine* **348**: 33–40. PMID 12510040.
197. Morphy, M. A., Feldman, J. A. & Kilburn, G. (1989). Hallervorden–Spatz disease in a psychiatric setting. *Journal of Clinical Psychiatry* **50**: 66–68. PMID 2914882.
198. Oner, O., Oner, P., Deda, G. & Icagasioglu, D. (2003). Psychotic disorder in a case with Hallervorden–Spatz disease. *Acta Psychiatrica Scandinavica* **108**: 394–397; discussion 397–398. PMID 14531762.
199. Hanna, P. A., Gerhardstein, B. L. & Garg, N. (2006). Hallervorden–Spatz disease. eMedicine. URL: http://www.emedicine.com/neuro/topic151.htm. Accessed 4 March 2008.
200. Chinnery, P. F. (2007). Neuroferritinopathy. GeneReviews (National Center for Biotechnology Information). URL: http://www.ncbi.nlm.nih.gov/bookshelf/br.fcgi?book=gene&part=neuroferritin. Accessed 2 September 2009.
201. Chinnery, P. F., Crompton, D. E., Birchall, D., Jackson, M. J., Coulthard, A., Lombes, A., Quinn, N., Wills, A., Fletcher, N., Mottershead, J. P., Cooper, P., Kellett, M., Bates, D. & Burn, J. (2007). Clinical features and natural history of

neuroferritinopathy caused by the FTL1 460InsA mutation. *Brain* **130**: 110–119. PMID 17142829.
202. Ferrer, I., Santpere, G. & van Leeuwen, F. W. (2008). Argyrophilic grain disease. *Brain* **131**: 1416–1432. PMID 18234698.
203. Deymeer, F., Smith, T. W., DeGirolami, U. & Drachman, D. A. (1989). Thalamic dementia and motor neuron disease. *Neurology* **39**: 58–61. PMID 2909915.
204. Jen, J., Cohen, A. H., Yue, Q., Stout, J. T., Vinters, H. V., Nelson, S. & Baloh, R. W. (1997). Hereditary endotheliopathy with retinopathy, nephropathy, and stroke (HERNS). *Neurology* **49**: 1322–1330. PMID 9371916.
205. Sasaki, A., Miyanaga, K., Ototsuji, M., Iwaki, A., Iwaki, T., Takahashi, S. & Nakazato, Y. (2000). Two autopsy cases with Pelizaeus–Merzbacher disease phenotype of adult onset, without mutation of proteolipid protein gene. *Acta Neuropathologica* **99**: 7–13. PMID 10651021.
206. Alagiakrishnan, K. & Masaki, K. (2007). Vascular dementia. eMedicine. URL: http://www.emedicine.com/med/topic3150.htm. Accessed 19 March 2008.
207. Ballard, C., Neill, D., O'Brien, J., McKeith, I. G., Ince, P. & Perry, R. (2000). Anxiety, depression and psychosis in vascular dementia: prevalence and associations. *Journal of Affective Disorders* **59**: 97–106. PMID 10837878.
208. UK National Institute for Health and Clinical Excellence, Social Care Institute for Excellence & British Psychological Society (2006). Dementia: a NICE-SCIE guideline on supporting people with dementia and their carers in health and social care. United Kingdom National Institute for Health and Clinical Excellence. URL: http://www.nice.org.uk/CG42. Accessed 18 March 2008.
209. Roman, G. C., Tatemichi, T. K., Erkinjuntti, T., Cummings, J. L., Masdeu, J. C., Garcia, J. H., Amaducci, L., Orgogozo, J. M., Brun, A., Hofman, A., Moody, D. M., O'Brien, M. D., Yamaguchi, T., Grafman, J., Drayer, B. P., Bennett, D. A., Fisher, M., Ogata, J., Kokmen, E., Bermejo, F., Wolf, P. A., Gorelick, P. B., Bick, K. L., Pajeau, A. K., Bell, M. A., DeCarli, C., Culebras, A., Korczyn, A. D., Bogousslavsky, J., Hartmann, A. & Scheinberg, P. (1993). Vascular dementia: diagnostic criteria for research studies. Report of the NINDS-AIREN International Workshop. *Neurology* **43**: 250–260. PMID 8094895.
210. Kumral, E. & Ozturk, O. (2004). Delusional state following acute stroke. *Neurology* **62**: 110–113. PMID 14718709.
211. Nishio, Y., Ishii, K., Kazui, H., Hosokai, Y. & Mori, E. (2007). Frontal-lobe syndrome and psychosis after damage to the brainstem dopaminergic nuclei. *Journal of the Neurological Sciences* **260**: 271–274. PMID 17512950.
212. Manford, M. & Andermann, F. (1998). Complex visual hallucinations. Clinical and neurobiological insights. *Brain* **121**: 1819–1840. PMID 9798740.
213. Behrendt, R. P. & Young, C. (2004). Hallucinations in schizophrenia, sensory impairment, and brain disease: a unifying model. *Behavioral and Brain Sciences* **27**: 771–787; discussion 787–830. PMID 16035402.
214. Douen, A. G. & Bourque, P. R. (1997). Musical auditory hallucinosis from Listeria rhombencephalitis. *Canadian Journal of Neurological Sciences* **24**: 70–72. PMID 9043753.
215. Low, J. A., Yap, K. B. & Chan, K. M. (1999). Posterior cerebral artery territory infarct presenting as acute psychosis. *Singapore Medical Journal* **40**: 702–703. PMID 10709410.
216. Kitabayashi, Y., Narumoto, J., Otakara, C., Hyungin, C., Fukui, K. & Yamada, K. (2006). Schizophrenia-like psychosis following right putaminal infarction. *Journal of Neuropsychiatry and Clinical Neurosciences* **18**: 561–562. PMID 17135392.
217. Narumoto, J., Matsushima, N., Oka, S., Shimizu, H., Kooguchi, Y., Kitabayashi, Y., Kunizawa, M., Ueda, H. & Fukui, K. (2005). Neurobehavioral changes associated with bilateral caudate nucleus infarctions. *Psychiatry and Clinical Neurosciences* **59**: 109–110. PMID 15679550.
218. Feinberg, W. M. & Rapcsak, S. Z. (1989). 'Peduncular hallucinosis' following paramedian thalamic infarction. *Neurology* **39**: 1535–1536. PMID 2812338.

219. McGilchrist, I., Goldstein, L. H., Jadresic, D. & Fenwick, P. (1993). Thalamo-frontal psychosis. *British Journal of Psychiatry* **163**: 113–115. PMID 8353678.
220. Price, B. H. & Mesulam, M. (1985). Psychiatric manifestations of right hemisphere infarctions. *Journal of Nervous and Mental Disease* **173**: 610–614. PMID 4031838.
221. Chemerinski, E. & Robinson, R. G. (2000). The neuropsychiatry of stroke. *Psychosomatics* **41**: 5–14. PMID 10665263.
222. Mobbs, R. J., Chandran, K. N. & Newcombe, R. L. (2001). Psychiatric presentation of aneurysmal subarachnoid haemorrhage. *ANZ Journal of Surgery* **71**: 69–70. PMID 11167606.
223. Gschwandtner, U., Borgwardt, S., Aston, J., Drewe, M., Radu, E. W. & Riecher-Rossler, A. (2004). [Chronic subdural hemorrhage in a patient with suspected schizophrenia prodrome]. *Nervenarzt* **75**: 691–693. PMID 15300326.
224. Tabet, N. & Fraser, C. (2001). Psychotic depression after a fall. *Journal of the Royal Society of Medicine* **94**: 83–84. PMID 11234206.
225. Feinberg, T. E. (2007). The "hard problem" of anosognosia: delusional confabulation and anosognosia. *Cortex* **43**: 1099–1101; discussion 1116–1021. PMID 18044673.
226. Turnbull, O. H. & Solms, M. (2007). Awareness, desire, and false beliefs: Freud in the light of modern neuropsychology. *Cortex* **43**: 1083–1090. PMID 18044668.
227. Joutel, A., Vahedi, K., Corpechot, C., Troesch, A., Chabriat, H., Vayssiere, C., Cruaud, C., Maciazek, J., Weissenbach, J., Bousser, M. G., Bach, J. F. & Tournier-Lasserve, E. (1997). Strong clustering and stereotyped nature of Notch3 mutations in CADASIL patients. *Lancet* **350**: 1511–1515. PMID 9388399.
228. Chabriat, H., Vahedi, K., Bousser, M. G., Iba-Zizen, M. T., Joutel, A., Nibbio, A., Nagy, T. G., Tournier-Lasserve, E., Krebs, M. O., Julien, J., Ducrocq, X., Levasseur, M., Mas, J. L., Dubois, B., Homeyer, P. & Lyon-Caen, O. (1995). Clinical spectrum of CADASIL: a study of 7 families. *Lancet* **346**: 934–939. PMID 7564728.
229. Chabriat, H. & Bousser, M. G. (2007). Neuropsychiatric manifestations in CADASIL. *Dialogues in Clinical Neuroscience* **9**: 199–208. PMID 17726918.
230. Hutchinson, M., O'Riordan, J., Javed, M., Quin, E., Macerlaine, D., Wilcox, T., Parfrey, N., Nagy, T. G. & Tournier-Lasserve, E. (1995). Familial hemiplegic migraine and autosomal dominant arteriopathy with leukoencephalopathy (CADASIL). *Annals of Neurology* **38**: 817–824. PMID 7486874.
231. Filley, C. M., Thompson, L. L., Sze, C. I., Simon, J. A., Paskavitz, J. F. & Kleinschmidt-DeMasters, B. K. (1999). White matter dementia in CADASIL. *Journal of the Neurological Sciences* **163**: 163–167. PMID 10371078.
232. Leyhe, T., Wiendl, H., Buchkremer, G. & Wormstall, H. (2005). CADASIL: underdiagnosed in psychiatric patients? *Acta Psychiatrica Scandinavica* **111**: 392–396; discussion 396–397. PMID 15819734.
233. Miller, B. L., Lesser, I. M., Boone, K., Goldberg, M., Hill, E., Miller, M. H., Benson, D. F. & Mehringer, M. (1989). Brain white-matter lesions and psychosis. *British Journal of Psychiatry* **155**: 73–78. PMID 2605435.
234. Razvi, S. S., Davidson, R., Bone, I. & Muir, K. W. (2005). The prevalence of cerebral autosomal dominant arteriopathy with subcortical infarcts and leucoencephalopathy (CADASIL) in the west of Scotland. *Journal of Neurology, Neurosurgery and Psychiatry* **76**: 739–741. PMID 15834040.
235. Kuriyama, S., Kusaka, Y., Fujimura, M., Wakai, K., Tamakoshi, A., Hashimoto, S., Tsuji, I., Inaba, Y. & Yoshimoto, T. (2008). Prevalence and clinicoepidemiological features of moyamoya disease in Japan: findings from a nationwide epidemiological survey. *Stroke* **39**: 42–47. PMID 18048855.
236. Klasen, H., Britton, J. & Newman, M. (1999). Moyamoya disease in a 12-year-old Caucasian boy presenting with acute transient psychosis. *European Child and Adolescent Psychiatry* **8**: 149–153. PMID 10435464.

237. Hanly, E. J., Meireles, O. R. & Cohn, E. J. (2009). Buerger disease (thromboangiitis obliterans). eMedicine. URL: http://emedicine.medscape.com/article/460027-overview. Accessed 12 June 2009.
238. Bozikas, V. P., Vlaikidis, N., Petrikis, P., Kourtis, A. & Karavatos, A. (2001). Schizophrenic-like symptoms in a patient with thrombo-angiitis obliterans (Winiwarter–Buerger's disease). *International Journal of Psychiatry in Medicine* **31**: 341–346. PMID 11841131.
239. Iizuka, T., Sakai, F., Kan, S. & Suzuki, N. (2003). Slowly progressive spread of the stroke-like lesions in MELAS. *Neurology* **61**: 1238–1244. PMID 14610127.
240. Guidetti, D., Casali, B., Mazzei, R. L. & Dotti, M. T. (2006). Cerebral autosomal dominant arteriopathy with subcortical infarcts and leukoencephalopathy. *Clinical and Experimental Hypertension* **28**: 271–277. PMID 16833034.
241. Masuhr, F., Mehraein, S. & Einhaupl, K. (2004). Cerebral venous and sinus thrombosis. *Journal of Neurology* **251**: 11–23. PMID 14999484.
242. Qin, P., Xu, H., Laursen, T. M., Vestergaard, M. & Mortensen, P. B. (2005). Risk for schizophrenia and schizophrenia-like psychosis among patients with epilepsy: population based cohort study. *British Medical Journal* **331**: 23. PMID 15964859.
243. Bancaud, J., Henriksen, O., Rubio-Donnadieu, F., Seino, M., Dreifuss, F. E. & Penry, J. K. (1981). Proposal for revised clinical and electroencephalographic classification of epileptic seizures. From the Commission on Classification and Terminology of the International League Against Epilepsy. *Epilepsia* **22**: 489–501. PMID 6790275.
244. Lowenstein, D. H., Bleck, T. & Macdonald, R. L. (1999). It's time to revise the definition of status epilepticus. *Epilepsia* **40**: 120–122. PMID 9924914.
245. Chen, D. K., So, Y. T. & Fisher, R. S. (2005). Use of serum prolactin in diagnosing epileptic seizures: report of the Therapeutics and Technology Assessment Subcommittee of the American Academy of Neurology. *Neurology* **65**: 668–675. PMID 16157897.
246. Phal, P. M., Usmanov, A., Nesbit, G. M., Anderson, J. C., Spencer, D., Wang, P., Helwig, J. A., Roberts, C. & Hamilton, B. E. (2008). Qualitative comparison of 3-T and 1.5-T MRI in the evaluation of epilepsy. *AJR: American Journal of Roentgenology* **191**: 890–895. PMID 18716125.
247. Duncan, J. (2008). Magnetic resonance imaging of the epilepsies. *Advances in Clinical Neurosciences and Rehabilitation* **8**: 5–8.
248. Nadkarni, S., Arnedo, V. & Devinsky, O. (2007). Psychosis in epilepsy patients. *Epilepsia* **48** Suppl 9: 17–19. PMID 18047594.
249. Riggio, S. (2006). Psychiatric manifestations of nonconvulsive status epilepticus. *Mount Sinai Journal of Medicine* **73**: 960–966. PMID 17195881.
250. Devinsky, O. (2008). Postictal psychosis: common, dangerous, and treatable. *Epilepsy Currents* **8**: 31–34. PMID 18330462.
251. Logsdail, S. J. & Toone, B. K. (1988). Post-ictal psychoses. A clinical and phenomenological description. *British Journal of Psychiatry* **152**: 246–252. PMID 3167343.
252. Adachi, N., Akanuma, N., Ito, M., Kato, M., Hara, T., Oana, Y., Matsuura, M., Okubo, Y. & Onuma, T. (2010). Epileptic, organic and genetic vulnerabilities for timing of the development of interictal psychosis. *British Journal of Psychiatry* **196**: 212–216. PMID 20194544.
253. Gatzonis, S. D., Stamboulis, E., Siafakas, Angelopoulos, E., Georgaculias, N., Sigounas, E. & Jekins, A. (2000). Acute psychosis and EEG normalisation after vagus nerve stimulation. *Journal of Neurology, Neurosurgery and Psychiatry* **69**: 278–279. PMID 10960292.
254. Sachdev, P. S. (2007). Alternating and postictal psychoses: review and a unifying hypothesis. *Schizophrenia Bulletin* **33**: 1029–1037. PMID 17337747.
255. Loder, E. (2010). Triptan therapy in migraine. *New England Journal of Medicine* **363**: 63–70. PMID 20592298.
256. Stiefel, F. C. & Ruttner, B. (1995). Migraine with aura and functional

psychosis: a rare differential diagnosis. *General Hospital Psychiatry* **17**: 389–391. PMID 8522155.

257. Liu, G. T., Schatz, N. J., Galetta, S. L., Volpe, N. J., Skobieranda, F. & Kosmorsky, G. S. (1995). Persistent positive visual phenomena in migraine. *Neurology* **45**: 664–668. PMID 7723952.

258. Fitzsimons, R. B. & Wolfenden, W. H. (1985). Migraine coma. Meningitic migraine with cerebral oedema associated with a new form of autosomal dominant cerebellar ataxia. *Brain* **108** (Part 3): 555–577. PMID 4041774.

259. Kors, E. E., Terwindt, G. M., Vermeulen, F. L., Fitzsimons, R. B., Jardine, P. E., Heywood, P., Love, S., van den Maagdenberg, A. M., Haan, J., Frants, R. R. & Ferrari, M. D. (2001). Delayed cerebral edema and fatal coma after minor head trauma: role of the CACNA1A calcium channel subunit gene and relationship with familial hemiplegic migraine. *Annals of Neurology* **49**: 753–760. PMID 11409427.

260. Silberstein, S. D., Niknam, R., Rozen, T. D. & Young, W. B. (2000). Cluster headache with aura. *Neurology* **54**: 219–221. PMID 10636152.

261. Martínez-Fernández, E., Alberca, R., Mir, P., Franco, E., Montes, E. & Lozano, P. (2002). Cluster headache with aura. *J Headache Pain* **3**: 105–110.

262. Bartynski, W. S. (2008). Posterior reversible encephalopathy syndrome, part 1: fundamental imaging and clinical features. *AJNR: American Journal of Neuroradiology* **29**: 1036–1042. PMID 18356474.

263. Hinchey, J., Chaves, C., Appignani, B., Breen, J., Pao, L., Wang, A., Pessin, M. S., Lamy, C., Mas, J. L. & Caplan, L. R. (1996). A reversible posterior leukoencephalopathy syndrome. *New England Journal of Medicine* **334**: 494–500. PMID 8559202.

264. Yildiz, O. K., Segmen, H., Oztoprak, I., Bolayir, E. & Topaktas, S. (2010). Posterior reversible encephalopathy and alexia without agraphia in a patient with Hashimoto's encephalopathy. *Neurological Sciences* **31**: 523–525. PMID 20119737.

265. Puy, H., Gouya, L. & Deybach, J. C. (2010). Porphyrias. *Lancet* **375**: 924–937. PMID 20226990.

266. Bartynski, W. S. (2008). Posterior reversible encephalopathy syndrome, part 2: controversies surrounding pathophysiology of vasogenic edema. *AJNR: American Journal of Neuroradiology* **29**: 1043–1049. PMID 18403560.

267. Fujii, D. E. & Ahmed, I. (2001). Risk factors in psychosis secondary to traumatic brain injury. *Journal of Neuropsychiatry and Clinical Neurosciences* **13**: 61–69. PMID 11207331.

268. David, A. S. & Prince, M. (2005). Psychosis following head injury: a critical review. *Journal of Neurology, Neurosurgery and Psychiatry* **76 Suppl 1**: i53–60. PMID 15718223.

269. Harrison, G., Whitley, E., Rasmussen, F., Lewis, G., Dalman, C. & Gunnell, D. (2006). Risk of schizophrenia and other non-affective psychosis among individuals exposed to head injury: case control study. *Schizophrenia Research* **88**: 119–126. PMID 16935470.

270. Kim, E., Lauterbach, E. C., Reeve, A., Arciniegas, D. B., Coburn, K. L., Mendez, M. F., Rummans, T. A. & Coffey, E. C. (2007). Neuropsychiatric complications of traumatic brain injury: a critical review of the literature (a report by the ANPA Committee on Research). *Journal of Neuropsychiatry and Clinical Neurosciences* **19**: 106–127. PMID 17431056.

271. Hoge, C. W., McGurk, D., Thomas, J. L., Cox, A. L., Engel, C. C. & Castro, C. A. (2008). Mild traumatic brain injury in U.S. soldiers returning from Iraq. *New England Journal of Medicine* **358**: 453–463. PMID 18234750.

272. Jellinger, K. A. (2004). Head injury and dementia. *Current Opinion in Neurology* **17**: 719–723. PMID 15542981.

273. Frank, J. (2005). Dementia due to head trauma. eMedicine. URL: http://www.emedicine.com/med/topic3152.htm. Accessed 11 September 2008.

274. Hord, E. (2006). Hydrocephalus. eMedicine. URL: http://www.emedicine.com/neuro/topic161.htm. Accessed 4 March 2008.

275. Dalvi, A. (2007). Normal pressure hydrocephalus. eMedicine. URL: http://www.emedicine.com/neuro/topic277.htm. Accessed 4 March 2008.
276. Pinner, G., Johnson, H., Bouman, W. P. & Isaacs, J. (1997). Psychiatric manifestations of normal-pressure hydrocephalus: a short review and unusual case. *International Psychogeriatrics* **9**: 465–470. PMID 9549596.
277. Lying-Tunell, U. (1979). Psychotic symptoms in normal-pressure hydrocephalus. *Acta Psychiatrica Scandinavica* **59**: 415–419. PMID 433632.
278. Galasko, D., Kwo-On-Yuen, P. F. & Thal, L. (1988). Intracranial mass lesions associated with late-onset psychosis and depression. *Psychiatric Clinics of North America* **11**: 151–166. PMID 3288979.
279. Pollak, L., Klein, C., Rabey, J. M. & Schiffer, J. (1996). Posterior fossa lesions associated with neuropsychiatric symptomatology. *International Journal of Neuroscience* **87**: 119–126. PMID 9003973.
280. Ouma, J. R. (2004). Psychotic manifestations in brain tumour patients: 2 case reports from South Africa. *African Health Sciences* **4**: 189–193. PMID 15687074.
281. Lisanby, S. H., Kohler, C., Swanson, C. L. & Gur, R. E. (1998). Psychosis secondary to brain tumor. *Seminars in Clinical Neuropsychiatry* **3**: 12–22. PMID 10085187.
282. Rueda-Lara, M. A., Buchert, S., Skotzko, C. & Clemow, L. P. (2003). Psychiatric symptoms masking pituitary adenoma in Spanish speaking immigrants. *General Hospital Psychiatry* **25**: 367–371. PMID 12972230.
283. Sumners, D. (1984). Believing your husband has been replaced by an impostor because you have a pituitary tumour. *British Medical Journal (Clinical Research Edition)* **289**: 699–700. PMID 6434047.
284. Kannabiran, M., Singh, V. & Grewal, S. (2006). Acromegaly presenting as psychotic disorder in a patient with familial autosomal dominant polycystic kidney disease. *German Journal of Psychiatry* **9**: 136–138.
285. Veendrick-Meekes, M. J., Verhoeven, W. M., van Erp, M. G., van Blarikom, W. & Tuinier, S. (2007). Neuropsychiatric aspects of patients with hypothalamic hamartomas. *Epilepsy & Behavior* **11**: 218–221. PMID 17606410.
286. Carson, B. S., Weingart, J. D., Guarnieri, M. & Fisher, P. G. (1997). Third ventricular choroid plexus papilloma with psychosis. Case report. *Journal of Neurosurgery* **87**: 103–105. PMID 9202274.
287. Vakis, A. F., Koutentakis, D. I., Karabetsos, D. A. & Kalostos, G. N. (2006). Psychosis-like syndrome associated with intermittent intracranial hypertension caused by a large arachnoid cyst of the left temporal lobe. *British Journal of Neurosurgery* **20**: 156–159. PMID 16801049.
288. Roberts, J. K., Trimble, M. R. & Robertson, M. (1983). Schizophrenic psychosis associated with aqueduct stenosis in adults. *Journal of Neurology, Neurosurgery and Psychiatry* **46**: 892–898. PMID 6644313.
289. Lazoff, M. (2008). Multiple sclerosis. eMedicine. URL: http://www.emedicine.com/emerg/topic321.htm. Accessed 5 March 2008.
290. Compston, A. & Coles, A. (2008). Multiple sclerosis. *Lancet* **372**: 1502–1517. PMID 18970977.
291. Ebers, G. C. (2008). Environmental factors and multiple sclerosis. *Lancet Neurology* **7**: 268–277. PMID 18275928.
292. Feinstein, A., du Boulay, G. & Ron, M. A. (1992). Psychotic illness in multiple sclerosis. A clinical and magnetic resonance imaging study. *British Journal of Psychiatry* **161**: 680–685. PMID 1422619.
293. McDonald, W. I., Compston, A., Edan, G., Goodkin, D., Hartung, H. P., Lublin, F. D., McFarland, H. F., Paty, D. W., Polman, C. H., Reingold, S. C., Sandberg-Wollheim, M., Sibley, W., Thompson, A., van den Noort, S., Weinshenker, B. Y. & Wolinsky, J. S. (2001). Recommended diagnostic criteria for multiple sclerosis: guidelines from the International Panel on the diagnosis of multiple sclerosis. *Annals of Neurology* **50**: 121–127. PMID 11456302.

294. Sa, M. J. (2007). Psychological aspects of multiple sclerosis. *Clinical Neurology and Neurosurgery* **110**: 868–877. PMID 18022759.
295. Reimer, J., Aderhold, V., Lambert, M. & Haasen, C. (2006). Manifestation of multiple sclerosis with paranoid-hallucinatory psychosis. *Journal of Neurology* **253**: 531–532. PMID 16435081.
296. Diaz-Olavarrieta, C., Cummings, J. L., Velazquez, J. & Garcia de la Cadena, C. (1999). Neuropsychiatric manifestations of multiple sclerosis. *Journal of Neuropsychiatry and Clinical Neurosciences* **11**: 51–57. PMID 9990556.
297. Patten, S. B., Svenson, L. W. & Metz, L. M. (2005). Psychotic disorders in MS: population-based evidence of an association. *Neurology* **65**: 1123–1125. PMID 16217073.
298. Luzzio, C. (2007). Central pontine myelinolysis. eMedicine. URL: http://www.emedicine.com/neuro/topic50.htm. Accessed 5 March 2008.
299. Lim, L. & Krystal, A. (2007). Psychotic disorder in a patient with central and extrapontine myelinolysis. *Psychiatry and Clinical Neurosciences* **61**: 320–322. PMID 17472602.
300. Franz, D. N. & Glauser, T. A. (2007). Tuberous sclerosis. eMedicine. URL: http://emedicine.medscape.com/article/1177711-overview. Accessed 15 May 2009.
301. Critchley, M. & Earl, C. J. C. (1932). Tuberose sclerosis and allied conditions. *Brain* **55**: 311–346.
302. Sedky, K., Hughes, T., Yusufzie, K. & Lippmann, S. (2003). Tuberous sclerosis with psychosis. *Psychosomatics* **44**: 521–522. PMID 14597689.
303. Hunt, A. & Dennis, J. (1987). Psychiatric disorder among children with tuberous sclerosis. *Developmental Medicine and Child Neurology* **29**: 190–198. PMID 3582788.
304. Clarke, D. J., Buckley, M. E. & Burns, B. H. (1987). Epilepsy and psychosis – ask the family. *British Journal of Psychiatry* **150**: 702–703. PMID 3651710.
305. Holschneider, D. P. & Szuba, M. P. (1992). Capgras' syndrome and psychosis in a patient with tuberous sclerosis. *Journal of Neuropsychiatry and Clinical Neurosciences* **4**: 352–353. PMID 1498593.
306. Raznahan, A., Joinson, C., O'Callaghan, F., Osborne, J. P. & Bolton, P. F. (2006). Psychopathology in tuberous sclerosis: an overview and findings in a population-based sample of adults with tuberous sclerosis. *Journal of Intellectual Disability Research* **50**: 561–569. PMID 16867063.
307. Schonfeldt-Lecuona, C., Freudenmann, R. W., Tumani, H., Kassubek, J. & Connemann, B. J. (2005). Acute psychosis with a mediastinal carcinoma metastasis. *Medical Science Monitor* **11**: CS6–8. PMID 15614198.
308. Turkel, S. B., Tishler, D. & Tavare, C. J. (2007). Late onset psychosis in survivors of pediatric central nervous system malignancies. *Journal of Neuropsychiatry and Clinical Neurosciences* **19**: 293–297. PMID 17827414.
309. Benabarre, A., Bosch, X., Plana, M. T., Lecube, A., Vieta, E., Cirera, E. & Valdes, M. (2005). Relapsing paranoid psychosis as the first manifestation of pheochromocytoma. *Journal of Clinical Psychiatry* **66**: 949–950. PMID 16013915.
310. Sweeney, A. T. & Blake, M. A. (2010). Pheochromocytoma. eMedicine. URL: http://emedicine.medscape.com/article/124059-overview. Accessed 18 Apr 2010.
311. Hanna, S. M. (1965). Carcinoid syndrome associated with psychosis. *Postgraduate Medical Journal* **41**: 566–567. PMID 5827675.
312. Santacroce, L., Diomede, L. & Balducci, L. (2009). Malignant carcinoid syndrome. eMedicine. URL: http://emedicine.medscape.com/article/282515-overview. Accessed 27 April 2010.
313. Kamangar, N. & O'Regan, A. W. (2009). Lymphomatoid granulomatosis. eMedicine. URL: http://emedicine.medscape.com/article/299751-overview. Accessed 16 April 2009.
314. Carone, D. A., Benedict, R. H., Zivadinov, R., Singh, B. & Ambrus, J. L. (2006). Progressive cerebral disease in lymphomatoid granulomatosis causes anterograde amnesia and neuropsychiatric disorder. *Journal*

of Neuroimaging **16**: 163–166. PMID 16629740.

315. Baehring, J. M., Henchcliffe, C., Ledezma, C. J., Fulbright, R. & Hochberg, F. H. (2005). Intravascular lymphoma: magnetic resonance imaging correlates of disease dynamics within the central nervous system. *Journal of Neurology, Neurosurgery and Psychiatry* **76**: 540–544. PMID 15774442.
316. Pless, M. L., Chen, Y. B., Copen, W. A. & Frosch, M. P. (2010). Case records of the Massachusetts General Hospital. Case 9–2010. A 37-year-old woman with paresthesias and ataxia. *New England Journal of Medicine* **362**: 1129–1138. PMID 20335590.
317. Higes-Pascual, F., Beroiz-Groh, P., Bravo-Guillen, A. I., Palomo-Martinez, V. & Cuevas-Santos, J. (2000). [Leptomeningeal carcinomatosis as presenting symptom of a gallbladder carcinoma]. *Revista de Neurologia* **30**: 841–844. PMID 10870198.
318. Wagner, A. L. (2010). Leptomeningeal carcinomatosis. eMedicine. URL: http://emedicine.medscape.com/article/341389-overview. Accessed 21 July 2010.
319. Sewell, R. A. & Recht, L. D. (2009). Leptomeningeal carcinomatosis. eMedicine. URL: http://emedicine.medscape.com/article/1156338-diagnosis. Accessed 21 July 2010.
320. Yolken, R. H. & Torrey, E. F. (2008). Are some cases of psychosis caused by microbial agents? A review of the evidence. *Molecular Psychiatry* **13**: 470–479. PMID 18268502.
321. Incesu, L. & Khosla, A. (2009). Meningitis, bacterial. eMedicine. URL: http://emedicine.medscape.com/article/341971-overview. Accessed 16 April 2009.
322. Chaudhuri, A. & Kennedy, P. G. (2002). Diagnosis and treatment of viral encephalitis. *Postgraduate Medical Journal* **78**: 575–583. PMID 12415078.
323. Lazoff, M. (2007). Encephalitis. eMedicine. URL: http://emedicine.medscape.com/article/791896-overview. Accessed 26 February 2009.
324. Razonable, R. R. & Keating, M. R. (2009). Meningitis. eMedicine. URL: http://emedicine.medscape.com/article/232915-overview. Accessed 27 April 2010.
325. Abrahao, A. L., Focaccia, R. & Gattaz, W. F. (2005). Childhood meningitis increases the risk for adult schizophrenia. *World Journal of Biological Psychiatry* **6 Suppl 2**: 44–48. PMID 16166023.
326. Leask, S. J., Done, D. J. & Crow, T. J. (2002). Adult psychosis, common childhood infections and neurological soft signs in a national birth cohort. *British Journal of Psychiatry* **181**: 387–392. PMID 12411263.
327. Rosenblum, D. & Ehrlich, V. (1995). Brain abscess and psychosis as a complication of a halo orthosis. *Archives of Physical Medicine and Rehabilitation* **76**: 865–867. PMID 7668959.
328. Swan, B. M. & Levine, N. (2005). Syphilis. eMedicine. URL: http://www.emedicine.com/derm/topic413.htm. Accessed 5 March 2008.
329. McGregor, T. A., Richard, A. J. & Pulver, B. (2006). Syphilis. eMedicine. URL: http://www.emedicine.com/emerg/topic563.htm. Accessed 5 March 2008.
330. McCalmont, T. (2009). Syphilis. eMedicine. URL: http://emedicine.medscape.com/article/1053426-overview. Accessed 15 November 2009.
331. Sivakumar, K. & Okocha, C. I. (1992). Neurosyphilis and schizophrenia. *British Journal of Psychiatry* **161**: 251–254. PMID 1521109.
332. Kohler, C. G., Pickholtz, J. & Ballas, C. (2000). Neurosyphilis presenting as schizophrenialike psychosis. *Neuropsychiatry, Neuropsychology, and Behavioral Neurology* **13**: 297–302. PMID 11186166.
333. Kararizou, E., Mitsonis, C., Dimopoulos, N., Gkiatas, K., Markou, I. & Kalfakis, N. (2006). Psychosis or simply a new manifestation of neurosyphilis? *Journal of International Medical Research* **34**: 335–337. PMID 16866029.
334. Estevez, R. F. (2006). Neurosyphilis presenting as rhabdomyolysis and acute renal failure with subsequent irreversible psychosis and dementia. *Psychosomatics* **47**: 538–539. PMID 17116961.

335. Cleare, A. J., Jacoby, R., Tovey, S. J. & Bergman, K. (1993). Syphilis, neither dead nor buried – a survey of psychogeriatric inpatients. *International Journal of Geriatric Psychiatry* **8**: 661–664.

336. Egglestone, S. I. & Turner, A. J. (2000). Serological diagnosis of syphilis. PHLS Syphilis Serology Working Group. *Communicable Disease and Public Health* **3**: 158–162. PMID 11014025.

337. Meyerhoff, J. (2007). Lyme disease. eMedicine. URL: http://www.emedicine.com/med/topic1346.htm. Accessed 14 November 2008.

338. Hurley, R. A. & Taber, K. H. (2008). Acute and chronic Lyme disease: controversies for neuropsychiatry. *Journal of Neuropsychiatry and Clinical Neurosciences* **20**: iv-6. PMID 18305280.

339. Bratton, R. L., Whiteside, J. W., Hovan, M. J., Engle, R. L. & Edwards, F. D. (2008). Diagnosis and treatment of Lyme disease. *Mayo Clinic Proceedings* **83**: 566–571. PMID 18452688.

340. Berglund, J., Eitrem, R., Ornstein, K., Lindberg, A., Ringer, A., Elmrud, H., Carlsson, M., Runehagen, A., Svanborg, C. & Norrby, R. (1995). An epidemiologic study of Lyme disease in southern Sweden. *New England Journal of Medicine* **333**: 1319–1327. PMID 7566023.

341. Feder, H. M., Jr., Johnson, B. J., O'Connell, S., Shapiro, E. D., Steere, A. C., Wormser, G. P., Agger, W. A., Artsob, H., Auwaerter, P., Dumler, J. S., Bakken, J. S., Bockenstedt, L. K., Green, J., Dattwyler, R. J., Munoz, J., Nadelman, R. B., Schwartz, I., Draper, T., McSweegan, E., Halperin, J. J., Klempner, M. S., Krause, P. J., Mead, P., Morshed, M., Porwancher, R., Radolf, J. D., Smith, R. P., Jr., Sood, S., Weinstein, A., Wong, S. J. & Zemel, L. (2007). A critical appraisal of "chronic Lyme disease". *New England Journal of Medicine* **357**: 1422–1430. PMID 17914043.

342. Hess, A., Buchmann, J., Zettl, U. K., Henschel, S., Schlaefke, D., Grau, G. & Benecke, R. (1999). Borrelia burgdorferi central nervous system infection presenting as an organic schizophrenialike disorder. *Biological Psychiatry* **45**: 795. PMID 10188012.

343. van den Bergen, H. A., Smith, J. P. & van der Zwan, A. (1993). [Lyme psychosis]. *Nederlands Tijdschrift voor Geneeskunde* **137**: 2098–2100. PMID 8413733.

344. Pfister, H. W., Preac-Mursic, V., Wilske, B., Rieder, G., Forderreuther, S., Schmidt, S. & Kapfhammer, H. P. (1993). Catatonic syndrome in acute severe encephalitis due to Borrelia burgdorferi infection. *Neurology* **43**: 433–435. PMID 8437717.

345. Hajek, T., Paskova, B., Janovska, D., Bahbouh, R., Hajek, P., Libiger, J. & Hoschl, C. (2002). Higher prevalence of antibodies to Borrelia burgdorferi in psychiatric patients than in healthy subjects. *American Journal of Psychiatry* **159**: 297–301. PMID 11823274.

346. Edlow, J. A. (2007). Tick-borne diseases, Lyme. eMedicine. URL: http://www.emedicine.com/emerg/topic588.htm. Accessed 14 November 2008.

347. Chan, S. S., Wong, Y. C. & Hodgkiss, I. J. (1996). A preliminary study of C-reactive protein in the diagnosis and monitoring of Lyme disease. *Biomedical and Environmental Sciences* **9**: 424–429. PMID 8988812.

348. Young, N. P. & Klein, C. J. (2007). Encephalopathy with seizures having PCR-positive Anaplasma phagocytophilum and Ehrlichia chaffeensis. *European Journal of Neurology* **14**: e3–4. PMID 17250712.

349. Adelson, M. E., Rao, R. V., Tilton, R. C., Cabets, K., Eskow, E., Fein, L., Occi, J. L. & Mordechai, E. (2004). Prevalence of Borrelia burgdorferi, Bartonella spp., Babesia microti, and Anaplasma phagocytophila in Ixodes scapularis ticks collected in Northern New Jersey. *Journal of Clinical Microbiology* **42**: 2799–2801. PMID 15184475.

350. Schraga, E. D. (2008). Catscratch disease. eMedicine. URL: http://www.emedicine.com/emerg/topic84.htm. Accessed 14 November 2008.

351. Rolain, J. M., Brouqui, P., Koehler, J. E., Maguina, C., Dolan, M. J. & Raoult, D. (2004). Recommendations for treatment of human infections caused by Bartonella species. *Antimicrobial Agents and Chemotherapy* **48**: 1921–1933. PMID 15155180.

Journal of Medicine **362**: 1993–2000. PMID 20505178.

393. Jarvis, M. R., Wasserman, A. L. & Todd, R. D. (1990). Acute psychosis in a patient with Epstein–Barr virus infection. *Journal of the American Academy of Child and Adolescent Psychiatry* **29**: 468–469. PMID 2347847.
394. Leavell, R., Ray, C. G., Ferry, P. C. & Minnich, L. L. (1986). Unusual acute neurologic presentations with Epstein–Barr virus infection. *Archives of Neurology* **43**: 186–188. PMID 3004399.
395. Klein, R. F., Betts, R., Horn, R. & Sullivan, J. L. (1984). Acute psychosis in a 45-year-old man with bipolar disorder and primary Epstein–Barr virus infection: a case report. *General Hospital Psychiatry* **6**: 13–15. PMID 6693024.
396. Gotlieb-Stematsky, T. & Arlazoroff, A. (1976). Antibodies to Epstein–Barr virus in neurological diseases. *Journal of the Neurological Sciences* **28**: 115–120. PMID 180262.
397. Gotlieb-Stematsky, T., Zonis, J., Arlazoroff, A., Mozes, T., Sigal, M. & Szekely, A. G. (1981). Antibodies to Epstein–Barr virus, herpes simplex type 1, cytomegalovirus and measles virus in psychiatric patients. *Archives of Virology* **67**: 333–339. PMID 6263228.
398. Srikanth, S., Ravi, V., Poornima, K. S., Shetty, K. T., Gangadhar, B. N. & Janakiramaiah, N. (1994). Viral antibodies in recent onset, nonorganic psychoses: correspondence with symptomatic severity. *Biological Psychiatry* **36**: 517–521. PMID 7827214.
399. Leweke, F. M., Gerth, C. W., Koethe, D., Klosterkotter, J., Ruslanova, I., Krivogorsky, B., Torrey, E. F. & Yolken, R. H. (2004). Antibodies to infectious agents in individuals with recent onset schizophrenia. *European Archives of Psychiatry and Clinical Neuroscience* **254**: 4–8. PMID 14991372.
400. Gultekin, S. H., Rosenfeld, M. R., Voltz, R., Eichen, J., Posner, J. B. & Dalmau, J. (2000). Paraneoplastic limbic encephalitis: neurological symptoms, immunological findings and tumour association in 50 patients. *Brain* **123**: 1481–1494. PMID 10869059.
401. Sharfstein, S. R., Gordon, M. F., Libman, R. B. & Malkin, E. S. (1999). Adult-onset MELAS presenting as herpes encephalitis. *Archives of Neurology* **56**: 241–243. PMID 10025431.
402. UNAIDS (2008). 2008 Report on the global AIDS epidemic. Joint United Nations Programme on HIV/AIDS. URL: http://www.unaids.org/en/KnowledgeCentre/HIVData/GlobalReport/2008/2008_Global_report.asp. Accessed 27 February 2009.
403. Hecht, F. M., Busch, M. P., Rawal, B., Webb, M., Rosenberg, E., Swanson, M., Chesney, M., Anderson, J., Levy, J. & Kahn, J. O. (2002). Use of laboratory tests and clinical symptoms for identification of primary HIV infection. *AIDS* **16**: 1119–1129. PMID 12004270.
404. Hazenberg, M. D., Hamann, D., Schuitemaker, H. & Miedema, F. (2000). T cell depletion in HIV-1 infection: how CD4+ T cells go out of stock. *Nature Immunology* **1**: 285–289. PMID 11017098.
405. Levy, R. M. & Bredesen, D. E. (1988). Central nervous system dysfunction in acquired immunodeficiency syndrome. *Journal of Acquired Immune Deficiency Syndromes* **1**: 41–64. PMID 3063805.
406. Harris, M. J., Jeste, D. V., Gleghorn, A. & Sewell, D. D. (1991). New-onset psychosis in HIV-infected patients. *Journal of Clinical Psychiatry* **52**: 369–376. PMID 1894589.
407. Bernhard, H., Frommberger, U., Weber, K. C., Philipp, M., Ramadori, G. & Meyer zum Buschenfelde, K. H. (1989). [Chronic paranoid-hallucinatory psychosis as the initial manifestation of an HIV infection?]. *Deutsche Medizinische Wochenschrift* **114**: 503–506. PMID 2924704.
408. Sewell, D. D. (1996). Schizophrenia and HIV. *Schizophrenia Bulletin* **22**: 465–473. PMID 8873297.
409. Lau, B., Sharrett, A. R., Kingsley, L. A., Post, W., Palella, F. J., Visscher, B. & Gange, S. J. (2006). C-reactive protein is a marker for human immunodeficiency

virus disease progression. *Archives of Internal Medicine* **166**: 64–70. PMID 16401812.
410. Navia, B. A. & Price, R. W. (1987). The acquired immunodeficiency syndrome dementia complex as the presenting or sole manifestation of human immunodeficiency virus infection. *Archives of Neurology* **44**: 65–69. PMID 3800724.
411. Herzlich, B. C. & Schiano, T. D. (1993). Reversal of apparent AIDS dementia complex following treatment with vitamin B12. *Journal of Internal Medicine* **233**: 495–497. PMID 8501420.
412. Nagasawa, H., Wada, M., Kurita, K., Iseki, C., Katagiri, T. & Kato, T. (2006). [A case of non-herpetic acute limbic encephalitis associated with a type-2 adenovirus infection]. *Rinsho Shinkeigaku (Clinical Neurology)* **46**: 322–327. PMID 16886798.
413. Althaus, J. (1893). On psychoses after influenza. *Journal of Mental Science* **39**: 163–176.
414. Neel, J. L. (2000). Neuropsychiatric sequelae in a case of St. Louis encephalitis. *General Hospital Psychiatry* **22**: 126–128. PMID 10896493.
415. Fry, W. F., Jr. & Tobin, A. (1967). Japanese B encephalitis. Symptom dynamics in an organic psychosis. *Psychiatric Quarterly* **41**: 91–107. PMID 4292103.
416. Hrabak, T., Yerkey, M. W., Callerame, K. & Graham, K. (2002). Eastern equine encephalitis presenting as psychosis. *Journal of the Mississippi State Medical Association* **43**: 109–110. PMID 11989192.
417. Stoler, M., Meshulam, B., Zoldan, J. & Sirota, P. (1987). Schizophreniform episode following measles infection. *British Journal of Psychiatry* **150**: 861–862. PMID 3651743.
418. Delage, J. (1955). [Moderate psychosis caused by mumps in a child of nine years]. *Laval Médical* **20**: 175–183. PMID 14382616.
419. Keddie, K. M. (1965). Toxic psychosis following mumps. *British Journal of Psychiatry* **111**: 691–696. PMID 14337417.
420. Koskiniemi, M., Donner, M. & Pettay, O. (1983). Clinical appearance and outcome in mumps encephalitis in children. *Acta Paediatrica Scandinavica* **72**: 603–609. PMID 6624436.
421. Paton, N. I., Leo, Y. S., Zaki, S. R., Auchus, A. P., Lee, K. E., Ling, A. E., Chew, S. K., Ang, B., Rollin, P. E., Umapathi, T., Sng, I., Lee, C. C., Lim, E. & Ksiazek, T. G. (1999). Outbreak of Nipah-virus infection among abattoir workers in Singapore. *Lancet* **354**: 1253–1256. PMID 10520634.
422. Gompf, S. G. & Somboonwit, C. (2008). Rabies. eMedicine. URL: http://emedicine.medscape.com/article/220967-overview. Accessed 27 February 2009.
423. de Wet, J. S. (1980). Rabies presenting as an acute psychiatric emergency. *South African Medical Journal* **58**: 297–298. PMID 7404238.
424. Goswami, U., Shankar, S. K., Channabasavanna, S. M. & Chattopadhyay, A. (1984). Psychiatric presentations in rabies. A clinico-pathologic report from South India with a review of literature. *Tropical and Geographical Medicine* **36**: 77–81. PMID 6375052.
425. Duncalf, C. M., Kent, J. N., Harbord, M. & Hicks, E. P. (1989). Subacute sclerosing panencephalitis presenting as schizophreniform psychosis. *British Journal of Psychiatry* **155**: 557–559. PMID 2611581.
426. Kayal, M., Varghese, S. T. & Balhara, Y. P. (2006). Psychiatric manifestation of SSPE. *Journal of Neuropsychiatry and Clinical Neurosciences* **18**: 560. PMID 17135391.
427. Brasic, J. R. (2008). Catatonia. eMedicine. URL: http://www.emedicine.com/neuro/topic708.htm. Accessed 16 December 2008.
428. Venna, N., Gonzalez, R. G. & Camelo-Piragua, S. I. (2010). Case records of the Massachusetts General Hospital. Case 11-2010. A 69-year-old woman with lethargy, confusion, and abnormalities on brain imaging. *New England Journal of Medicine* **362**: 1431–1437. PMID 20393180.
429. Aribandi, M. & Aribandi, A. K. (2009). Progressive multifocal leukodystrophy. eMedicine. URL: http://emedicine.

469. Dimitri, D., Jehel, L., Durr, A., Levy-Soussan, M., Andreux, V., Laplanche, J. L., Fossati, P. & Cohen, D. (2006). Fatal familial insomnia presenting as psychosis in an 18-year-old man. *Neurology* **67**: 363–364. PMID 16864846.
470. Mohamed, I. & Moorjani, B. I. (2007). Chorea in children. eMedicine. URL: http://www.emedicine.com/neuro/topic644.htm. Accessed 4 March 2008.
471. Berman, S. A., Dinnerstein, E., Herrera, M. A. & Galvez-Jimenez, N. (2006). Chorea in adults. eMedicine. URL: http://www.emedicine.com/neuro/topic62.htm. Accessed 4 March 2008.
472. Dale, R. C., Church, A. J., Surtees, R. A., Lees, A. J., Adcock, J. E., Harding, B., Neville, B. G. & Giovannoni, G. (2004). Encephalitis lethargica syndrome: 20 new cases and evidence of basal ganglia autoimmunity. *Brain* **127**: 21–33. PMID 14570817.
473. Teixeira, A. L., Jr., Maia, D. P. & Cardoso, F. (2007). Psychosis following acute Sydenham's chorea. *European Child and Adolescent Psychiatry* **16**: 67–69. PMID 16791540.
474. Hu, M. T. M., Butterworth, R., Giovannoni, G., Church, A. & Logsdail, S. (2009). Lesson of the month: chorea. *Clinical Medicine* **9**: 188–189.
475. Brockington, I. (2006). Psychosis complicating chorea gravidarum. *Archives of Women's Mental Health* **9**: 113–114. PMID 16429327.
476. Wilcox, J. A. & Nasrallah, H. A. (1986). Sydenham's chorea and psychosis. *Neuropsychobiology* **15**: 13–14. PMID 3014370.
477. American Heart Association (1992). Guidelines for the diagnosis of rheumatic fever. Jones Criteria, 1992 update. Special Writing Group of the Committee on Rheumatic Fever, Endocarditis, and Kawasaki Disease of the Council on Cardiovascular Disease in the Young of the American Heart Association. *Journal of the American Medical Association* **268**: 2069–2073. PMID 1404745.
478. Swedo, S. E., Leonard, H. L., Garvey, M., Mittleman, B., Allen, A. J., Perlmutter, S., Lougee, L., Dow, S., Zamkoff, J. & Dubbert, B. K. (1998). Pediatric autoimmune neuropsychiatric disorders associated with streptococcal infections: clinical description of the first 50 cases. *American Journal of Psychiatry* **155**: 264–271. PMID 9464208.
479. Bennetto, L. & Scolding, N. (2004). Inflammatory/post-infectious encephalomyelitis. *Journal of Neurology, Neurosurgery and Psychiatry* **75 Suppl 1**: i22–28. PMID 14978147.
480. Nasr, J. T., Andriola, M. R. & Coyle, P. K. (2000). ADEM: literature review and case report of acute psychosis presentation. *Pediatric Neurology* **22**: 8–18. PMID 10669199.
481. Smith, A. L. & Beattie, R. M. (1998). Child psychosis due to hypothyroidism. *Journal of the Royal Society of Medicine* **91**: 537–538. PMID 10070376.
482. Bharaktiya, S., Orlander, P. R., Woodhouse, W. R. & Bhalla Davis, A. (2007). Hypothyroidism. eMedicine. URL: http://www.emedicine.com/med/topic1145.htm. Accessed 6 January 2008.
483. Benvenga, S., Lapa, D. & Trimarchi, F. (2003). Don't forget the thyroid in the etiology of psychoses. *American Journal of Medicine* **115**: 159–160. PMID 12893408.
484. Kudrjavcev, T. (1978). Neurologic complications of thyroid dysfunction. *Advances in Neurology* **19**: 619–636. PMID 742545.
485. Leigh, H. (1990). Cerebral effects of endocrine disease (chapter 199). In *Principles and Practice of Endocrinology and Metabolism* (Becker, K. L., Bilezikian, J. P., Bremner, W. J., Hung, W., Kahn, C. R., Loriaux, D. L., Rebar, R. W., Robertson, G. L. & Wartofsky, L., Eds.), pp. 1479–1483. Philadelphia, PA: Lippincott.
486. Roberts, C. G. & Ladenson, P. W. (2004). Hypothyroidism. *Lancet* **363**: 793–803. PMID 15016491.
487. Stowell, C. P. & Barnhill, J. W. (2005). Acute mania in the setting of severe hypothyroidism. *Psychosomatics* **46**: 259–261. PMID 15883148.
488. Schraga, E. D. & Manifold, C. A. (2006). Hyperthyroidism, thyroid storm, and Graves disease. eMedicine. URL: http://www.emedicine.com/emerg/topic269.htm. Accessed 6 January 2008.

489. Fenton, B. W. & Barnes, W. (2007). Struma ovarii. eMedicine. URL: http://www.emedicine.com/med/topic2191.htm. Accessed 6 January 2008.
490. Josephson, A. M. & Mackenzie, T. B. (1980). Thyroid-induced mania in hypothyroid patients. *British Journal of Psychiatry* **137**: 222–228. PMID 7437657.
491. Josephson, A. M. & Mackenzie, T. B. (1979). Appearance of manic psychosis following rapid normalization of thyroid status. *American Journal of Psychiatry* **136**: 846–847. PMID 443476.
492. El-Kaissi, S., Kotowicz, M. A., Berk, M. & Wall, J. R. (2005). Acute delirium in the setting of primary hypothyroidism: the role of thyroid hormone replacement therapy. *Thyroid* **15**: 1099–1101. PMID 16187922.
493. Marshall, W. J. & Bangert, S. K. (2004). *Clinical Chemistry*. Fifth edition, London: Mosby.
494. Toft, A. D. (2001). Clinical practice. Subclinical hyperthyroidism. *New England Journal of Medicine* **345**: 512–516. PMID 11519506.
495. Wenzel, K. W., Meinhold, H., Raffenberg, M., Adlkofer, F. & Schleusener, H. (1974). Classification of hypothyroidism in evaluating patients after radioiodine therapy by serum cholesterol, T3-uptake. Total T4, FT4-index, total T3, basal TSH and TRH-test. *European Journal of Clinical Investigation* **4**: 141–148. PMID 4208979.
496. Lehrmann, J. A. & Jain, S. (2002). Myxedema psychosis with grade II hypothyroidism. *General Hospital Psychiatry* **24**: 275–277. PMID 12100840.
497. Haggerty, J. J., Jr., Evans, D. L. & Prange, A. J., Jr. (1986). Organic brain syndrome associated with marginal hypothyroidism. *American Journal of Psychiatry* **143**: 785–786. PMID 3717406.
498. Targum, S. D., Sullivan, A. C. & Byrnes, S. M. (1982). Neuroendocrine interrelationships in major depressive disorder. *American Journal of Psychiatry* **139**: 282–286. PMID 6800269.
499. Kusalic, M. (1992). Grade II and grade III hypothyroidism in rapid-cycling bipolar patients. *Neuropsychobiology* **25**: 177–181. PMID 1454157.
500. Gyulai, L., Bauer, M., Bauer, M. S., Garcia-Espana, F., Cnaan, A. & Whybrow, P. C. (2003). Thyroid hypofunction in patients with rapid-cycling bipolar disorder after lithium challenge. *Biological Psychiatry* **53**: 899–905. PMID 12742677.
501. Oomen, H. A., Schipperijn, A. J. & Drexhage, H. A. (1996). The prevalence of affective disorder and in particular of a rapid cycling of bipolar disorder in patients with abnormal thyroid function tests. *Clinical Endocrinology* **45**: 215–223. PMID 8881455.
502. Cooper, D. S. (2001). Clinical practice. Subclinical hypothyroidism. *New England Journal of Medicine* **345**: 260–265. PMID 11474665.
503. Cooper, D. S. (2004). Subclinical thyroid disease: consensus or conundrum? *Clinical Endocrinology* **60**: 410–412. PMID 15049953.
504. Surks, M. I., Ortiz, E., Daniels, G. H., Sawin, C. T., Col, N. F., Cobin, R. H., Franklyn, J. A., Hershman, J. M., Burman, K. D., Denke, M. A., Gorman, C., Cooper, R. S. & Weissman, N. J. (2004). Subclinical thyroid disease: scientific review and guidelines for diagnosis and management. *Journal of the American Medical Association* **291**: 228–238. PMID 14722150.
505. Shrier, D. K. & Burman, K. D. (2002). Subclinical hyperthyroidism: controversies in management. *American Family Physician* **65**: 431–438. PMID 11858626.
506. Adler, G. & Dipp, S. L. (2006). Cushing syndrome. eMedicine. URL: http://www.emedicine.com/med/topic485.htm. Accessed 6 January 2008.
507. Smith, C. K., Barish, J., Correa, J. & Williams, R. H. (1972). Psychiatric disturbance in endocrinologic disease. *Psychosomatic Medicine* **34**: 69–86. PMID 4335737.
508. Odeke, S. & Nagelberg, S. B. (2006). Addison disease. eMedicine. URL: http://www.emedicine.com/med/topic42.htm. Accessed 6 January 2008.
509. Laureti, S., Aubourg, P., Calcinaro, F., Rocchiccioli, F., Casucci, G., Angeletti, G., Brunetti, P., Lernmark,

A., Santeusanio, F. & Falorni, A. (1998). Etiological diagnosis of primary adrenal insufficiency using an original flowchart of immune and biochemical markers. *Journal of Clinical Endocrinology and Metabolism* **83**: 3163–3168. PMID 9745420.

510. Anglin, R. E., Rosebush, P. I. & Mazurek, M. F. (2006). The neuropsychiatric profile of Addison's disease: revisiting a forgotten phenomenon. *Journal of Neuropsychiatry and Clinical Neurosciences* **18**: 450–459. PMID 17135373.
511. Mills, L. S. (2008). Hypopituitarism. eMedicine. URL: http://emedicine.medscape.com/article/767828-overview. Accessed 5 March 2010.
512. Jacobs, J. K. & Merritt, C. R., 2nd (1966). Magnesium deficiency in hyperparathyroidism: case report of toxic psychosis. *Annals of Surgery* **163**: 260–262. PMID 5906615.
513. Velasco, P. J., Manshadi, M., Breen, K. & Lippmann, S. (1999). Psychiatric aspects of parathyroid disease. *Psychosomatics* **40**: 486–490. PMID 10581976.
514. Watson, L. C. & Marx, C. E. (2002). New onset of neuropsychiatric symptoms in the elderly: possible primary hyperparathyroidism. *Psychosomatics* **43**: 413–417. PMID 12297611.
515. Denko, J. D. & Kaelbling, R. (1962). The psychiatric aspects of hypoparathyroidism. *Acta Psychiatrica Scandinavica. Supplementum* **38**: 1–70. PMID 14027013.
516. Seeman, M. V. (1997). Psychopathology in women and men: focus on female hormones. *American Journal of Psychiatry* **154**: 1641–1647. PMID 9396940.
517. Riecher-Rossler, A., Hafner, H., Stumbaum, M., Maurer, K. & Schmidt, R. (1994). Can estradiol modulate schizophrenic symptomatology? *Schizophrenia Bulletin* **20**: 203–214. PMID 8197416.
518. Hafner, H., Behrens, S., De Vry, J. & Gattaz, W. F. (1991). Oestradiol enhances the vulnerability threshold for schizophrenia in women by an early effect on dopaminergic neurotransmission. Evidence from an epidemiological study and from animal experiments. *European Archives of Psychiatry and Clinical Neuroscience* **241**: 65–68. PMID 1653619.
519. Riecher-Rossler, A., Hafner, H., Dutsch-Strobel, A., Oster, M., Stumbaum, M., van Gulick-Bailer, M. & Loffler, W. (1994). Further evidence for a specific role of estradiol in schizophrenia? *Biological Psychiatry* **36**: 492–494. PMID 7811850.
520. Hafner, H., Behrens, S., De Vry, J. & Gattaz, W. F. (1991). An animal model for the effects of estradiol on dopamine-mediated behavior: implications for sex differences in schizophrenia. *Psychiatry Research* **38**: 125–134. PMID 1754627.
521. Riecher-Rossler, A. & Hafner, H. (1993). Schizophrenia and oestrogens – is there an association? *European Archives of Psychiatry and Clinical Neuroscience* **242**: 323–328. PMID 8323981.
522. Harrison, P. J. & Tunbridge, E. M. (2008). Catechol-O-methyltransferase (COMT): a gene contributing to sex differences in brain function, and to sexual dimorphism in the predisposition to psychiatric disorders. *Neuropsychopharmacology* **33**: 3037–3045. PMID 17805313.
523. Huber, T. J., Rollnik, J., Wilhelms, J., von zur Muhlen, A., Emrich, H. M. & Schneider, U. (2001). Estradiol levels in psychotic disorders. *Psychoneuroendocrinology* **26**: 27–35. PMID 11070332.
524. Hafner, H., an der Heiden, W., Behrens, S., Gattaz, W. F., Hambrecht, M., Loffler, W., Maurer, K., Munk-Jorgensen, P., Nowotny, B., Riecher-Rossler, A. & Stein, A. (1998). Causes and consequences of the gender difference in age at onset of schizophrenia. *Schizophrenia Bulletin* **24**: 99–113. PMID 9502549.
525. Huber, T. J., Borsutzky, M., Schneider, U. & Emrich, H. M. (2004). Psychotic disorders and gonadal function: evidence supporting the oestrogen hypothesis. *Acta Psychiatrica Scandinavica* **109**: 269–274. PMID 15008800.
526. Oades, R. D. & Schepker, R. (1994). Serum gonadal steroid hormones in young schizophrenic patients.

Psychoneuroendocrinology **19**: 373–385. PMID 8047641.
527. Gattaz, W. F., Vogel, P., Riecher-Rossler, A. & Soddu, G. (1994). Influence of the menstrual cycle phase on the therapeutic response in schizophrenia. *Biological Psychiatry* **36**: 137–139. PMID 7948447.
528. Huber, T. J., Tettenborn, C., Leifke, E. & Emrich, H. M. (2005). Sex hormones in psychotic men. *Psychoneuroendocrinology* **30**: 111–114. PMID 15358449.
529. Howes, O. D., Wheeler, M. J., Pilowsky, L. S., Landau, S., Murray, R. M. & Smith, S. (2007). Sexual function and gonadal hormones in patients taking antipsychotic treatment for schizophrenia or schizoaffective disorder. *Journal of Clinical Psychiatry* **68**: 361–367. PMID 17388704.
530. Sharma, V. (2003). Pharmacotherapy of postpartum psychosis. *Expert Opinion on Pharmacotherapy* **4**: 1651–1658. PMID 14521476.
531. Kendell, R. E., Chalmers, J. C. & Platz, C. (1987). Epidemiology of puerperal psychoses. *British Journal of Psychiatry* **150**: 662–673. PMID 3651704.
532. Viguera, A. C., Nonacs, R., Cohen, L. S., Tondo, L., Murray, A. & Baldessarini, R. J. (2000). Risk of recurrence of bipolar disorder in pregnant and nonpregnant women after discontinuing lithium maintenance. *American Journal of Psychiatry* **157**: 179–184. PMID 10671384.
533. Viguera, A. C., Emmerich, A. D. & Cohen, L. S. (2008). Case records of the Massachusetts General Hospital. Case 24–2008. A 35-year-old woman with postpartum confusion, agitation, and delusions. *New England Journal of Medicine* **359**: 509–515. PMID 18669430.
534. Saigusa, T., Takada, K., Baker, S. C., Kumar, R. & Stephenson, J. D. (1997). Dopamine efflux in the rat nucleus accumbens evoked by dopamine receptor stimulation in the entorhinal cortex is modulated by oestradiol and progesterone. *Synapse* **25**: 37–43. PMID 8987146.
535. Wieck, A., Kumar, R., Hirst, A. D., Marks, M. N., Campbell, I. C. & Checkley, S. A. (1991). Increased sensitivity of dopamine receptors and recurrence of affective psychosis after childbirth. *British Medical Journal* **303**: 613–616. PMID 1805821.
536. Ahokas, A. & Aito, M. (1999). Role of estradiol in puerperal psychosis. *Psychopharmacology* **147**: 108–110. PMID 10591876.
537. Gentile, S. (2005). The role of estrogen therapy in postpartum psychiatric disorders: an update. *CNS Spectrums* **10**: 944–952. PMID 16344831.
538. Kumar, C., McIvor, R. J., Davies, T., Brown, N., Papadopoulos, A., Wieck, A., Checkley, S. A., Campbell, I. C. & Marks, M. N. (2003). Estrogen administration does not reduce the rate of recurrence of affective psychosis after childbirth. *Journal of Clinical Psychiatry* **64**: 112–118. PMID 12633118.
539. Mahe, V. & Dumaine, A. (2001). Oestrogen withdrawal associated psychoses. *Acta Psychiatrica Scandinavica* **104**: 323–331. PMID 11722312.
540. Brockington, I. F. (2007). Cerebral vascular disease as a cause of postpartum psychosis. *Archives of Women's Mental Health* **10**: 177–178. PMID 17541703.
541. Busby, G. & Bancroft, K. (2007). Encephalopathy and psychosis following administration of the combined oral contraceptive pill in an 11-year-old female. *Gynecological Endocrinology* **23**: 361–362. PMID 17616863.
542. Sale, I. & Kalucy, R. (1981). Psychosis associated with oral contraceptive-induced chorea. *Medical Journal of Australia* **1**: 79–80. PMID 7194963.
543. Miranda, M., Cardoso, F., Giovannoni, G. & Church, A. (2004). Oral contraceptive induced chorea: another condition associated with anti-basal ganglia antibodies. *Journal of Neurology, Neurosurgery and Psychiatry* **75**: 327–328. PMID 14742621.
544. Vessey, M. P., McPherson, K., Lawless, M. & Yeates, D. (1985). Oral contraception and serious psychiatric illness: absence of an association. *British Journal of Psychiatry* **146**: 45–49. PMID 3978343.
545. Majeed, K. I. (2007). Hyperammonemia. eMedicine. URL: http://www.emedicine.com/neuro/topic162.htm. Accessed 18 January 2008.

546. Wolf, D. C. (2007). Encephalopathy, hepatic. eMedicine. URL: http://www.emedicine.com/med/topic3185.htm. Accessed 18 January 2008.
547. Roth, K. S. (2007). Hyperammonemia. eMedicine. URL: http://www.emedicine.com/ped/topic1057.htm. Accessed 18 January 2008.
548. Lee, P. J. & Lachmann, R. H. (2008). Acute presentations of inherited metabolic disease in adulthood. *Clinical Medicine* **8**: 621–624.
549. Enns, G. M., O'Brien, W. E., Kobayashi, K., Shinzawa, H. & Pellegrino, J. E. (2005). Postpartum "psychosis" in mild argininosuccinate synthetase deficiency. *Obstetrics and Gynecology* **105**: 1244–1246. PMID 15863597.
550. Belanger-Quintana, A., Martinez-Pardo, M., Garcia, M. J., Wermuth, B., Torres, J., Pallares, E. & Ugarte, M. (2003). Hyperammonaemia as a cause of psychosis in an adolescent. *European Journal of Pediatrics* **162**: 773–775. PMID 12942317.
551. Peterson, D. E. (2003). Acute postpartum mental status change and coma caused by previously undiagnosed ornithine transcarbamylase deficiency. *Obstetrics and Gynecology* **102**: 1212–1215. PMID 14607061.
552. Carr, R. B. & Shrewsbury, K. (2007). Hyperammonemia due to valproic acid in the psychiatric setting. *American Journal of Psychiatry* **164**: 1020–1027. PMID 17606652.
553. Yanai, S., Minami, T., Sonoda, K., Gondo, K., Tasaki, K., Hijii, T., Fukushige, J., Ueda, K., Hirata, T., Hayashi, T. & Hasuo, K. (1995). Patent ductus venosus associated with a hyperintense globus pallidum on T1-weighted magnetic resonance imaging and pulmonary hypertension. *European Journal of Pediatrics* **154**: 526–529. PMID 7556316.
554. Croarkin, P. (2002). From King George to neuroglobin: the psychiatric aspects of acute intermittent porphyria. *Journal of Psychiatric Practice* **8**: 398–405. PMID 15985908.
555. Gonzalez-Arriaza, H. L. & Bostwick, J. M. (2003). Acute porphyrias: a case report and review. *American Journal of Psychiatry* **160**: 450–459. PMID 12611823.
556. Mustajoki, P., Kauppinen, R., Lannfelt, L., Lilius, L. & Koistinen, J. (1992). Frequency of low erythrocyte porphobilinogen deaminase activity in Finland. *Journal of Internal Medicine* **231**: 389–395. PMID 1588264.
557. Gibney, G. N., Jones, I. H. & Meek, J. H. (1972). Schizophrenia in association with erythropoietic protoporphyria – report of a case. *British Journal of Psychiatry* **121**: 79–81. PMID 5047175.
558. Crimlisk, H. L. (1997). The little imitator – porphyria: a neuropsychiatric disorder. *Journal of Neurology, Neurosurgery and Psychiatry* **62**: 319–328. PMID 9120442.
559. Bonkovsky, H. L., Siao, P., Roig, Z., Hedley-Whyte, E. T. & Flotte, T. J. (2008). Case records of the Massachusetts General Hospital. Case 20-2008. A 57-year-old woman with abdominal pain and weakness after gastric bypass surgery. *New England Journal of Medicine* **358**: 2813–2825. PMID 18579817.
560. Burgovne, K., Swartz, R. & Ananth, J. (1995). Porphyria: reexamination of psychiatric implications. *Psychotherapy and Psychosomatics* **64**: 121–130. PMID 8657842.
561. Roth, K. S. (2007). Tyrosinemia. eMedicine. URL: http://www.emedicine.com/ped/topic2339.htm. Accessed 17 February 2008.
562. Mitchell, G., Larochelle, J., Lambert, M., Michaud, J., Grenier, A., Ogier, H., Gauthier, M., Lacroix, J., Vanasse, M., Larbrisseau, A., Paradis, K., Weber, A., Lefevre, Y., Melançon, S. & Dallaire, L. (1990). Neurologic crises in hereditary tyrosinemia. *New England Journal of Medicine* **322**: 432–437. PMID 2153931.
563. Sniderman King, L., Trahms, C. & Scott, C. R. (2006). Tyrosinemia type 1. GeneReviews (National Center for Biotechnology Information). URL: http://www.ncbi.nlm.nih.gov/books/bv.fcgi?rid=gene.chapter.tyrosinemia. Accessed 17 February 2008.
564. Finkelstein, J. D. & Gahl, W. A. (1990). Heritable diseases of amino acid

metabolism. In *Principles and Practice of Endocrinology and Metabolism* (Becker, K. L., Bilezikian, J. P., Bremner, W. J., Hung, W., Kahn, C. R., Loriaux, D. L., Rebar, R. W., Robertson, G. L. & Wartofsky, L., Eds.), pp. 1422–1430. Philadelphia, PA: Lippincott.

565. Baloghova, J. & Schwartz, R. A. (2006). Homocystinuria. eMedicine. URL: http://www.emedicine.com/derm/topic708.htm. Accessed 17 February 2008.

566. Selhub, J. (1999). Homocysteine metabolism. *Annual Review of Nutrition* **19**: 217–246. PMID 10448523.

567. Leclerc, D. & Rozen, R. (2007). [Molecular genetics of MTHFR: polymorphisms are not all benign]. *Médecine Sciences (Paris)* **23**: 297–302. PMID 17349292.

568. Gilbody, S., Lewis, S. & Lightfoot, T. (2007). Methylenetetrahydrofolate reductase (MTHFR) genetic polymorphisms and psychiatric disorders: a HuGE review. *American Journal of Epidemiology* **165**: 1–13. PMID 17074966.

569. Muntjewerff, J. W., Kahn, R. S., Blom, H. J. & den Heijer, M. (2006). Homocysteine, methylenetetrahydrofolate reductase and risk of schizophrenia: a meta-analysis. *Molecular Psychiatry* **11**: 143–149. PMID 16172608.

570. Lewis, S. J., Zammit, S., Gunnell, D. & Smith, G. D. (2005). A meta-analysis of the MTHFR C677T polymorphism and schizophrenia risk. *American Journal of Medical Genetics. Part B, Neuropsychiatric Genetics* **135**: 2–4. PMID 15729744.

571. Kempisty, B., Bober, A., Luczak, M., Czerski, P., Szczepankiewicz, A., Hauser, J. & Jagodzinski, P. P. (2007). Distribution of 1298A>C polymorphism of methylenetetrahydrofolate reductase gene in patients with bipolar disorder and schizophrenia. *European Psychiatry* **22**: 39–43. PMID 17188847.

572. Freeman, J. M., Finkelstein, J. D. & Mudd, S. H. (1975). Folate-responsive homocystinuria and "schizophrenia". A defect in methylation due to deficient 5,10-methylenetetrahydrofolate reductase activity. *New England Journal of Medicine* **292**: 491–496. PMID 1117892.

573. Regland, B., Johansson, B. V. & Gottfries, C. G. (1994). Homocysteinemia and schizophrenia as a case of methylation deficiency. *Journal of Neural Transmission. General Section* **98**: 143–152. PMID 7734111.

574. Roffman, J. L., Weiss, A. P., Deckersbach, T., Freudenreich, O., Henderson, D. C., Purcell, S., Wong, D. H., Halsted, C. H. & Goff, D. C. (2007). Effects of the methylenetetrahydrofolate reductase (MTHFR) C677T polymorphism on executive function in schizophrenia. *Schizophrenia Research* **92**: 181–188. PMID 17344026.

575. Roffman, J. L., Weiss, A. P., Deckersbach, T., Freudenreich, O., Henderson, D. C., Wong, D. H., Halsted, C. H. & Goff, D. C. (2008). Interactive effects of COMT Val108/158Met and MTHFR C677T on executive function in schizophrenia. *American Journal of Medical Genetics. Part B, Neuropsychiatric Genetics* **147**: 990–995. PMID 18186041.

576. Muntjewerff, J. W., van der Put, N., Eskes, T., Ellenbroek, B., Steegers, E., Blom, H. & Zitman, F. (2003). Homocysteine metabolism and B-vitamins in schizophrenic patients: low plasma folate as a possible independent risk factor for schizophrenia. *Psychiatry Research* **121**: 1–9. PMID 14572619.

577. Wyatt, R. J., Termini, B. A. & Davis, J. (1971). Biochemical and sleep studies of schizophrenia: a review of the literature – 1960–1970. Part 1. Biochemical studies. *Schizophrenia Bulletin* **4**: 10–44.

578. Sekulovic, L. K., Karadaglic, D. & Stojanov, L. (2006). Hartnup disease. eMedicine. URL: http://www.emedicine.com/derm/topic713.htm. Accessed 4 March 2008.

579. Kleta, R., Romeo, E., Ristic, Z., Ohura, T., Stuart, C., Arcos-Burgos, M., Dave, M. H., Wagner, C. A., Camargo, S. R., Inoue, S., Matsuura, N., Helip-Wooley, A., Bockenhauer, D., Warth, R., Bernardini, I., Visser, G., Eggermann, T., Lee, P., Chairoungdua, A., Jutabha, P., Babu, E., Nilwarangkoon, S., Anzai, N., Kanai, Y., Verrey, F., Gahl, W. A. & Koizumi, A. (2004). Mutations in SLC6A19, encoding B0AT1, cause Hartnup disorder. *Nature Genetics* **36**: 999–1002. PMID 15286787.

580. Bodamer, O. A. & Lee, B. (2008). Maple syrup urine disease. eMedicine. URL: http://emedicine.medscape.com/article/946234-overview. Accessed 30 April 2010.
581. Holmgren, G., Brundin, A., Gustavson, K. H., Sjogren, S., Kleijer, W. J. & Niermeijer, M. F. (1980). Intermittent neurological symptoms in a girl with a maple syrup urine disease (MSUD) variant. *Neuropediatrics* **11**: 377–383. PMID 7207707.
582. Dening, T. R. & Berrios, G. E. (1989). Wilson's disease: a prospective study of psychopathology in 31 cases. *British Journal of Psychiatry* **155**: 206–213. PMID 2597916.
583. Kumawat, B. L., Sharma, C. M., Tripathi, G., Ralot, T. & Dixit, S. (2007). Wilson's disease presenting as isolated obsessive-compulsive disorder. *Indian Journal of Medical Sciences* **61**: 607–610. PMID 18025747.
584. Akil, M. & Brewer, G. J. (1995). Psychiatric and behavioral abnormalities in Wilson's disease. *Advances in Neurology* **65**: 171–178. PMID 7872138.
585. Rathbun, J. K. (1996). Neuropsychological aspects of Wilson's disease. *International Journal of Neuroscience* **85**: 221–229. PMID 8734560.
586. McDonald, L. V. & Lake, C. R. (1995). Psychosis in an adolescent patient with Wilson's disease: effects of chelation therapy. *Psychosomatic Medicine* **57**: 202–204. PMID 7792379.
587. Dening, T. R. & Berrios, G. E. (1989). Wilson's disease. Psychiatric symptoms in 195 cases. *Archives of General Psychiatry* **46**: 1126–1134. PMID 2589927.
588. Taly, A. B., Meenakshi-Sundaram, S., Sinha, S., Swamy, H. S. & Arunodaya, G. R. (2007). Wilson disease: description of 282 patients evaluated over 3 decades. *Medicine* **86**: 112–121. PMID 17435591.
589. Sullivan, C. A., Chopdar, A. & Shun-Shin, G. A. (2002). Dense Kayser–Fleischer ring in asymptomatic Wilson's disease (hepatolenticular degeneration). *British Journal of Ophthalmology* **86**: 114. PMID 11801516.
590. Josephson, S. A., Schmidt, R. E., Millsap, P., McManus, D. Q. & Morris, J. C. (2001). Autosomal dominant Kufs' disease: a cause of early onset dementia. *Journal of the Neurological Sciences* **188**: 51–60. PMID 11489285.
591. Meikle, P. J., Hopwood, J. J., Clague, A. E. & Carey, W. F. (1999). Prevalence of lysosomal storage disorders. *JAMA* **281**: 249–254. PMID 9918480.
592. Shen, Y. C., Haw-Ming, L., Lin, C. C. & Chen, C. H. (2007). Psychosis in a patient with Fabry's disease and treatment with aripiprazole. *Progress in Neuro-Psychopharmacology and Biological Psychiatry* **31**: 779–780. PMID 17188413.
593. Vargas-Diez, E., Chabas, A., Coll, M. J., Sanchez-Perez, J., Garcia-Diez, A. & Fernandez-Herrera, J. M. (2002). Angiokeratoma corporis diffusum in a Spanish patient with aspartylglucosaminuria. *British Journal of Dermatology* **147**: 760–764. PMID 12366426.
594. Black, D. N., Taber, K. H. & Hurley, R. A. (2003). Metachromatic leukodystrophy: a model for the study of psychosis. *Journal of Neuropsychiatry and Clinical Neurosciences* **15**: 289–293. PMID 12928504.
595. Hyde, T. M., Ziegler, J. C. & Weinberger, D. R. (1992). Psychiatric disturbances in metachromatic leukodystrophy. Insights into the neurobiology of psychosis. *Archives of Neurology* **49**: 401–406. PMID 1532712.
596. Propping, P., Friedl, W., Huschka, M., Schlor, K. H., Reimer, F., Lee-Vaupel, M., Conzelmann, E. & Sandhoff, K. (1986). The influence of low arylsulfatase A activity on neuropsychiatric morbidity: a large-scale screening in patients. *Human Genetics* **74**: 244–248. PMID 2877931.
597. Moore, T. & Steiner, R. D. (2006). Metachromatic leukodystrophy. eMedicine. URL: http://www.emedicine.com/ped/topic2893.htm. Accessed 29 December 2007.
598. Rosebush, P. I., Garside, S., Levinson, A. J. & Mazurek, M. F. (1999). The neuropsychiatry of adult-onset adrenoleukodystrophy. *Journal of Neuropsychiatry and Clinical Neurosciences* **11**: 315–327. PMID 10440007.

599. Chedrawi, A. & Clark, G. D. (2007). Peroxisomal disorders. eMedicine. URL: http://www.emedicine.com/neuro/topic309.htm. Accessed 29 February 2008.
600. Berginer, V. M., Foster, N. L., Sadowsky, M., Townsend, J. A., 3rd, Siegel, G. J. & Salen, G. (1988). Psychiatric disorders in patients with cerebrotendinous xanthomatosis. *American Journal of Psychiatry* **145**: 354–357. PMID 3344851.
601. Malm, D., Pantel, J. & Linaker, O. M. (2005). Psychiatric symptoms in alpha-mannosidosis. *Journal of Intellectual Disability Research* **49**: 865–871. PMID 16207285.
602. Seidl, U., Giesel, F. L., Cantz, M., Schmidbauer, M., Schroder, J. & Pantel, J. (2005). [Unusual course of alpha-mannosidosis with symptoms of paranoid-hallucinatory psychosis]. *Nervenarzt* **76**: 335–338. PMID 15759164.
603. Wenger, D. A. (2008). Krabbe disease. GeneReviews (National Center for Biotechnology Information). URL: http://www.ncbi.nlm.nih.gov/bookshelf/br.fcgi?book=gene&part=krabbe. Accessed 2 September 2009.
604. Kolodny, E. H., Raghavan, S. & Krivit, W. (1991). Late-onset Krabbe disease (globoid cell leukodystrophy): clinical and biochemical features of 15 cases. *Developmental Neuroscience* **13**: 232–239. PMID 1817026.
605. Hagberg, B. (1984). Krabbe's disease: clinical presentation of neurological variants. *Neuropediatrics* **15 Suppl**: 11–15. PMID 6546163.
606. Fluharty, A. L., Neidengard, L., Holtzman, D. & Kihara, H. (1986). Late-onset Krabbe disease initially diagnosed as cerebroside sulfatase activator deficiency. *Metabolic Brain Disease* **1**: 187–195. PMID 2907603.
607. Cox, T. M. (2001). Gaucher disease: understanding the molecular pathogenesis of sphingolipidoses. *Journal of Inherited Metabolic Disease* **24 Suppl 2**: 106–121; discussion 187–108. PMID 11758671.
608. Pastores, G. M. (2008). Gaucher disease. GeneReviews (National Center for Biotechnology Information). URL: http://www.ncbi.nlm.nih.gov/bookshelf/br.fcgi?book=gene&part=gaucher. Accessed 2 September 2009.
609. Guimaraes, J., Amaral, O. & Sa Miranda, M. C. (2003). Adult-onset neuronopathic form of Gaucher's disease: a case report. *Parkinsonism and Related Disorders* **9**: 261–264. PMID 12781591.
610. Neil, J. F., Glew, R. H. & Peters, S. P. (1979). Familial psychosis and diverse neurologic abnormalities in adult-onset Gaucher's disease. *Archives of Neurology* **36**: 95–99. PMID 420629.
611. Ohtake, H., Shimohata, T., Terajima, K., Kimura, T., Jo, R., Kaseda, R., Iizuka, O., Takano, M., Akaiwa, Y., Goto, H., Kobayashi, H., Sugai, T., Muratake, T., Hosoki, T., Shioiri, T., Okamoto, K., Onodera, O., Tanaka, K., Someya, T., Nakada, T. & Tsuji, S. (2004). Adult-onset leukoencephalopathy with vanishing white matter with a missense mutation in EIF2B5. *Neurology* **62**: 1601–1603. PMID 15136690.
612. Denier, C., Orgibet, A., Roffi, F., Jouvent, E., Buhl, C., Niel, F., Boespflug-Tanguy, O., Said, G. & Ducreux, D. (2007). Adult-onset vanishing white matter leukoencephalopathy presenting as psychosis. *Neurology* **68**: 1538–1539. PMID 17470759.
613. Rust, R. S. (2008). Diffuse sclerosis. eMedicine. URL: http://emedicine.medscape.com/article/1145927-overview. Accessed 3 April 2009.
614. Martin, J. J. & Guazzi, G. C. (1991). Schilder's diffuse sclerosis. *Developmental Neuroscience* **13**: 267–273. PMID 1817032.
615. Kirkman, M. A., Yu-Wai-Man, P. & Chinnery, P. F. (2008). The clinical spectrum of mitochondrial genetic disorders. *Clinical Medicine* **8**: 601–606. PMID 19149282.
616. Hammans, S. R. (2008). Mitochondrial disease: old and new. *Advances in Clinical Neuroscience and Rehabilitation* **7**: 12–16.
617. Kiejna, A., DiMauro, S., Adamowski, T., Rymaszewska, J., Leszek, J. & Pachalska, M. (2002). Psychiatric symptoms in a patient with the clinical features of MELAS. *Medical Science Monitor* **8**: CS66–72. PMID 12118207.

618. Sartor, H., Loose, R., Tucha, O., Klein, H. E. & Lange, K. W. (2002). MELAS: a neuropsychological and radiological follow-up study. Mitochondrial encephalomyopathy, lactic acidosis and stroke. *Acta Neurologica Scandinavica* **106**: 309–313. PMID 12371926.
619. Suzuki, T., Koizumi, J., Shiraishi, H., Ishikawa, N., Ofuku, K., Sasaki, M., Hori, T., Ohkoshi, N. & Anno, I. (1990). Mitochondrial encephalomyopathy (MELAS) with mental disorder. CT, MRI and SPECT findings. *Neuroradiology* **32**: 74–76. PMID 2333139.
620. Thomeer, E. C., Verhoeven, W. M., van de Vlasakker, C. J. & Klompenhouwer, J. L. (1998). Psychiatric symptoms in MELAS; a case report. *Journal of Neurology, Neurosurgery and Psychiatry* **64**: 692–693. PMID 9598702.
621. Carter, S. M. & Gross, S. J. (2008). Glucose-6-phosphate dehydrogenase deficiency. eMedicine. URL: http://emedicine.medscape.com/article/200390-overview. Accessed 8 November 2009.
622. Bocchetta, A. (2003). Psychotic mania in glucose-6-phosphate-dehydrogenase-deficient subjects. *Annals of General Hospital Psychiatry* **2**: 6. PMID 12844366.
623. Nguyen-Khoa, D.-T., Cope, D. W., Busschots, G. V. & Vallee, P. A. (2006). Beriberi (thiamine deficiency). eMedicine. URL: http://www.emedicine.com/med/topic221.htm. Accessed 18 January 2008.
624. Donnino, M. W., Vega, J., Miller, J. & Walsh, M. (2007). Myths and misconceptions of Wernicke's encephalopathy: what every emergency physician should know. *Annals of Emergency Medicine* **50**: 715–721. PMID 17681641.
625. Cook, C. C., Hallwood, P. M. & Thomson, A. D. (1998). B Vitamin deficiency and neuropsychiatric syndromes in alcohol misuse. *Alcohol and Alcoholism* **33**: 317–336. PMID 9719389.
626. Sivolap, Y. P. (2005). The current state of S. S. Korsakov's concept of alcoholic polyneuritic psychosis. *Neuroscience and Behavioral Physiology* **35**: 977–982. PMID 16270181.
627. Thomson, A. D. & Marshall, E. J. (2006). The natural history and pathophysiology of Wernicke's Encephalopathy and Korsakoff's Psychosis. *Alcohol and Alcoholism* **41**: 151–158. PMID 16384871.
628. Agabio, R. (2005). Thiamine administration in alcohol-dependent patients. *Alcohol and Alcoholism* **40**: 155–156. PMID 15550446.
629. Rajakumar, K. (2006). Pellagra. eMedicine. URL: http://www.emedicine.com/ped/topic1755.htm. Accessed 18 January 2008.
630. Frye, R. E. & Jabbour, S. A. (2008). Pyridoxine deficiency. eMedicine. URL: http://emedicine.medscape.com/article/124947-overview. Accessed 29 October 2009.
631. Alao, A. O. & Yolles, J. C. (1998). Isoniazid-induced psychosis. *Annals of Pharmacotherapy* **32**: 889–891. PMID 9762376.
632. Ryan, M. M., Sidhu, R. K., Alexander, J. & Megerian, J. T. (2002). Homocystinuria presenting as psychosis in an adolescent. *Journal of Child Neurology* **17**: 859–860. PMID 12585732.
633. Sandyk, R. & Pardeshi, R. (1990). Pyridoxine improves drug-induced parkinsonism and psychosis in a schizophrenic patient. *International Journal of Neuroscience* **52**: 225–232. PMID 2269609.
634. Lerner, V., Miodownik, C., Kaptsan, A., Cohen, H., Matar, M., Loewenthal, U. & Kotler, M. (2001). Vitamin B(6) in the treatment of tardive dyskinesia: a double-blind, placebo-controlled, crossover study. *American Journal of Psychiatry* **158**: 1511–1514. PMID 11532741.
635. Lerner, V., Miodownik, C., Kaptsan, A., Cohen, H., Loewenthal, U. & Kotler, M. (2002). Vitamin B6 as add-on treatment in chronic schizophrenic and schizoaffective patients: a double-blind, placebo-controlled study. *Journal of Clinical Psychiatry* **63**: 54–58. PMID 11838627.
636. Singh, N. N., Thomas, F. P., Diamond, A. L. & Diamond, R. (2006). Vitamin B-12 associated neurological diseases. eMedicine. URL: http://www.emedicine.com/neuro/topic439.htm. Accessed 18 January 2008.

637. Andres, E., Federici, L., Affenberger, S., Vidal-Alaball, J., Loukili, N. H., Zimmer, J. & Kaltenbach, G. (2007). B12 deficiency: a look beyond pernicious anemia. *Journal of Family Practice* **56**: 537–542. PMID 17605945.
638. de Jager, J., Kooy, A., Lehert, P., Wulffele, M. G., van der Kolk, J., Bets, D., Verburg, J., Donker, A. J. & Stehouwer, C. D. (2010). Long term treatment with metformin in patients with type 2 diabetes and risk of vitamin B-12 deficiency: randomised placebo controlled trial. *British Medical Journal* **340**: c2181. PMID 20488910.
639. Sethi, N. K., Mullin, P., Torgovnick, J. & Capasso, G. (2006). Nitrous oxide "whippit" abuse presenting with cobalamin responsive psychosis. *Journal of Medical Toxicology* **2**: 71–74. PMID 18072118.
640. Healton, E. B., Savage, D. G., Brust, J. C., Garrett, T. J. & Lindenbaum, J. (1991). Neurologic aspects of cobalamin deficiency. *Medicine* **70**: 229–245. PMID 1648656.
641. Andres, E., Vidal-Alaball, J., Federici, L., Loukili, N. H., Zimmer, J. & Kaltenbach, G. (2007). Clinical aspects of cobalamin deficiency in elderly patients. Epidemiology, causes, clinical manifestations, and treatment with special focus on oral cobalamin therapy. *European Journal of Internal Medicine* **18**: 456–462. PMID 17822656.
642. Lindenbaum, J., Healton, E. B., Savage, D. G., Brust, J. C., Garrett, T. J., Podell, E. R., Marcell, P. D., Stabler, S. P. & Allen, R. H. (1988). Neuropsychiatric disorders caused by cobalamin deficiency in the absence of anemia or macrocytosis. *New England Journal of Medicine* **318**: 1720–1728. PMID 3374544.
643. Devalia, V. (2006). Diagnosing vitamin B-12 deficiency on the basis of serum B-12 assay. *British Medical Journal* **333**: 385–386. PMID 16916826.
644. Snow, C. F. (1999). Laboratory diagnosis of vitamin B12 and folate deficiency: a guide for the primary care physician. *Archives of Internal Medicine* **159**: 1289–1298. PMID 10386505.
645. Roze, E., Gervais, D., Demeret, S., Ogier de Baulny, H., Zittoun, J., Benoist, J. F., Said, G., Pierrot-Deseilligny, C. & Bolgert, F. (2003). Neuropsychiatric disturbances in presumed late-onset cobalamin C disease. *Archives of Neurology* **60**: 1457–1462. PMID 14568819.
646. Herbert, V. (1964). Studies of folate deficiency in man. *Proceedings of the Royal Society of Medicine* **57**: 377–384. PMID 14168843.
647. Gentili, A., Vohra, M., Vij, S., Chen, D. K.-H. & Siddiqi, W. (2009). Folic acid deficiency. eMedicine. URL: http://emedicine.medscape.com/article/200184-overview. Accessed 21 July 2010.
648. Herbert, V. (1973). The five possible causes of all nutrient deficiency: illustrated by deficiencies of vitamin B12 and folic acid. *American Journal of Clinical Nutrition* **26**: 77–86. PMID 4577371.
649. Hutto, B. R. (1997). Folate and cobalamin in psychiatric illness. *Comprehensive Psychiatry* **38**: 305–314. PMID 9406735.
650. Godfrey, P. S., Toone, B. K., Carney, M. W., Flynn, T. G., Bottiglieri, T., Laundy, M., Chanarin, I. & Reynolds, E. H. (1990). Enhancement of recovery from psychiatric illness by methylfolate. *Lancet* **336**: 392–395. PMID 1974941.
651. Levine, J., Stahl, Z., Sela, B. A., Ruderman, V., Shumaico, O., Babushkin, I., Osher, Y., Bersudsky, Y. & Belmaker, R. H. (2006). Homocysteine-reducing strategies improve symptoms in chronic schizophrenic patients with hyperhomocysteinemia. *Biological Psychiatry* **60**: 265–269. PMID 16412989.
652. Galloway, M. & Rushworth, L. (2003). Red cell or serum folate? Results from the National Pathology Alliance benchmarking review. *Journal of Clinical Pathology* **56**: 924–926. PMID 14645351.
653. British Medical Association & Royal Pharmaceutical Society of Great Britain (2008). *British National Formulary (BNF) 55 [March 2008]*. London: BMJ Publishing Group Ltd & RPS Publishing.
654. Ramaekers, V. T. & Blau, N. (2004). Cerebral folate deficiency. *Developmental Medicine and Child Neurology* **46**: 843–851. PMID 15581159.
655. Ramaekers, V. T., Rothenberg, S. P., Sequeira, J. M., Opladen, T., Blau, N.,

Quadros, E. V. & Selhub, J. (2005). Autoantibodies to folate receptors in the cerebral folate deficiency syndrome. *New England Journal of Medicine* **352**: 1985–1991. PMID 15888699.
656. Ho, A., Michelson, D., Aaen, G. & Ashwal, S. (2010). Cerebral folate deficiency presenting as adolescent catatonic schizophrenia: a case report. *Journal of Child Neurology* **25**: 898–900. PMID 20445197.
657. Henkin, R. I., Patten, B. M., Re, P. K. & Bronzert, D. A. (1975). A syndrome of acute zinc loss. Cerebellar dysfunction, mental changes, anorexia, and taste and smell dysfunction. *Archives of Neurology* **32**: 745–751. PMID 1180744.
658. Strassnig, M., Singh Brar, J. & Ganguli, R. (2005). Dietary fatty acid and antioxidant intake in community-dwelling patients suffering from schizophrenia. *Schizophrenia Research* **76**: 343–351. PMID 15949667.
659. Fenton, W. S., Hibbeln, J. & Knable, M. (2000). Essential fatty acids, lipid membrane abnormalities, and the diagnosis and treatment of schizophrenia. *Biological Psychiatry* **47**: 8–21. PMID 10650444.
660. Peet, M., Brind, J., Ramchand, C. N., Shah, S. & Vankar, G. K. (2001). Two double-blind placebo-controlled pilot studies of eicosapentaenoic acid in the treatment of schizophrenia. *Schizophrenia Research* **49**: 243–251. PMID 11356585.
661. Berger, G. E., Proffitt, T. M., McConchie, M., Yuen, H., Wood, S. J., Amminger, G. P., Brewer, W. & McGorry, P. D. (2007). Ethyl-eicosapentaenoic acid in first-episode psychosis: a randomized, placebo-controlled trial. *Journal of Clinical Psychiatry* **68**: 1867–1875. PMID 18162017.
662. Meerloo, J. A. & Klauber, L. D. (1952). Clinical significance of starvation and oral deprivation. *Psychosomatic Medicine* **14**: 491–497. PMID 13014226.
663. Kopala, L. C., Good, K. P. & Honer, W. G. (1994). Olfactory hallucinations and olfactory identification ability in patients with schizophrenia and other psychiatric disorders. *Schizophrenia Research* **12**: 205–211. PMID 8054312.
664. Mavrogiorgou, P., Juckel, G. & Bauer, M. (2001). [Recurrence of paranoid hallucinatory psychoses after beginning a fasting period in a patient with anorexia nervosa]. *Fortschritte der Neurologie-Psychiatrie* **69**: 211–214. PMID 11417260.
665. Grounds, A. (1982). Transient psychoses in anorexia nervosa: a report of 7 cases. *Psychological Medicine* **12**: 107–113. PMID 7079419.
666. Lempert, T., Bauer, M. & Schmidt, D. (1994). Syncope: a videometric analysis of 56 episodes of transient cerebral hypoxia. *Annals of Neurology* **36**: 233–237. PMID 8053660.
667. Brugger, P., Regard, M., Landis, T. & Oelz, O. (1999). Hallucinatory experiences in extreme-altitude climbers. *Neuropsychiatry, Neuropsychology, and Behavioral Neurology* **12**: 67–71. PMID 10082335.
668. Howard, J. S., 3rd (1993). The psychosis of metabolic alkalosis. *Integrative Physiological and Behavioral Science* **28**: 353–357. PMID 8117580.
669. Weatherall, D. J., Ledingham, J. G. G. & Warrell, D. A., Eds. (1996). *Oxford Textbook of Medicine*. Third edition. Oxford: Oxford University Press.
670. Quinn, A. & Sinert, R. H. (2009). Metabolic acidosis. eMedicine. URL: http://emedicine.medscape.com/article/768268-overview. Accessed 30 April 2010.
671. Nicks, B. A., McGinnis, H. D., Borron, S. W. & Mégarbane, B. (2010). Lactic acidosis. URL: http://emedicine.medscape.com/article/768159-overview. Accessed 30 April 2010.
672. Brady, W. J., Jr. & Duncan, C. W. (1999). Hypoglycemia masquerading as acute psychosis and acute cocaine intoxication. *American Journal of Emergency Medicine* **17**: 318–319. PMID 10337905.
673. Longmore, M., Wilkinson, I. B. & Rajagopalan, S. (2004). *Oxford Handbook of Clinical Medicine*. Sixth edition. Oxford: Oxford University Press.
674. Smeeks, F. C. (2008). Hypoglycemia. eMedicine. URL: http://emedicine.medscape.com/article/767359-overview. Accessed 2 September 2009.
675. Raghavan, V. A., Srinivasan, V. A. R. & Snow, K. (2010). Hypoglycemia.

eMedicine. URL: http://emedicine.medscape.com/article/122122-overview. Accessed 27 April 2010.
676. Meyer, T. W. & Hostetter, T. H. (2007). Uremia. *New England Journal of Medicine* **357**: 1316–1325. PMID 17898101.
677. Brown, T. M. & Brown, R. L. (1995). Neuropsychiatric consequences of renal failure. *Psychosomatics* **36**: 244–253. PMID 7638311.
678. Brouns, R. & De Deyn, P. P. (2004). Neurological complications in renal failure: a review. *Clinical Neurology and Neurosurgery* **107**: 1–16. PMID 15567546.
679. Bucurescu, G. (2006). Uremic encephalopathy. eMedicine. URL: http://www.emedicine.com/neuro/topic388.htm. Accessed 6 January 2008.
680. Moe, S. M. & Sprague, S. M. (1994). Uremic encephalopathy. *Clinical Nephrology* **42**: 251–256. PMID 7834918.
681. Slatopolsky, E., Martin, K. & Hruska, K. (1980). Parathyroid hormone metabolism and its potential as a uremic toxin. *American Journal of Physiology* **239**: F1–12. PMID 6994509.
682. Akmal, M., Goldstein, D. A., Multani, S. & Massry, S. G. (1984). Role of uremia, brain calcium, and parathyroid hormone on changes in electroencephalogram in chronic renal failure. *American Journal of Physiology* **246**: F575–579. PMID 6720963.
683. Klahr, S. & Slatopolsky, E. (1986). Toxicity of parathyroid hormone in uremia. *Annual Review of Medicine* **37**: 71–78. PMID 3010810.
684. Sood, G. K. (2009). Acute liver failure. eMedicine. URL: http://emedicine.medscape.com/article/177354-overview. Accessed 2 September 2009.
685. Wolf, D. C. (2008). Encephalopathy, hepatic. eMedicine. URL: http://emedicine.medscape.com/article/186101-overview. Accessed 2 September 2009.
686. Ardizzone, G., Arrigo, A., Schellino, M. M., Stratta, C., Valzan, S., Skurzak, S., Andruetto, P., Panio, A., Ballaris, M. A., Lavezzo, B., Salizzoni, M. & Cerutti, E. (2006). Neurological complications of liver cirrhosis and orthotopic liver transplant. *Transplantation Proceedings* **38**: 789–792. PMID 16647471.
687. Wolf, D. C. (2008). Cirrhosis. eMedicine. URL: http://emedicine.medscape.com/article/185856-overview. Accessed 2 September 2009.
688. Muller, N., Klages, U. & Gunther, W. (1994). Hepatic encephalopathy presenting as delirium and mania. The possible role of bilirubin. *General Hospital Psychiatry* **16**: 138–140. PMID 8039693.
689. Seebach, J. & Jost, R. (1992). Flumazenil-induced psychotic disorder in hepatic encephalopathy. *Lancet* **339**: 488–489. PMID 1346834.
690. Ruggieri, R. M., Lupo, I. & Piccoli, F. (2002). Pancreatic encephalopathy: a 7-year follow-up case report and review of the literature. *Neurological Sciences* **23**: 203–205. PMID 12536291.
691. Ding, X., Liu, C. A., Gong, J. P. & Li, S. W. (2004). Pancreatic encephalopathy in 24 patients with severe acute pancreatitis. *Hepatobiliary and Pancreatic Diseases International* **3**: 608–611. PMID 15567756.
692. Weiner, D. L. (2009). Pediatrics, Reye syndrome. eMedicine. URL: http://emedicine.medscape.com/article/803683-overview. Accessed 2 September 2009.
693. Fleisher, G. R., Ludwig, S., Henretig, F. M., Ruddy, R. M. & Silverman, B. K., Eds. (2005). *Textbook of Pediatric Emergency Medicine*. Fifth edition. Philadelphia, PA: Lippincott Williams & Wilkins.
694. Anderson, R. J., Chung, H. M., Kluge, R. & Schrier, R. W. (1985). Hyponatremia: a prospective analysis of its epidemiology and the pathogenetic role of vasopressin. *Annals of Internal Medicine* **102**: 164–168. PMID 3966753.
695. Simon, E. E. & Hamrahian, S. M. (2007). Hyponatremia. eMedicine. URL: http://www.emedicine.com/med/topic1130.htm. Accessed 29 December 2007.
696. Craig, S. (2007). Hyponatremia. eMedicine. URL: http://www.emedicine.com/emerg/topic275.htm. Accessed 29 December 2007.
697. Cooper, D. H., Krainik, A. J., Lubner, S. J., Reno, H. E. & Micek, S. (2007). *The Washington Manual of Medical Therapeutics*. Philadelphia, PA: Lippincott Williams & Wilkins.

698. Wachter, R. M., Goldman, L. & Hollander, H. (2005). *Hospital Medicine*. Philadelphia, PA: Lippincott Williams & Wilkins.
699. Deshmukh, S. & Thomas, C. (2007). Syndrome of inappropriate secretion of antidiuretic hormone. eMedicine. URL: http://www.emedicine.com/med/topic3541.htm. Accessed 6 January 2008.
700. Ferry, R. J. & Pascual-y-Baralt, J. F. (2008). Syndrome of inappropriate antidiuretic hormone secretion. eMedicine. URL: http://www.emedicine.com/ped/topic2190.htm. Accessed 31 October 2008.
701. Ellis, S. J. (1995). Severe hyponatraemia: complications and treatment. *QJM* **88**: 905–909. PMID 8593551.
702. Verghese, C., de Leon, J. & Josiassen, R. C. (1996). Problems and progress in the diagnosis and treatment of polydipsia and hyponatremia. *Schizophrenia Bulletin* **22**: 455–464. PMID 8873296.
703. Goldman, M. B., Luchins, D. J. & Robertson, G. L. (1988). Mechanisms of altered water metabolism in psychotic patients with polydipsia and hyponatremia. *New England Journal of Medicine* **318**: 397–403. PMID 3340117.
704. Shutty, M. S., Jr., Briscoe, L., Sautter, S. & Leadbetter, R. A. (1993). Neuropsychological manifestations of hyponatremia in chronic schizophrenic patients with the syndrome of psychosis, intermittent hyponatremia and polydipsia (PIP). *Schizophrenia Research* **10**: 125–130. PMID 8398944.
705. Goldman, M. B., Robertson, G. L., Luchins, D. J., Hedeker, D. & Pandey, G. N. (1997). Psychotic exacerbations and enhanced vasopressin secretion in schizophrenic patients with hyponatremia and polydipsia. *Archives of General Psychiatry* **54**: 443–449. PMID 9152098.
706. Stephanides, S. L. (2007). Hypernatremia. eMedicine. URL: http://www.emedicine.com/emerg/topic263.htm. Accessed 29 December 2007.
707. Tisdall, M., Crocker, M., Watkiss, J. & Smith, M. (2006). Disturbances of sodium in critically ill adult neurologic patients: a clinical review. *Journal of Neurosurgical Anesthesiology* **18**: 57–63. PMID 16369141.
708. Arieff, A. I. & Guisado, R. (1976). Effects on the central nervous system of hypernatremic and hyponatremic states. *Kidney International* **10**: 104–116. PMID 7702.
709. Jana, D. K. & Romano-Jana, L. (1973). Hypernatremic psychosis in the elderly: case reports. *Journal of the American Geriatrics Society* **21**: 473–477. PMID 4729012.
710. Farley, P. C., Lau, K. Y. & Suba, S. (1986). Severe hypernatremia in a patient with psychiatric illness. *Archives of Internal Medicine* **146**: 1214–1215. PMID 3718109.
711. Aidley, D. J. (1989). *The Physiology of Excitable Cells*. Third edition. Cambridge: Cambridge University Press.
712. Beach, C. B. (2007). Hypocalcemia. eMedicine. URL: http://www.emedicine.com/emerg/topic271.htm. Accessed 29 December 2007.
713. Juan, D. (1979). Hypocalcemia. Differential diagnosis and mechanisms. *Archives of Internal Medicine* **139**: 1166–1171. PMID 226022.
714. Hemphill, R. R. (2007). Hypercalcemia. eMedicine. URL: http://www.emedicine.com/emerg/topic260.htm. Accessed 29 December 2007.
715. Hafez, H., Strauss, J. S., Aronson, M. D. & Holt, C. (1984). Hypokalemia-induced psychosis in a chronic schizophrenic patient. *Journal of Clinical Psychiatry* **45**: 277–279. PMID 6725222.
716. Garth, D. (2007). Hypokalemia. eMedicine. URL: http://www.emedicine.com/emerg/topic273.htm. Accessed 29 December 2007.
717. Hatta, K., Takahashi, T., Nakamura, H., Yamashiro, H., Asukai, N. & Yonezawa, Y. (1999). Hypokalemia and agitation in acute psychotic patients. *Psychiatry Research* **86**: 85–88. PMID 10359485.
718. Novello, N. P. & Blumstein, H. A. (2007). Hypomagnesemia. eMedicine. URL: http://www.emedicine.com/emerg/topic274.htm. Accessed 29 December 2007.

719. Ang, A. W., Ko, S. M. & Tan, C. H. (1995). Calcium, magnesium, and psychotic symptoms in a girl with idiopathic hypoparathyroidism. *Psychosomatic Medicine* **57**: 299–302. PMID 7652132.
720. Gitelman, H. J. & Welt, L. G. (1969). Magnesium deficiency. *Annual Review of Medicine* **20**: 233–242. PMID 4893400.
721. Kramp, P., Hemmingsen, R. & Rafaelsen, O. J. (1979). Magnesium concentrations in blood and cerebrospinal fluid during delirium tremens. *Psychiatry Research* **1**: 161–171. PMID 298346.
722. Zakhari, S. & Altura, B. M. (1994). Alcohol and magnesium. Introduction to the symposium. *Alcoholism, Clinical and Experimental Research* **18**: 1037–1039. PMID 7847585.
723. Mota de Freitas, D., Castro, M. M. & Geraldes, C. F. (2006). Is competition between Li+ and Mg2+ the underlying theme in the proposed mechanisms for the pharmacological action of lithium salts in bipolar disorder? *Accounts of Chemical Research* **39**: 283–291. PMID 16618096.
724. Gould, T. D., Quiroz, J. A., Singh, J., Zarate, C. A. & Manji, H. K. (2004). Emerging experimental therapeutics for bipolar disorder: insights from the molecular and cellular actions of current mood stabilizers. *Molecular Psychiatry* **9**: 734–755. PMID 15136794.
725. Weisinger, J. R. & Bellorin-Font, E. (1998). Magnesium and phosphorus. *Lancet* **352**: 391–396. PMID 9717944.
726. Moore, D. J. & Rosh, A. J. (2009). Hypophosphatemia. eMedicine. URL: http://emedicine.medscape.com/article/767955-overview. Accessed 15 November 2009.
727. Nanji, A. A. (1984). The psychiatric aspect of hypophosphatemia. *Canadian Journal of Psychiatry* **29**: 599–600. PMID 6391648.
728. Di Comite, G. & Sabbadini, M. G. (2005). Neurological involvement in rheumatological diseases. *Neurological Sciences* **26 Suppl 1**: S9–14. PMID 15883701.
729. Sofat, N., Malik, O. & Higgens, C. S. (2006). Neurological involvement in patients with rheumatic disease. *QJM* **99**: 69–79. PMID 16434469.
730. Patel, M., Clarke, A. M., Bruce, I. N. & Symmons, D. P. (2006). The prevalence and incidence of biopsy-proven lupus nephritis in the UK: evidence of an ethnic gradient. *Arthritis and Rheumatism* **54**: 2963–2969. PMID 16947632.
731. Sanna, G., Bertolaccini, M. L., Cuadrado, M. J., Laing, H., Khamashta, M. A., Mathieu, A. & Hughes, G. R. (2003). Neuropsychiatric manifestations in systemic lupus erythematosus: prevalence and association with antiphospholipid antibodies. *Journal of Rheumatology* **30**: 985–992. PMID 12734893.
732. Joseph, F. G., Lammie, G. A. & Scolding, N. J. (2007). CNS lupus: a study of 41 patients. *Neurology* **69**: 644–654. PMID 17698785.
733. Ainiala, H., Loukkola, J., Peltola, J., Korpela, M. & Hietaharju, A. (2001). The prevalence of neuropsychiatric syndromes in systemic lupus erythematosus. *Neurology* **57**: 496–500. PMID 11502919.
734. Appenzeller, S., Cendes, F. & Costallat, L. T. (2008). Acute psychosis in systemic lupus erythematosus. *Rheumatology International* **28**: 237–243. PMID 17634902.
735. American College of Rheumatology (1999). The American College of Rheumatology nomenclature and case definitions for neuropsychiatric lupus syndromes. *Arthritis and Rheumatism* **42**: 599–608. PMID 10211873.
736. Fricchione, G. L., Kaufman, L. D., Gruber, B. L. & Fink, M. (1990). Electroconvulsive therapy and cyclophosphamide in combination for severe neuropsychiatric lupus with catatonia. *American Journal of Medicine* **88**: 442–443. PMID 2327432.
737. Wang, H. Y. & Huang, T. L. (2006). Benzodiazepines in catatonia associated with systemic lupus erythematosus. *Psychiatry and Clinical Neurosciences* **60**: 768–770. PMID 17109714.
738. Kengne, F. G. & Decaux, G. (2006). Inappropriate secretion of ADH and central diabetes insipidus are related to antiphospholipid antibodies in SLE – case

report and review of the literature. *Nephrology, Dialysis, Transplantation* **21**: 3311–3315. PMID 16935893.

739. Tan, E. M., Cohen, A. S., Fries, J. F., Masi, A. T., McShane, D. J., Rothfield, N. F., Schaller, J. G., Talal, N. & Winchester, R. J. (1982). The 1982 revised criteria for the classification of systemic lupus erythematosus. *Arthritis and Rheumatism* **25**: 1271–1277. PMID 7138600.
740. Solomon, D. H., Kavanaugh, A. J. & Schur, P. H. (2002). Evidence-based guidelines for the use of immunologic tests: antinuclear antibody testing. *Arthritis and Rheumatism* **47**: 434–444. PMID 12209492.
741. McHardy, K. C., Horne, C. H. & Rennie, J. (1982). Antinuclear antibody-negative systemic lupus erythematosus – how common? *Journal of Clinical Pathology* **35**: 1118–1121. PMID 6982285.
742. American College of Rheumatology (1999). Guidelines for referral and management of systemic lupus erythematosus in adults. *Arthritis and Rheumatism* **42**: 1785–1796. PMID 10513791.
743. Faria, A. C., Barcellos, K. S. & Andrade, L. E. (2005). Longitudinal fluctuation of antibodies to extractable nuclear antigens in systemic lupus erythematosus. *Journal of Rheumatology* **32**: 1267–1272. PMID 15996063.
744. Kurien, B. T. & Scofield, R. H. (2006). Autoantibody determination in the diagnosis of systemic lupus erythematosus. *Scandinavian Journal of Immunology* **64**: 227–235. PMID 16918691.
745. Tikly, M., Burgin, S., Mohanlal, P., Bellingan, A. & George, J. (1996). Autoantibodies in black South Africans with systemic lupus erythematosus: spectrum and clinical associations. *Clinical Rheumatology* **15**: 143–147. PMID 8777847.
746. Camilleri, F. & Mallia, C. (1999). RNP positivity in Maltese SLE patients. *Advances in Experimental Medicine and Biology* **455**: 161–166. PMID 10599338.
747. Zandi, M. (2010). Advances and challenges in neuropsychiatric systemic lupus erythematosus. *Advances in Clinical Neuroscience and Rehabilitation* **10**: 8–13.
748. Vincent, A., Lang, B. & Kleopa, K. A. (2006). Autoimmune channelopathies and related neurological disorders. *Neuron* **52**: 123–138. PMID 17015231.
749. Vernino, S. (2007). Autoimmune and paraneoplastic channelopathies. *Neurotherapeutics* **4**: 305–314. PMID 17395141.
750. Kowal, C., Degiorgio, L. A., Lee, J. Y., Edgar, M. A., Huerta, P. T., Volpe, B. T. & Diamond, B. (2006). Human lupus autoantibodies against NMDA receptors mediate cognitive impairment. *Proceedings of the National Academy of Sciences of the United States of America* **103**: 19854–19859. PMID 17170137.
751. Matus, S., Burgos, P. V., Bravo-Zehnder, M., Kraft, R., Porras, O. H., Farias, P., Barros, L. F., Torrealba, F., Massardo, L., Jacobelli, S. & Gonzalez, A. (2007). Antiribosomal-P autoantibodies from psychiatric lupus target a novel neuronal surface protein causing calcium influx and apoptosis. *Journal of Experimental Medicine* **204**: 3221–3234. PMID 18056288.
752. Vincent, A. (2010). An update on antibody-mediated diseases. *Advances in Clinical Neuroscience and Rehabilitation* **10**: 8–11.
753. Hochberg, M. C. (1997). Updating the American College of Rheumatology revised criteria for the classification of systemic lupus erythematosus. *Arthritis and Rheumatism* **40**: 1725. PMID 9324032.
754. Hughes, G. R. (1998). Is it lupus? The St. Thomas' Hospital "alternative" criteria. *Clinical and Experimental Rheumatology* **16**: 250–252. PMID 9631744.
755. Abreu, M. R., Jakosky, A., Folgerini, M., Brenol, J. C., Xavier, R. M. & Kapczinsky, F. (2005). Neuropsychiatric systemic lupus erythematosus: correlation of brain MR imaging, CT, and SPECT. *Clinical Imaging* **29**: 215–221. PMID 15855069.
756. Scolding, N. J. & Joseph, F. G. (2002). The neuropathology and pathogenesis of systemic lupus erythematosus. *Neuropathology and Applied Neurobiology* **28**: 173–189. PMID 12060342.
757. Peterson, P. L., Axford, J. S. & Isenberg, D. (2005). Imaging in CNS lupus. *Best Practice and Research Clinical*

Rheumatology **19**: 727–739. PMID 16150400.

758. Kauffman, C. L. & Fredeking, A. E. (2009). Lupus erythematosus, drug-induced. eMedicine. URL: http://emedicine.medscape.com/article/1065086-overview. Accessed 12 November 2009.

759. Vedove, C. D., Del Giglio, M., Schena, D. & Girolomoni, G. (2009). Drug-induced lupus erythematosus. *Archives of Dermatological Research (Archiv für Dermatologische Forschung)* **301**: 99–105. PMID 18797892.

760. Rand, J. H. (2007). The antiphospholipid syndrome. *Hematology American Society of Hematology Education Program* **2007**: 136–142. PMID 18024621.

761. Sanna, G., Bertolaccini, M. L. & Hughes, G. R. (2005). Hughes syndrome, the antiphospholipid syndrome: a new chapter in neurology. *Annals of the New York Academy of Sciences* **1051**: 465–486. PMID 16126988.

762. Pusterla, S., Previtali, S., Marziali, S., Cortelazzo, S., Rossi, A., Barbui, T. & Galli, M. (2004). Antiphospholipid antibodies in lymphoma: prevalence and clinical significance. *Hematology Journal* **5**: 341–346. PMID 15297851.

763. Shi, W., Krilis, S. A., Chong, B. H., Gordon, S. & Chesterman, C. N. (1990). Prevalence of lupus anticoagulant and anticardiolipin antibodies in a healthy population. *Australian and New Zealand Journal of Medicine* **20**: 231–236. PMID 2115326.

764. Raza, H., Epstein, S. A., Pao, M. & Rosenstein, D. L. (2008). Mania: psychiatric manifestations of the antiphospholipid syndrome. *Psychosomatics* **49**: 438–441.

765. Cardinal, R. N., Shah, D. N., Edwards, C. J., Hughes, G. R. & Fernandez-Egea, E. (2009). Psychosis and catatonia as a first presentation of antiphospholipid syndrome. *British Journal of Psychiatry* **195**: 272. PMID 19721128.

766. Sanna, G., Bertolaccini, M. L., Cuadrado, M. J., Khamashta, M. A. & Hughes, G. R. (2003). Central nervous system involvement in the antiphospholipid (Hughes) syndrome. *Rheumatology* **42**: 200–213. PMID 12595612.

767. Schwartz, M., Rochas, M., Weller, B., Sheinkman, A., Tal, I., Golan, D., Toubi, N., Eldar, I., Sharf, B. & Attias, D. (1998). High association of anticardiolipin antibodies with psychosis. *Journal of Clinical Psychiatry* **59**: 20–23. PMID 9491061.

768. Sneddon, I. B. (1965). Cerebro-vascular lesions and livedo reticularis. *British Journal of Dermatology* **77**: 180–185. PMID 14278790.

769. Atkinson, J. C., Royce, L. S., Wellner, R., Pillemer, S. R., Bermudez, D. & Fox, P. C. (1995). Anti-salivary antibodies in primary Sjogren's syndrome. *Journal of Oral Pathology and Medicine* **24**: 206–212. PMID 7616459.

770. Spezialetti, R., Bluestein, H. G., Peter, J. B. & Alexander, E. L. (1993). Neuropsychiatric disease in Sjogren's syndrome: anti-ribosomal P and anti-neuronal antibodies. *American Journal of Medicine* **95**: 153–160. PMID 8356981.

771. Francis, M. L. & Ranatunga, S. M. (2006). Sjögren syndrome. eMedicine. URL: http://www.emedicine.com/med/topic2136.htm. Accessed 9 December 2008.

772. Steen, V. D., Oddis, C. V., Conte, C. G., Janoski, J., Casterline, G. Z. & Medsger, T. A., Jr. (1997). Incidence of systemic sclerosis in Allegheny County, Pennsylvania. A twenty-year study of hospital-diagnosed cases, 1963–1982. *Arthritis and Rheumatism* **40**: 441–445. PMID 9082931.

773. Hietaharju, A., Jaaskelainen, S., Hietarinta, M. & Frey, H. (1993). Central nervous system involvement and psychiatric manifestations in systemic sclerosis (scleroderma): clinical and neurophysiological evaluation. *Acta Neurologica Scandinavica* **87**: 382–387. PMID 8333243.

774. Wise, T. N. & Ginzler, E. M. (1975). Scleroderma cerebritis, an unusual manifestation of progressive systemic sclerosis. *Diseases of the Nervous System* **36**: 60–62. PMID 1116415.

775. Shiraishi, H., Koizumi, J., Suzuki, T., Mizukami, K., Tanaka, Y. & Sato, T. (1991). Progressive systemic sclerosis with mental disorder. *Japanese Journal of Psychiatry and Neurology* **45**: 855–860. PMID 1813680.

776. Muller, N., Gizycki-Nienhaus, B., Botschev, C. & Meurer, M. (1993). Cerebral involvement of scleroderma presenting as schizophrenia-like psychosis. *Schizophrenia Research* **10**: 179–181. PMID 8398950.
777. Bennett, R. M., Bong, D. M. & Spargo, B. H. (1978). Neuropsychiatric problems in mixed connective tissue disease. *American Journal of Medicine* **65**: 955–962. PMID 217265.
778. Kallenberg, C. G. (2008). The last classification of vasculitis. *Clinical Reviews in Allergy and Immunology* **35**: 5–10. PMID 18172778.
779. Scott, D. G. & Watts, R. A. (1994). Classification and epidemiology of systemic vasculitis. *British Journal of Rheumatology* **33**: 897–899. PMID 7646607.
780. Abramsky, O., Compston, D. A. S., Miller, A. & Said, G., Eds. (2001). *Brain Disease: Therapeutic strategies and repair.* London: Informa Healthcare.
781. Tabarki, B., Mahdhaoui, A., Selmi, H., Yacoub, M. & Essoussi, A. S. (2001). Kawasaki disease with predominant central nervous system involvement. *Pediatric Neurology* **25**: 239–241. PMID 11587880.
782. Zandi, M. S. & Coles, A. J. (2007). Notes on the kidney and its diseases for the neurologist. *Journal of Neurology, Neurosurgery and Psychiatry* **78**: 444–449. PMID 17435183.
783. Meusser, S., Rubbert, A., Manger, B., Bock, E., Platsch, G., Feistel, H., Engelhardt, A., Wolf, F. & Kalden, J. R. (1996). 99m-Tc-HMPAO-SPECT in diagnosis of early cerebral vasculitis. *Rheumatology International* **16**: 37–42. PMID 8783421.
784. Johnson, H., Bouman, W. & Pinner, G. (1997). Psychiatric aspects of temporal arteritis: a case report and review of the literature. *Journal of Geriatric Psychiatry and Neurology* **10**: 142–145. PMID 9453679.
785. Chung, S. (2006). Polyarteritis nodosa. eMedicine. URL: http://www.emedicine.com/neuro/topic314.htm. Accessed 17 October 2008.
786. Fernandes, S. R., Coimbra, I. B., Costallat, L. T. & Ribeiro Filho, J. E. (1998). Uncommon features of polyarteritis nodosa: psychosis and angio-oedema. *Clinical Rheumatology* **17**: 353–356. PMID 9776125.
787. Rose, N. R. & Mackay, I. R. (2006). *The Autoimmune Diseases.* Fourth edition, San Diego, CA: Academic Press.
788. Cush, J. J., Kavanaugh, A. & Stein, C. M. (2004). *Rheumatology: Diagnosis and therapeutics.* Second edition. Philadelphia, PA: Lippincott Williams & Wilkins.
789. Scott, T. (2006). Wegener granulomatosis. eMedicine. URL: http://www.emedicine.com/neuro/topic396.htm. Accessed 12 October 2008.
790. Sharma, S. (2006). Wegener granulomatosis. eMedicine. URL: http://www.emedicine.com/med/topic2401.htm. Accessed 12 October 2008.
791. Spisek, R., Kolouchova, E., Jensovsky, J., Rusina, R., Fendrych, P., Plas, J. & Bartunkova, J. (2006). Combined CNS and pituitary involvement as a primary manifestation of Wegener granulomatosis. *Clinical Rheumatology* **25**: 739–742. PMID 16322901.
792. Lim, I. G., Spira, P. J. & McNeil, H. P. (2002). Headache as the initial presentation of Wegener's granulomatosis. *Annals of the Rheumatic Diseases* **61**: 571–572. PMID 12006344.
793. Seo, P., Min, Y. I., Holbrook, J. T., Hoffman, G. S., Merkel, P. A., Spiera, R., Davis, J. C., Ytterberg, S. R., St Clair, E. W., McCune, W. J., Specks, U., Allen, N. B., Luqmani, R. A. & Stone, J. H. (2005). Damage caused by Wegener's granulomatosis and its treatment: prospective data from the Wegener's Granulomatosis Etanercept Trial (WGET). *Arthritis and Rheumatism* **52**: 2168–2178. PMID 15986348.
794. Farid-Moayer, M. (2006). Microscopic polyangiitis. eMedicine. URL: http://www.emedicine.com/med/topic2931.htm. Accessed 12 October 2008.
795. Askari, A., Saadeh, A. & Buheis, N. I. (1999). Microscopic polyangiitis presenting as schizophrenia. *Rheumatology International* **18**: 215–217. PMID 10399798.
796. Rust, R. (2006). Churg–Strauss disease. eMedicine. URL: http://www.emedicine.

com/neuro/topic501.htm. Accessed 12 October 2008.
797. Leone, J. C. & Swigar, M. E. (1986). Marfan's syndrome and neuropsychiatric symptoms: case report and literature review. *Comprehensive Psychiatry* **27**: 247–250. PMID 2872016.
798. Zwaneveld, H. L. (1958). [An organic psychosis associated with pseudoxanthoma elasticum]. *Nederlands Tijdschrift voor Geneeskunde* **102**: 191–193. PMID 13517349.
799. Albayram, M. S., Wityk, R., Yousem, D. M. & Zinreich, S. J. (2001). The cerebral angiographic findings in Cogan syndrome. *AJNR: American Journal of Neuroradiology* **22**: 751–754. PMID 11290493.
800. Majmudar, P. A. (2007). Keratitis, interstitial. eMedicine. URL: http://emedicine.medscape.com/article/1194376-overview. Accessed 8 November 2009.
801. Bicknell, J. M. & Holland, J. V. (1978). Neurologic manifestations of Cogan syndrome. *Neurology* **28**: 278–281. PMID 305011.
802. Pandey, R. S., Srinivas, K. N. & Khanna, S. (1988). Mania in a case of Eale's disease. *British Journal of Psychiatry* **153**: 129–130. PMID 3224245.
803. Borth, D. B. (2007). Eales disease. URL: http://emedicine.medscape.com/article/1225636-overview. Accessed 8 November 2009.
804. Kleffner, I., Ringelstein, E. B., Stupp, N., Niederstadt, T. U. & Young, P. (2006). Neurological picture. Susac's syndrome: effective combination of immunosuppression and antiplatelet treatment. *Journal of Neurology, Neurosurgery and Psychiatry* **77**: 1335. PMID 17110748.
805. Saenz, R., Quan, A. W., Magalhaes, A. & Kish, K. (2005). MRI of Susac's syndrome. *AJR: American Journal of Roentgenology* **184**: 1688–1690. PMID 15855140.
806. Hahn, J. S., Lannin, W. C. & Sarwal, M. M. (2004). Microangiopathy of brain, retina, and inner ear (Susac's syndrome) in an adolescent female presenting as acute disseminated encephalomyelitis. *Pediatrics* **114**: 276–281. PMID 15231946.
807. Fialho, D., Holmes, P., Riordan-Eva, P. & Silber, E. (2002). A blinding headache falling on deaf ears (Susac's syndrome). *Practical Neurology* **2**: 358–361.
808. International Study Group for Behçet's Disease (1990). Criteria for diagnosis of Behçet's disease. *Lancet* **335**: 1078–1080. PMID 1970380.
809. Kikuchi, H., Aramaki, K. & Hirohata, S. (2008). Effect of infliximab in progressive neuro-Behçet's syndrome. *Journal of the Neurological Sciences* **272**: 99–105. PMID 18550081.
810. Farah, S., Al-Shubaili, A., Montaser, A., Hussein, J. M., Malaviya, A. N., Mukhtar, M., Al-Shayeb, A., Khuraibet, A. J., Khan, R. & Trontelj, J. V. (1998). Behçet's syndrome: a report of 41 patients with emphasis on neurological manifestations. *Journal of Neurology, Neurosurgery and Psychiatry* **64**: 382–384. PMID 9527155.
811. Celik, Y., Tugly, C., Utku, U. & Abay, E. (2008). Behçet's disease presented with isolated peduncular hallucinosis: a case report. *The Internet Journal of Neurology* **9**.
812. Good, A. E. (1974). Reiter's disease: a review with special attention to cardiovascular and neurologic sequellae. *Seminars in Arthritis and Rheumatism* **3**: 253–286.
813. Scoggins, T. (2007). Reactive arthritis. eMedicine. URL: http://www.emedicine.com/emerg/topic498.htm. Accessed 21 October 2008.
814. Yakobi, R. (2007). Sarcoidosis. eMedicine. URL: http://www.emedicine.com/emerg/topic516.htm. Accessed 18 April 2008.
815. Newman, L. S., Rose, C. S. & Maier, L. A. (1997). Sarcoidosis. *New England Journal of Medicine* **336**: 1224–1234. PMID 9110911.
816. Allen, R. K., Sellars, R. E. & Sandstrom, P. A. (2003). A prospective study of 32 patients with neurosarcoidosis. *Sarcoidosis, Vasculitis, and Diffuse Lung Diseases* **20**: 118–125. PMID 12870721.
817. O'Brien, G. M., Baughman, R. P., Broderick, J. P., Arnold, L. & Lower, E. E. (1994). Paranoid psychosis due to

neurosarcoidosis. *Sarcoidosis* **11**: 34–36. PMID 8036341.

818. Westhout, F. D. & Linskey, M. E. (2008). Obstructive hydrocephalus and progressive psychosis: rare presentations of neurosarcoidosis. *Surgical Neurology* **69**: 288–292; discussion 292. PMID 17976699.
819. Sabaawi, M., Gutierrez-Nunez, J. & Fragala, M. R. (1992). Neurosarcoidosis presenting as schizophreniform disorder. *International Journal of Psychiatry in Medicine* **22**: 269–274. PMID 1487390.
820. Friedman, S. H. & Gould, D. J. (2002). Neurosarcoidosis presenting as psychosis and dementia: a case report. *International Journal of Psychiatry in Medicine* **32**: 401–403. PMID 12779189.
821. Thompson, C. & Checkley, S. (1981). Short term memory deficit in a patient with cerebral sarcoidosis. *British Journal of Psychiatry* **139**: 160–161. PMID 7306755.
822. Bourgeois, J. A., Maddock, R. J., Rogers, L., Greco, C. M., Mangrulkar, R. S. & Saint, S. (2005). Neurosarcoidosis and delirium. *Psychosomatics* **46**: 148–150. PMID 15774954.
823. Stiller, J., Goodman, A., Komhi, L. M., Sacher, M. & Bender, M. B. (1984). Neurosarcoidosis presenting as major depression. *Journal of Neurology, Neurosurgery and Psychiatry* **47**: 1050–1051. PMID 6481378.
824. Johnstone, E. C., Macmillan, J. F. & Crow, T. J. (1987). The occurrence of organic disease of possible or probable aetiological significance in a population of 268 cases of first episode schizophrenia. *Psychological Medicine* **17**: 371–379. PMID 3602229.
825. Cokonis Georgakis, C. D., Falasca, G., Georgakis, A. & Heymann, W. R. (2006). Scleromyxedema. *Clinics in Dermatology* **24**: 493–497. PMID 17113967.
826. Wun, T. & Bahou, W. F. (2006). Thrombotic thrombocytopenic purpura. eMedicine. URL: http://emedicine.medscape.com/article/206598-overview. Accessed 12 June 2009.
827. Kwok, S. K., Ju, J. H., Cho, C. S., Kim, H. Y. & Park, S. H. (2009). Thrombotic thrombocytopenic purpura in systemic lupus erythematosus: risk factors and clinical outcome: a single centre study. *Lupus* **18**: 16–21. PMID 19074164.
828. Kapfhammer, H. P. & Heigl, F. (1993). [Bipolar affective disorder and neuropsychiatric complications in a chronic course of thrombotic thrombocytopenic purpura. A case report]. *Nervenarzt* **64**: 612–617. PMID 8413764.
829. Leach, J. W., Pham, T., Diamandidis, D. & George, J. N. (1999). Thrombotic thrombocytopenic purpura-hemolytic uremic syndrome (TTP-HUS) following treatment with deoxycoformycin in a patient with cutaneous T-cell lymphoma (Sezary syndrome): a case report. *American Journal of Hematology* **61**: 268–270. PMID 10440915.
830. Gomez, E., Roncero, C., De Pablo, J., Rovira, M., Mazzarra, R., Blade, J. & Cirera, E. (2000). [Hyperviscosity syndrome and mental disorders]. *Actas Espanolas de Psiquiatria* **28**: 263–266. PMID 11116798.
831. Gertz, M. A. & Kyle, R. A. (1995). Hyperviscosity syndrome. *Journal of Intensive Care Medicine* **10**: 128–141. PMID 10155178.
832. Ainsworth, C., Edgerton, C. C. & Oglesby, R. J. (2009). Cryoglobulinemia. eMedicine. URL: http://emedicine.medscape.com/article/329255-overview. Accessed 29 October 2009.
833. Pines, A., Kaplinsky, N., Goldhammer, E. & Frankl, O. (1982). Cerebral involvement in primary mixed cryoglobulinaemia. *Postgraduate Medical Journal* **58**: 359–361. PMID 7122371.
834. Fatourechi, V. (2005). Hashimoto's encephalopathy: myth or reality? An endocrinologist's perspective. *Best Practice and Research. Clinical Endocrinology and Metabolism* **19**: 53–66. PMID 15826922.
835. Castillo, P., Woodruff, B., Caselli, R., Vernino, S., Lucchinetti, C., Swanson, J., Noseworthy, J., Aksamit, A., Carter, J., Sirven, J., Hunder, G., Fatourechi, V., Mokri, B., Drubach, D., Pittock, S., Lennon, V. & Boeve, B. (2006). Steroid-responsive encephalopathy associated

with autoimmune thyroiditis. *Archives of Neurology* **63**: 197–202. PMID 16476807.

836. Mijajlovic, M., Mirkovic, M., Dackovic, J., Zidverc-Trajkovic, J. & Sternic, N. (2010). Clinical manifestations, diagnostic criteria and therapy of Hashimoto's encephalopathy: report of two cases. *Journal of the Neurological Sciences* **288**: 194–196. PMID 19846119.
837. Arrojo, M., Perez-Rodriguez, M. M., Mota, M., Moreira, R., Azevedo, A., Oliveira, A., Abreu, P., Marques, P., Silva, A., Pereira, J. G., Palha, A. P. & Baca-Garcia, E. (2007). Psychiatric presentation of Hashimoto's encephalopathy. *Psychosomatic Medicine* **69**: 200–201. PMID 17327214.
838. Mocellin, R., Lubman, D. I., Lloyd, J., Tomlinson, E. B. & Velakoulis, D. (2006). Reversible dementia with psychosis: Hashimoto's encephalopathy. *Psychiatry and Clinical Neurosciences* **60**: 761–763. PMID 17109712.
839. Garrard, P., Hodges, J. R., De Vries, P. J., Hunt, N., Crawford, A. & Balan, K. (2000). Hashimoto's encephalopathy presenting as "myxodematous madness". *Journal of Neurology, Neurosurgery and Psychiatry* **68**: 102–103. PMID 10671115.
840. Lawn, N. D., Westmoreland, B. F., Kiely, M. J., Lennon, V. A. & Vernino, S. (2003). Clinical, magnetic resonance imaging, and electroencephalographic findings in paraneoplastic limbic encephalitis. *Mayo Clinic Proceedings* **78**: 1363–1368. PMID 14601695.
841. Ances, B. M., Vitaliani, R., Taylor, R. A., Liebeskind, D. S., Voloschin, A., Houghton, D. J., Galetta, S. L., Dichter, M., Alavi, A., Rosenfeld, M. R. & Dalmau, J. (2005). Treatment-responsive limbic encephalitis identified by neuropil antibodies: MRI and PET correlates. *Brain* **128**: 1764–1777. PMID 15888538.
842. Dalmau, J. & Rosenfeld, M. R. (2008). Paraneoplastic syndromes of the CNS. *Lancet Neurology* 7: 327–340. PMID 18339348.
843. Bataller, L., Kleopa, K. A., Wu, G. F., Rossi, J. E., Rosenfeld, M. R. & Dalmau, J. (2007). Autoimmune limbic encephalitis in 39 patients: immunophenotypes and outcomes. *Journal of Neurology, Neurosurgery and Psychiatry* **78**: 381–385. PMID 16980333.
844. Tomimitsu, H., Arimura, K., Nagado, T., Watanabe, O., Otsuka, R., Kurono, A., Sonoda, Y., Osame, M. & Kameyama, M. (2004). Mechanism of action of voltage-gated K+ channel antibodies in acquired neuromyotonia. *Annals of Neurology* **56**: 440–444. PMID 15349875.
845. Hudson, L. A., Rollins, Y. D., Anderson, C. A., Johnston-Brooks, C., Tyler, K. L. & Filley, C. M. (2007). Reduplicative paramnesia in Morvan's syndrome. *Journal of the Neurological Sciences*. PMID 17928004.
846. McKeon, A., Marnane, M., O'Connell, M., Stack, J. P., Kelly, P. J. & Lynch, T. (2007). Potassium channel antibody associated encephalopathy presenting with a frontotemporal dementia like syndrome. *Archives of Neurology* **64**: 1528–1530. PMID 17923638.
847. Buckley, C., Oger, J., Clover, L., Tuzun, E., Carpenter, K., Jackson, M. & Vincent, A. (2001). Potassium channel antibodies in two patients with reversible limbic encephalitis. *Annals of Neurology* **50**: 73–78. PMID 11456313.
848. Parthasarathi, U. D., Harrower, T., Tempest, M., Hodges, J. R., Walsh, C., McKenna, P. J. & Fletcher, P. C. (2006). Psychiatric presentation of voltage-gated potassium channel antibody-associated encephalopathy. Case report. *British Journal of Psychiatry* **189**: 182–183. PMID 16880491.
849. Sansing, L. H., Tuzun, E., Ko, M. W., Baccon, J., Lynch, D. R. & Dalmau, J. (2007). A patient with encephalitis associated with NMDA receptor antibodies. *Nature Clinical Practice. Neurology* **3**: 291–296. PMID 17479076.
850. Florance, N. R., Davis, R. L., Lam, C., Szperka, C., Zhou, L., Ahmad, S., Campen, C. J., Moss, H., Peter, N., Gleichman, A. J., Glaser, C. A., Lynch, D. R., Rosenfeld, M. R. & Dalmau, J. (2009). Anti-N-methyl-D-aspartate receptor (NMDAR) encephalitis in children and adolescents. *Annals of Neurology* **66**: 11–18. PMID 19670433.
851. Dalmau, J., Tuzun, E., Wu, H. Y., Masjuan, J., Rossi, J. E., Voloschin, A.,

Baehring, J. M., Shimazaki, H., Koide, R., King, D., Mason, W., Sansing, L. H., Dichter, M. A., Rosenfeld, M. R. & Lynch, D. R. (2007). Paraneoplastic anti-N-methyl-D-aspartate receptor encephalitis associated with ovarian teratoma. *Annals of Neurology* **61**: 25–36. PMID 17262855.

852. Sabin, T. D., Jednacz, J. A. & Staats, P. N. (2008). Case records of the Massachusetts General Hospital. Case 26–2008. A 26-year-old woman with headache and behavioral changes. *New England Journal of Medicine* **359**: 842–853. PMID 18716302.

853. Dalmau, J., Gleichman, A. J., Hughes, E. G., Rossi, J. E., Peng, X., Lai, M., Dessain, S. K., Rosenfeld, M. R., Balice-Gordon, R. & Lynch, D. R. (2008). Anti-NMDA-receptor encephalitis: case series and analysis of the effects of antibodies. *Lancet Neurology* 7: 1091–1098. PMID 18851928.

854. Irani, S. R., Bera, K., Waters, P., Zuliani, L., Maxwell, S., Zandi, M. S., Friese, M. A., Galea, I., Kullmann, D. M., Beeson, D., Lang, B., Bien, C. G. & Vincent, A. (2010). N-methyl-D-aspartate antibody encephalitis: temporal progression of clinical and paraclinical observations in a predominantly non-paraneoplastic disorder of both sexes. *Brain* **133**: 1655–1667. PMID 20511282.

855. Graus, F., Saiz, A., Lai, M., Bruna, J., Lopez, F., Sabater, L., Blanco, Y., Rey, M. J., Ribalta, T. & Dalmau, J. (2008). Neuronal surface antigen antibodies in limbic encephalitis: clinical-immunologic associations. *Neurology* **71**: 930–936. PMID 18794496.

856. Vitaliani, R., Mason, W., Ances, B., Zwerdling, T., Jiang, Z. & Dalmau, J. (2005). Paraneoplastic encephalitis, psychiatric symptoms, and hypoventilation in ovarian teratoma. *Annals of Neurology* **58**: 594–604. PMID 16178029.

857. Rees, J. H. (2004). Paraneoplastic syndromes: when to suspect, how to confirm, and how to manage. *Journal of Neurology, Neurosurgery and Psychiatry* 75 **Suppl 2**: ii43–50. PMID 15146039.

858. Boylan, L. S. (2000). Limbic encephalitis and late-onset psychosis. *American Journal of Psychiatry* **157**: 1343–1344. PMID 10910808.

859. Dalmau, J., Graus, F., Rosenblum, M. K. & Posner, J. B. (1992). Anti-Hu–associated paraneoplastic encephalomyelitis/sensory neuronopathy. A clinical study of 71 patients. *Medicine* **71**: 59–72. PMID 1312211.

860. Honnorat, J. & Antoine, J. C. (2007). Paraneoplastic neurological syndromes. *Orphanet Journal of Rare Diseases* **2**: 22. PMID 17480225.

861. Mata, S., Muscas, G. C., Naldi, I., Rosati, E., Paladini, S., Cruciatti, B., Bisulli, F., Paganini, M., Mazzi, G., Sorbi, S. & Tinuper, P. (2008). Non-paraneoplastic limbic encephalitis associated with anti-glutamic acid decarboxylase antibodies. *Journal of Neuroimmunology* **199**: 155–159. PMID 18586329.

862. Hadjivassiliou, M. (2010). Primary autoimmune cerebellar ataxia (PACA). *Advances in Clinical Neuroscience and Rehabilitation* **9**: 8–11.

863. Caselli, R. J., Boeve, B. F., Scheithauer, B. W., O'Duffy, J. D. & Hunder, G. G. (1999). Nonvasculitic autoimmune inflammatory meningoencephalitis (NAIM): a reversible form of encephalopathy. *Neurology* **53**: 1579–1581. PMID 10534272.

864. Josephs, K. A., Rubino, F. A. & Dickson, D. W. (2004). Nonvasculitic autoimmune inflammatory meningoencephalitis. *Neuropathology* **24**: 149–152. PMID 15139593.

865. Lyons, M. K., Caselli, R. J. & Parisi, J. E. (2008). Nonvasculitic autoimmune inflammatory meningoencephalitis as a cause of potentially reversible dementia: report of 4 cases. *Journal of Neurosurgery* **108**: 1024–1027. PMID 18447724.

866. Hoffman Snyder, C., Mishark, K. J., Caviness, J. N., Drazkowski, J. F. & Caselli, R. J. (2006). Nonvasculitic autoimmune inflammatory meningoencephalitis imitating Creutzfeldt–Jakob disease. *Archives of Neurology* **63**: 766–768. PMID 16682549.

867. Trzepacz, P. T. & Francis, J. (1990). Low serum albumin levels and risk of delirium. *American Journal of Psychiatry* **147**: 675. PMID 2327504.

868. Hsu, C. W., Chu, K. A., Lu, T., Lai, R. S. & Lu, J. Y. (1999). Ethambutol-induced psychosis: a case report. *Zhonghua Yi Xue Za Zhi (Chinese Medical Journal, Taipei)* **62**: 724–727. PMID 10533303.
869. Araskiewicz, A. & Rybakowski, J. K. (1994). Hoigne's syndrome: a procaine-induced limbic kindling. *Medical Hypotheses* **42**: 261–264. PMID 8072433.
870. Rao, R. (1999). Penicillin psychosis in later life: Hoigne's syndrome revisited. *Journal of Neuropsychiatry and Clinical Neurosciences* **11**: 517–518. PMID 10570770.
871. Kossoff, E. H., Bergey, G. K., Freeman, J. M. & Vining, E. P. (2001). Levetiracetam psychosis in children with epilepsy. *Epilepsia* **42**: 1611–1613. PMID 11879376.
872. Motamedi, M., Nguyen, D. K., Zaatreh, M., Singh, S. P., Westerveld, M., Thompson, J. L., Mattson, R., Blumenfeld, H., Novotny, E. & Spencer, S. S. (2003). Levetiracetam efficacy in refractory partial-onset seizures, especially after failed epilepsy surgery. *Epilepsia* **44**: 211–214. PMID 12558576.
873. Kober, D. & Gabbard, G. O. (2005). Topiramate-induced psychosis. *American Journal of Psychiatry* **162**: 1542. PMID 16055782.
874. Levinson, D. F. & Devinsky, O. (1999). Psychiatric adverse events during vigabatrin therapy. *Neurology* **53**: 1503–1511. PMID 10534259.
875. Kantrowitz, J. T. & Tampi, R. R. (2008). Risk of psychosis exacerbation by tricyclic antidepressants in unipolar Major Depressive Disorder with psychotic features. *Journal of Affective Disorders* **106**: 279–284. PMID 17764752.
876. Dilsaver, S. C. (1994). Withdrawal phenomena associated with antidepressant and antipsychotic agents. *Drug Safety* **10**: 103–114. PMID 7912078.
877. Dilsaver, S. C. (1988). Monoamine oxidase inhibitor withdrawal phenomena: symptoms and pathophysiology. *Acta Psychiatrica Scandinavica* **78**: 1–7. PMID 2845711.
878. Parker, G. & Blennerhassett, J. (1998). Withdrawal reactions associated with venlafaxine. *Australian and New Zealand Journal of Psychiatry* **32**: 291–294. PMID 9588310.
879. Bruns, J. J. (2006). Toxicity, anticholinergic. eMedicine. URL: http://www.emedicine.com/emerg/topic36.htm. Accessed 11 January 2008.
880. Moncrieff, J. (2006). Why is it so difficult to stop psychiatric drug treatment? It may be nothing to do with the original problem. *Medical Hypotheses* **67**: 517–523. PMID 16632226.
881. Lu, M. L., Pan, J. J., Teng, H. W., Su, K. P. & Shen, W. W. (2002). Metoclopramide-induced supersensitivity psychosis. *Annals of Pharmacotherapy* **36**: 1387–1390. PMID 12196057.
882. Hellden, A., Odar-Cederlof, I., Larsson, K., Fehrman-Ekholm, I. & Linden, T. (2007). Death delusion. *British Medical Journal* **335**: 1305. PMID 18156240.
883. Foster, R., Olajide, D. & Everall, I. P. (2003). Antiretroviral therapy-induced psychosis: case report and brief review of the literature. *HIV Medicine* **4**: 139–144. PMID 12702135.
884. Cullis, P. A. & Cushing, R. (1984). Vidarabine encephalopathy. *Journal of Neurology, Neurosurgery and Psychiatry* **47**: 1351–1354. PMID 6512557.
885. Maxwell, S., Scheftner, W. A., Kessler, H. A. & Busch, K. (1988). Manic syndrome associated with zidovudine treatment. *Journal of the American Medical Association* **259**: 3406–3407. PMID 3163740.
886. Chawla, J. M. & Sagar, R. (2006). Baclofen-induced psychosis. *Annals of Pharmacotherapy* **40**: 2071–2073. PMID 17047139.
887. Rivas, D. A., Chancellor, M. B., Hill, K. & Freedman, M. K. (1993). Neurological manifestations of baclofen withdrawal. *Journal of Urology* **150**: 1903–1905. PMID 8230532.
888. Duncan, J. (1988). Neuropsychiatric aspects of sedative drug withdrawal. *Human Psychopharmacology* **3**: 171–180.
889. Mackay, J. (1969). A case of bromism. *Canadian Medical Association Journal* **100**: 730–731. PMID 5778961.
890. Adler, L. E., Bell, J., Kirch, D., Friedrich, E. & Freedman, R. (1982). Psychosis associated with clonidine withdrawal.

Journal of the American Medical Directors Association **6**: 265–269. PMID 16005413.

931. Rosebraugh, C. J., Flockhart, D. A., Yasuda, S. U. & Woosley, R. L. (2001). Visual hallucination and tremor induced by sertraline and oxycodone in a bone marrow transplant patient. *Journal of Clinical Pharmacology* **41**: 224–227. PMID 11210406.
932. Bastani, J. B., Troester, M. M. & Bastani, A. J. (1996). Serotonin syndrome and fluvoxamine: a case study. *Nebraska Medical Journal* **81**: 107–109. PMID 8628448.
933. Feldman, R. S., Meyer, J. S. & Quenzer, L. F. (1997). *Principles of Neuropsychopharmacology*. Sunderland, MA: Sinauer, Sunderland.
934. Perry, P. J., Alexander, B. & Ellingrod, V. L. (1996). Stimulant psychosis. Virtual Hospital, University of Iowa. URL: http://www.janela1.com/vh/docs/v0002510.htm. Accessed 11 January 2008.
935. Snyder, S. H. (1972). Catecholamines in the brain as mediators of amphetamine psychosis. *Archives of General Psychiatry* **27**: 169–179. PMID 4339577.
936. Bell, D. S. (1965). Comparison of amphetamine psychosis and schizophrenia. *British Journal of Psychiatry* **111**: 701–707. PMID 14337419.
937. Bell, D. S. (1973). The experimental reproduction of amphetamine psychosis. *Archives of General Psychiatry* **29**: 35–40. PMID 4711131.
938. Laruelle, M., Abi-Dargham, A., van Dyck, C. H., Gil, R., D'Souza, C. D., Erdos, J., McCance, E., Rosenblatt, W., Fingado, C., Zoghbi, S. S., Baldwin, R. M., Seibyl, J. P., Krystal, J. H., Charney, D. S. & Innis, R. B. (1996). Single photon emission computerized tomography imaging of amphetamine-induced dopamine release in drug-free schizophrenic subjects. *Proceedings of the National Academy of Sciences of the United States of America* **93**: 9235–9240. PMID 8799184.
939. Abi-Dargham, A., Gil, R., Krystal, J., Baldwin, R. M., Seibyl, J. P., Bowers, M., van Dyck, C. H., Charney, D. S., Innis, R. B. & Laruelle, M. (1998). Increased striatal dopamine transmission in schizophrenia: confirmation in a second cohort. *American Journal of Psychiatry* **155**: 761–767. PMID 9619147.
940. Curran, C., Byrappa, N. & McBride, A. (2004). Stimulant psychosis: systematic review. *British Journal of Psychiatry* **185**: 196–204. PMID 15339823.
941. Yui, K., Goto, K., Ikemoto, S., Ishiguro, T. & Kamada, Y. (1999). Increased sensitivity to stress and episode recurrence in spontaneous recurrence of methamphetamine psychosis. *Psychopharmacology* **145**: 267–272. PMID 10494575.
942. Lucas, P. B., Pickar, D., Kelsoe, J., Rapaport, M., Pato, C. & Hommer, D. (1990). Effects of the acute administration of caffeine in patients with schizophrenia. *Biological Psychiatry* **28**: 35–40. PMID 2375945.
943. Lande, R. G. (2007). Caffeine-related psychiatric disorders. eMedicine. URL: http://www.emedicine.com/med/topic3115.htm. Accessed 29 December 2007.
944. Winston, A. P., Hardwick, E. & Jaberi, N. (2005). Neuropsychiatric effects of caffeine. *Advances in Psychiatric Treatment* **11**: 432–439.
945. Nickell, P. V. & Uhde, T. W. (1994). Dose-response effects of intravenous caffeine in normal volunteers. *Anxiety* **1**: 161–168. PMID 9160568.
946. Perry, P. J., Alexander, B. & Ellingrod, V. L. (1996). Marijuana mental disturbances. Virtual Hospital, University of Iowa. URL: http://www.janela1.com/vh/docs/v0002514.htm. Accessed 11 January 2008.
947. D'Souza, D. C., Perry, E., MacDougall, L., Ammerman, Y., Cooper, T., Wu, Y. T., Braley, G., Gueorguieva, R. & Krystal, J. H. (2004). The psychotomimetic effects of intravenous delta-9-tetrahydrocannabinol in healthy individuals: implications for psychosis. *Neuropsychopharmacology* **29**: 1558–1572. PMID 15173844.
948. D'Souza, D. C., Abi-Saab, W. M., Madonick, S., Forselius-Bielen, K., Doersch, A., Braley, G., Gueorguieva, R., Cooper, T. B. & Krystal, J. H. (2005). Delta-9-tetrahydrocannabinol effects

in schizophrenia: implications for cognition, psychosis, and addiction. *Biological Psychiatry* **57**: 594–608. PMID 15780846.

949. Barnett, J. H., Werners, U., Secher, S. M., Hill, K. E., Brazil, R., Masson, K., Pernet, D. E., Kirkbride, J. B., Murray, G. K., Bullmore, E. T. & Jones, P. B. (2007). Substance use in a population-based clinic sample of people with first-episode psychosis. *British Journal of Psychiatry* **190**: 515–520. PMID 17541112.
950. Zammit, S., Moore, T. H., Lingford-Hughes, A., Barnes, T. R., Jones, P. B., Burke, M. & Lewis, G. (2008). Effects of cannabis use on outcomes of psychotic disorders: systematic review. *British Journal of Psychiatry* **193**: 357–363. PMID 18978312.
951. Moore, T. H., Zammit, S., Lingford-Hughes, A., Barnes, T. R., Jones, P. B., Burke, M. & Lewis, G. (2007). Cannabis use and risk of psychotic or affective mental health outcomes: a systematic review. *Lancet* **370**: 319–328. PMID 17662880.
952. Di Forti, M., Morgan, C., Dazzan, P., Pariante, C., Mondelli, V., Marques, T. R., Handley, R., Luzi, S., Russo, M., Paparelli, A., Butt, A., Stilo, S. A., Wiffen, B., Powell, J. & Murray, R. M. (2009). High-potency cannabis and the risk of psychosis. *British Journal of Psychiatry* **195**: 488–491. PMID 19949195.
953. Morgan, C. J. & Curran, H. V. (2008). Effects of cannabidiol on schizophrenia-like symptoms in people who use cannabis. *British Journal of Psychiatry* **192**: 306–307. PMID 18378995.
954. Machado Rocha, F. C., Stefano, S. C., De Cassia Haiek, R., Rosa Oliveira, L. M. & Da Silveira, D. X. (2008). Therapeutic use of Cannabis sativa on chemotherapy-induced nausea and vomiting among cancer patients: systematic review and meta-analysis. *European Journal of Cancer Care* **17**: 431–443. PMID 18625004.
955. Floyd, A. G., Boutros, N. N., Struve, F. A., Wolf, E. & Oliwa, G. M. (2006). Risk factors for experiencing psychosis during cocaine use: a preliminary report. *Journal of Psychiatric Research* **40**: 178–182. PMID 16048728.
956. Brady, K. T., Lydiard, R. B., Malcolm, R. & Ballenger, J. C. (1991). Cocaine-induced psychosis. *Journal of Clinical Psychiatry* **52**: 509–512. PMID 1752853.
957. Miller, N. S., Gold, M. S. & Mahler, J. C. (1991). Violent behaviors associated with cocaine use: possible pharmacological mechanisms. *International Journal of the Addictions* **26**: 1077–1088. PMID 1683859.
958. Satel, S. L., Southwick, S. M. & Gawin, F. H. (1991). Clinical features of cocaine-induced paranoia. *American Journal of Psychiatry* **148**: 495–498. PMID 2006696.
959. Siegel, R. K. (1978). Cocaine hallucinations. *American Journal of Psychiatry* **135**: 309–314. PMID 626219.
960. Bartlett, E., Hallin, A., Chapman, B. & Angrist, B. (1997). Selective sensitization to the psychosis-inducing effects of cocaine: a possible marker for addiction relapse vulnerability? *Neuropsychopharmacology* **16**: 77–82. PMID 8981391.
961. Fontanilla, D., Johannessen, M., Hajipour, A. R., Cozzi, N. V., Jackson, M. B. & Ruoho, A. E. (2009). The hallucinogen N, N-dimethyltryptamine (DMT) is an endogenous sigma-1 receptor regulator. *Science* **323**: 934–937. PMID 19213917.
962. Larson, M. (2006). Alcohol-related psychosis. eMedicine. URL: http://www.emedicine.com/med/topic3113.htm. Accessed 11 January 2008.
963. Bayard, M., McIntyre, J., Hill, K. R. & Woodside, J., Jr. (2004). Alcohol withdrawal syndrome. *American Family Physician* **69**: 1443–1450. PMID 15053409.
964. Michael, A., Mirza, S., Mirza, K. A., Babu, V. S. & Vithayathil, E. (1995). Morbid jealousy in alcoholism. *British Journal of Psychiatry* **167**: 668–672. PMID 8564326.
965. Kaufman, T., Jauch, E. C. & Cadena, R. S. (2007). Inhalants. eMedicine. URL: http://www.emedicine.com/neuro/topic173.htm. Accessed 11 January 2008.
966. Snead, O. C., 3rd & Gibson, K. M. (2005). Gamma-hydroxybutyric acid. *New England Journal of Medicine* **352**: 2721–2732. PMID 15987921.

967. Constantinides, P. & Vincent, P. (2009). Chronic gamma-hydroxybutyric-acid use followed by gamma-hydroxybutyric-acid withdrawal mimic schizophrenia: a case report. *Cases Journal* **2**: 7520. PMID 19829990.
968. Catalano, M. C., Glass, J. M., Catalano, G., Burrows, S. L., Lynn, W. A. & Weitzner, B. S. (2001). Gamma butyrolactone (GBL) withdrawal syndromes. *Psychosomatics* **42**: 83–88. PMID 11161128.
969. Zvosec, D. L., Smith, S. W., McCutcheon, J. R., Spillane, J., Hall, B. J. & Peacock, E. A. (2001). Adverse events, including death, associated with the use of 1,4-butanediol. *New England Journal of Medicine* **344**: 87–94. PMID 11150358.
970. Nichols, D. E. (2004). Hallucinogens. *Pharmacology and Therapeutics* **101**: 131–181. PMID 14761703.
971. Perry, P. J., Alexander, B. & Ellingrod, V. L. (1996). LSD psychosis. Virtual Hospital, University of Iowa. URL: http://www.janela1.com/vh/docs/v0002512.htm. Accessed 11 January 2008.
972. Toxbase (2010). Mephedrone. UK National Poisons Information Service. URL: http://www.toxbase.org/Poisons-Index-A-Z/M-Products/Mephedrone/. Accessed 27 April 2010.
973. Wood, D. M., Davies, S., Puchnarewicz, M., Button, J., Archer, R., Ovaska, H., Ramsey, J., Lee, T., Holt, D. W. & Dargan, P. I. (2010). Recreational use of mephedrone (4-methylmethcathinone, 4-MMC) with associated sympathomimetic toxicity. *Journal of Medical Toxicology* **6**: 327–330. PMID 20358417.
974. Emerson, T. S. & Cisek, J. E. (1993). Methcathinone: a Russian designer amphetamine infiltrates the rural midwest. *Annals of Emergency Medicine* **22**: 1897–1903. PMID 8239113.
975. O'Reilly, R. L. & Davis, B. A. (1994). Phenylethylamine and schizophrenia. *Progress in Neuro-Psychopharmacology and Biological Psychiatry* **18**: 63–75. PMID 7906896.
976. Iwanami, A., Sugiyama, A., Kuroki, N., Toda, S., Kato, N., Nakatani, Y., Horita, N. & Kaneko, T. (1994). Patients with methamphetamine psychosis admitted to a psychiatric hospital in Japan. A preliminary report. *Acta Psychiatrica Scandinavica* **89**: 428–432. PMID 8085475.
977. Kimko, H. C., Cross, J. T. & Abernethy, D. R. (1999). Pharmacokinetics and clinical effectiveness of methylphenidate. *Clinical Pharmacokinetics* **37**: 457–470. PMID 10628897.
978. Volkow, N. D., Ding, Y. S., Fowler, J. S., Wang, G. J., Logan, J., Gatley, J. S., Dewey, S., Ashby, C., Liebermann, J., Hitzemann, R. & Wolf, A. P. (1995). Is methylphenidate like cocaine? Studies on their pharmacokinetics and distribution in the human brain. *Archives of General Psychiatry* **52**: 456–463. PMID 7771915.
979. Yew, D. & Hahn, I. (2005). Toxicity, MDMA. eMedicine. URL: http://www.emedicine.com/emerg/topic927.htm. Accessed 11 January 2008.
980. Stephens, E. (2007). Toxicity, narcotics. eMedicine. URL: http://www.emedicine.com/emerg/topic330.htm. Accessed 11 January 2008.
981. Perry, P. J., Alexander, B. & Ellingrod, V. L. (1996). Phencyclidine intoxication. Virtual Hospital, University of Iowa. URL: http://www.janela1.com/vh/docs/v0002513.htm. Accessed 11 January 2008.
982. Wilkins, C., Girling, M. & Sweetsur, P. (2007). The prevalence of use, dependency and harms of legal 'party pills' containing benzylpiperazine (BZP) and trifluorophenylmethylpiperazine (TFMPP) in New Zealand. *Journal of Substance Use* **12**: 213–224.
983. Pope, H. G., Jr. & Katz, D. L. (1988). Affective and psychotic symptoms associated with anabolic steroid use. *American Journal of Psychiatry* **145**: 487–490. PMID 3279830.
984. Perry, P. J., Alexander, B. & Ellingrod, V. L. (1996). Steroid-induced mental disturbances. Virtual Hospital, University of Iowa. URL: http://www.janela1.com/vh/docs/v0002511.htm. Accessed 11 January 2008.
985. Fitzgerald, G. M. & Sole, D. P. (2009). CBRNE – incapacitating agents, Agent 15. eMedicine. URL: http://emedicine.medscape.com/article/833238-overview. Accessed 27 April 2010.

986. Raedler, T. J., Knable, M. B., Jones, D. W., Urbina, R. A., Gorey, J. G., Lee, K. S., Egan, M. F., Coppola, R. & Weinberger, D. R. (2003). In vivo determination of muscarinic acetylcholine receptor availability in schizophrenia. *American Journal of Psychiatry* **160**: 118–127. PMID 12505810.

987. Perry, P. J., Alexander, B. & Ellingrod, V. L. (1996). Anticholinergic psychosis. Virtual Hospital, University of Iowa. URL: http://www.janela1.com/vh/docs/v0002509.htm. Accessed 11 January 2008.

988. Tune, L. & Coyle, J. T. (1980). Serum levels of anticholinergic drugs in treatment of acute extrapyramidal side effects. *Archives of General Psychiatry* **37**: 293–297. PMID 6102457.

989. Mach, J. R., Jr., Dysken, M. W., Kuskowski, M., Richelson, E., Holden, L. & Jilk, K. M. (1995). Serum anticholinergic activity in hospitalized older persons with delirium: a preliminary study. *Journal of the American Geriatrics Society* **43**: 491–495. PMID 7730529.

990. Tune, L. E., Damlouji, N. F., Holland, A., Gardner, T. J., Folstein, M. F. & Coyle, J. T. (1981). Association of postoperative delirium with raised serum levels of anticholinergic drugs. *Lancet* **2**: 651–653. PMID 6116042.

991. Weil, A. T. & Davis, W. (1994). Bufo alvarius: a potent hallucinogen of animal origin. *Journal of Ethnopharmacology* **41**: 1–8. PMID 8170151.

992. Costa, T. O., Morales, R. A., Brito, J. P., Gordo, M., Pinto, A. C. & Bloch, C., Jr. (2005). Occurrence of bufotenin in the Osteocephalus genus (Anura: Hylidae). *Toxicon* **46**: 371–375. PMID 16054186.

993. de Haro, L. & Pommier, P. (2006). Hallucinatory fish poisoning (ichthyoallyeinotoxism): two case reports from the Western Mediterranean and literature review. *Clinical Toxicology (Philadelphia, Pa.)* **44**: 185–188. PMID 16615678.

994. Gable, R. S. (2007). Risk assessment of ritual use of oral dimethyltryptamine (DMT) and harmala alkaloids. *Addiction* **102**: 24–34. PMID 17207120.

995. Blackledge, R. D. & Taylor, C. M. (2003). Psychotria viridis – a botanical source of dimethyltryptamine (DMT). *Microgram Journal (US Drug Enforcement Administration, Office of Forensic Sciences)* **1**: 18–22.

996. Przekop, P. & Lee, T. (2009). Persistent psychosis associated with salvia divinorum use. *American Journal of Psychiatry* **166**: 832. PMID 19570943.

997. Willmore-Fordham, C. B., Krall, D. M., McCurdy, C. R. & Kinder, D. H. (2007). The hallucinogen derived from Salvia divinorum, salvinorin A, has kappa-opioid agonist discriminative stimulus effects in rats. *Neuropharmacology* **53**: 481–486. PMID 17681558.

998. Paulzen, M. & Grunder, G. (2008). Toxic psychosis after intake of the hallucinogen salvinorin A. *Journal of Clinical Psychiatry* **69**: 1501–1502. PMID 19193352.

999. Valdes, L. J., 3rd (1994). Salvia divinorum and the unique diterpene hallucinogen, Salvinorin (divinorin) A. *Journal of Psychoactive Drugs* **26**: 277–283. PMID 7844657.

1000. Bucheler, R., Gleiter, C. H., Schwoerer, P. & Gaertner, I. (2005). Use of nonprohibited hallucinogenic plants: increasing relevance for public health? A case report and literature review on the consumption of Salvia divinorum (Diviner's Sage). *Pharmacopsychiatry* **38**: 1–5. PMID 15706458.

1001. Siebert, D. J. (1994). Salvia divinorum and salvinorin A: new pharmacologic findings. *Journal of Ethnopharmacology* **43**: 53–56. PMID 7526076.

1002. Albertson, D. N. & Grubbs, L. E. (2009). Subjective effects of Salvia divinorum: LSD- or marijuana-like? *Journal of Psychoactive Drugs* **41**: 213–217. PMID 19999674.

1003. Eadie, M. J. (2003). Convulsive ergotism: epidemics of the serotonin syndrome? *Lancet Neurology* **2**: 429–434. PMID 12849122.

1004. Waldron, H. A. (1983). Did the Mad Hatter have mercury poisoning? *British Medical Journal (Clinical Research Edition)* **287**: 1961. PMID 6418283.

1005. Agency for Toxic Substances and Disease Registry (1999). Toxicological profile for mercury. US Department of Health and Human Services, Public Health Service, Agency for Toxic Substances and Disease Registry, Atlanta, Georgia.

1006. McAlpine, D. & Araki, S. (1958). Minamata disease: an unusual neurological disorder caused by contaminated fish. *Lancet* **2**: 629–631. PMID 13588955.

1007. Clarkson, T. W., Magos, L. & Myers, G. J. (2003). The toxicology of mercury – current exposures and clinical manifestations. *New England Journal of Medicine* **349**: 1731–1737. PMID 14585942.

1008. Padlewska, K. K. & Schwartz, R. A. (2007). Acrodynia. eMedicine. URL: http://www.emedicine.com/derm/topic592.htm. Accessed 20 December 2007.

1009. Olson, D. A. (2006). Mercury. eMedicine. URL: http://www.emedicine.com/neuro/topic617.htm. Accessed 20 December 2007.

1010. Michaeli-Yossef, Y., Berkovitch, M. & Goldman, M. (2007). Mercury intoxication in a 2-year-old girl: a diagnostic challenge for the physician. *Pediatric Nephrology* **22**: 903–906. PMID 17310361.

1011. Agency for Toxic Substances and Disease Registry (2007). Toxicological profile for arsenic. US Department of Health and Human Services, Public Health Service, Agency for Toxic Substances and Disease Registry, Atlanta, Georgia.

1012. Soghoian, S. & Sinert, R. (2006). Toxicity, heavy metals. eMedicine. URL: http://www.emedicine.com/emerg/topic237.htm. Accessed 20 December 2007.

1013. Agency for Toxic Substances and Disease Registry (1992). Toxicological profile for thallium. US Department of Health and Human Services, Public Health Service, Agency for Toxic Substances and Disease Registry, Atlanta, Georgia.

1014. Jha, S. & Kumar, R. (2006). Thallium poisoning presenting as paresthesias, paresis, psychosis and pain in abdomen. *Journal of the Association of Physicians of India* **54**: 53–55. PMID 16649741.

1015. Tsai, Y. T., Huang, C. C., Kuo, H. C., Wang, H. M., Shen, W. S., Shih, T. S. & Chu, N. S. (2006). Central nervous system effects in acute thallium poisoning. *Neurotoxicology* **27**: 291–295. PMID 16337004.

1016. Moss, M. A. & Cooper, P. J. (1986). Gasoline sniffing and lead poisoning. *Acta Pharmacologica et Toxicologica* **59 Suppl 7**: 48–51. PMID 3776613.

1017. Morgan, B. W., Barnes, L., Parramore, C. S. & Kaufmann, R. B. (2003). Elevated blood lead levels associated with the consumption of moonshine among emergency department patients in Atlanta, Georgia. *Annals of Emergency Medicine* **42**: 351–358. PMID 12944887.

1018. Wiwanitkit, V. & Suwansaksri, J. (2006). Lead intoxication: a summary of the clinical presentation among Thai patients. *Biometals* **19**: 345–348. PMID 16841244.

1019. Badawy, M. & Conners, G. P. (2006). Toxicity, lead. eMedicine. URL: http://www.emedicine.com/ped/topic1285.htm. Accessed 14 December 2007.

1020. Needleman, H. L. (1997). Clamped in a straitjacket: the insertion of lead into gasoline. *Environmental Research* **74**: 95–103. PMID 9339221.

1021. Agency for Toxic Substances and Disease Registry (2007). Toxicological profile for lead. US Department of Health and Human Services, Public Health Service, Agency for Toxic Substances and Disease Registry, Atlanta, Georgia.

1022. Mani, J., Chaudhary, N., Kanjalkar, M. & Shah, P. U. (1998). Cerebellar ataxia due to lead encephalopathy in an adult. *Journal of Neurology, Neurosurgery and Psychiatry* **65**: 797. PMID 9810963.

1023. Sinha, S., Gascon, P., Schwartz, R. A. & Shumate, M. J. (2006). ALA dehydratase deficiency porphyria. eMedicine. URL: http://www.emedicine.com/med/topic90.htm. Accessed 18 January 2008.

1024. Marcus, S. (2007). Toxicity, lead. eMedicine. URL: http://www.emedicine.com/emerg/topic293.htm. Accessed 14 December 2007.

1025. Finkelstein, Y., Milatovic, D. & Aschner, M. (2007). Modulation of cholinergic systems by manganese. *Neurotoxicology* **28**: 1003–1014. PMID 17920128.
1026. Meral, H., Kutukcu, Y., Atmaca, B., Ozer, F. & Hamamcioglu, K. (2007). Parkinsonism caused by chronic usage of intravenous potassium permanganate. *Neurologist* **13**: 92–94. PMID 17351530.
1027. Rahelic, D., Kujundzic, M., Romic, Z., Brkic, K. & Petrovecki, M. (2006). Serum concentration of zinc, copper, manganese and magnesium in patients with liver cirrhosis. *Collegium Antropologicum* **30**: 523–528. PMID 17058518.
1028. Fitsanakis, V. A., Zhang, N., Avison, M. J., Gore, J. C., Aschner, J. L. & Aschner, M. (2006). The use of magnetic resonance imaging (MRI) in the study of manganese neurotoxicity. *Neurotoxicology* **27**: 798–806. PMID 16620989.
1029. Agency for Toxic Substances and Disease Registry (2000). Toxicological profile for manganese. US Department of Health and Human Services, Public Health Service, Agency for Toxic Substances and Disease Registry, Atlanta, Georgia.
1030. Reynolds, N., Blumsohn, A., Baxter, J. P., Houston, G. & Pennington, C. R. (1998). Manganese requirement and toxicity in patients on home parenteral nutrition. *Clinical Nutrition* **17**: 227–230. PMID 10205343.
1031. Alves, G., Thiebot, J., Tracqui, A., Delangre, T., Guedon, C. & Lerebours, E. (1997). Neurologic disorders due to brain manganese deposition in a jaundiced patient receiving long-term parenteral nutrition. *JPEN: Journal of Parenteral and Enteral Nutrition* **21**: 41–45. PMID 9002084.
1032. Shin, Y. C., Kim, E., Cheong, H. K., Cho, S., Sakong, J., Kim, K. S., Yang, J. S., Jin, Y. W., Kang, S. K. & Kim, Y. (2007). High signal intensity on magnetic resonance imaging as a predictor of neurobehavioral performance of workers exposed to manganese. *Neurotoxicology* **28**: 257–262. PMID 16647136.
1033. Herrero Hernandez, E., Discalzi, G., Valentini, C., Venturi, F., Chio, A., Carmellino, C., Rossi, L., Sacchetti, A. & Pira, E. (2006). Follow-up of patients affected by manganese-induced Parkinsonism after treatment with CaNa2EDTA. *Neurotoxicology* **27**: 333–339. PMID 16271769.
1034. Akintonwa, A., Mabadeje, A. F. & Odutola, T. A. (1989). Fatal poisonings by copper sulfate ingested from "spiritual water". *Veterinary and Human Toxicology* **31**: 453–454. PMID 2603365.
1035. Beer, S. T., Bradberry, S. M. & Vale, J. A. (1998). Copper sulphate [UKPID monograph]. UK National Poisons Information Service. URL: http://www.intox.org/databank/documents/chemical/copsulf/ukpid56.htm. Accessed 20 December 2007.
1036. Hoveyda, N., Yates, B., Bond, C. R. & Hunter, P. R. (2003). A cluster of cases of abdominal pain possibly associated with high copper levels in a private water supply. *Journal of Environmental Health* **66**: 29–32. PMID 12971043.
1037. Agency for Toxic Substances and Disease Registry (2004). Toxicological profile for copper. US Department of Health and Human Services, Public Health Service, Agency for Toxic Substances and Disease Registry, Atlanta, Georgia.
1038. Eife, R., Weiss, M., Barros, V., Sigmund, B., Goriup, U., Komb, D., Wolf, W., Kittel, J., Schramel, P. & Reiter, K. (1999). Chronic poisoning by copper in tap water: I. Copper intoxications with predominantly gastointestinal symptoms. *European Journal of Medical Research* **4**: 219–223. PMID 10383875.
1039. Eife, R., Weiss, M., Muller-Hocker, M., Lang, T., Barros, V., Sigmund, B., Thanner, F., Welling, P., Lange, H., Wolf, W., Rodeck, B., Kittel, J., Schramel, P. & Reiter, K. (1999). Chronic poisoning by copper in tap water: II. Copper intoxications with predominantly systemic symptoms. *European Journal of Medical Research* **4**: 224–228. PMID 10383876.

1040. Burn, D. J. & Bates, D. (1998). Neurology and the kidney. *Journal of Neurology, Neurosurgery and Psychiatry* **65**: 810–821. PMID 9854955.

1041. Bradberry, S. M., Beer, S. T. & Vale, J. A. (2006). Bismuth [UKPID monograph]. UK National Poisons Information Service. URL: http://www.intox.org/databank/documents/chemical/bismuth/ukpid49.htm. Accessed 18 April 2008.

1042. Momcilovic, B. (1999). A case report of acute human molybdenum toxicity from a dietary molybdenum supplement – a new member of the "Lucor metallicum" family. *Arhiv za Higijenu Rada i Toksikologiju* **50**: 289–297. PMID 10649845.

1043. Olson, K. R. (1984). Carbon monoxide poisoning: mechanisms, presentation, and controversies in management. *Journal of Emergency Medicine* **1**: 233–243. PMID 6491241.

1044. Prockop, L. D. & Chichkova, R. I. (2007). Carbon monoxide intoxication: an updated review. *Journal of the Neurological Sciences* **262**: 122–130. PMID 17720201.

1045. Smith, J. S. & Brandon, S. (1973). Morbidity from acute carbon monoxide poisoning at three-year follow-up. *British Medical Journal* **1**: 318–321.

1046. Pae, C. U., Kim, T. S., Lee, C. & Paik, I. H. (2006). Effect of aripiprazole for a patient with psychotic symptoms and parkinsonism associated with delayed-sequelae of carbon monoxide intoxication. *Journal of Neuropsychiatry and Clinical Neurosciences* **18**: 130–131. PMID 16525083.

1047. Thacker, A. K., Asthana, A. B. & Sarkari, N. B. (1995). Delayed post-anoxic encephalopathy. *Postgraduate Medical Journal* **71**: 373–374. PMID 7644404.

1048. Mizutani, T., Shiozawa, R., Takemori, S., Tsurumaru, M. & Akiyama, H. (1993). Delayed post-anoxic encephalopathy without relation to carbon monoxide poisoning. *Internal Medicine* **32**: 430–433. PMID 8400510.

1049. Agency for Toxic Substances and Disease Registry (1992). Toxicological profile for bromomethane. US Department of Health and Human Services, Public Health Service, Agency for Toxic Substances and Disease Registry, Atlanta, Georgia.

1050. Zatuchni, J. & Hong, K. (1981). Methyl bromide poisoning seen initially as psychosis. *Archives of Neurology* **38**: 529–530. PMID 7247792.

1051. Agency for Toxic Substances and Disease Registry (1996). Toxicological profile for carbon disulfide. US Department of Health and Human Services, Public Health Service, Agency for Toxic Substances and Disease Registry, Atlanta, Georgia.

1052. US Environmental Protection Agency (2004). Carbon disulfide: interim acute exposure guideline levels (AEGLs). US Environmental Protection Agency, Atlanta, Georgia.

1053. Dumont, M. P. (1989). Psychotoxicology: the return of the mad hatter. *Social Science and Medicine* **29**: 1077–1082. PMID 2683123.

1054. Agency for Toxic Substances and Disease Registry (2000). Toxicological profile for endosulfan. US Department of Health and Human Services, Public Health Service, Agency for Toxic Substances and Disease Registry, Atlanta, Georgia.

1055. Agency for Toxic Substances and Disease Registry (2005). Toxicological profile for alpha-, beta-, gamma-, and delta-hexachlorocyclohexane. US Department of Health and Human Services, Public Health Service, Agency for Toxic Substances and Disease Registry, Atlanta, Georgia.

1056. Agency for Toxic Substances and Disease Registry (1995). Toxicological profile for mirex and chlordecone. US Department of Health and Human Services, Public Health Service, Agency for Toxic Substances and Disease Registry, Atlanta, Georgia.

1057. Bradberry, S. M., Watt, B. E., Proudfoot, A. T. & Vale, J. A. (2000). Mechanisms of toxicity, clinical features, and management of acute chlorophenoxy herbicide poisoning: a review. *Journal of Toxicology. Clinical Toxicology* **38**: 111–122. PMID 10778907.

1058. Agency for Toxic Substances and Disease Registry (2006). Toxicological profile for cyanide. US Department of Health and Human Services, Public Health Service, Agency for Toxic Substances and Disease Registry, Atlanta, Georgia.

1059. Agency for Toxic Substances and Disease Registry (1990). Toxicological profile for acrylonitrile. US Department of Health and Human Services, Public Health Service, Agency for Toxic Substances and Disease Registry, Atlanta, Georgia.

1060. Keyes, D. C. (2010). Toxicity, ethylene glycol. eMedicine. URL: http://emedicine.medscape.com/article/814701-overview. Accessed 30 April 2010.

1061. Scalley, R. D., Ferguson, D. R., Piccaro, J. C., Smart, M. L. & Archie, T. E. (2002). Treatment of ethylene glycol poisoning. *American Family Physician* **66**: 807–812. PMID 12322772.

1062. Piagnerelli, M., Lejeune, P. & Vanhaeverbeek, M. (1999). Diagnosis and treatment of an unusual cause of metabolic acidosis: ethylene glycol poisoning. *Acta Clinica Belgica* **54**: 351–356. PMID 10686708.

1063. Agency for Toxic Substances and Disease Registry (2006). Toxicological profile for hydrogen sulfide. US Department of Health and Human Services, Public Health Service, Agency for Toxic Substances and Disease Registry, Atlanta, Georgia.

1064. Rey, C., Reinecke, H. J. & Besser, R. (1984). Methyltin intoxication in six men; toxicologic and clinical aspects. *Veterinary and Human Toxicology* **26**: 121–122. PMID 6730297.

1065. Agency for Toxic Substances and Disease Registry (2004). DEET (N, N-diethylmeta-toluamide) [consultation]. US Department of Health and Human Services, Public Health Service, Agency for Toxic Substances and Disease Registry. URL: http://www.atsdr.cdc.gov/consultations/deet/index.html. Accessed 4 November 2010.

1066. Hampers, L. C., Oker, E. & Leikin, J. B. (1999). Topical use of DEET insect repellent as a cause of severe encephalopathy in a healthy adult male. *Academic Emergency Medicine* **6**: 1295–1297. PMID 10609933.

1067. Snyder, J. W., Poe, R. O., Stubbins, J. F. & Garrettson, L. K. (1986). Acute manic psychosis following the dermal application of N, N-diethyl-m-toluamide (DEET) in an adult. *Journal of Toxicology. Clinical Toxicology* **24**: 429–439. PMID 3783806.

1068. Katz, K. D., Brooks, D. E., Furtado, M. C. & Chan, L. (2008). Toxicity, organophosphorus. eMedicine. URL: http://www.emedicine.com/med/topic1677.htm. Accessed 21 October 2008.

1069. Merrill, D. G. & Mihm, F. G. (1982). Prolonged toxicity of organophosphate poisoning. *Critical Care Medicine* **10**: 550–551. PMID 7094603.

1070. Agency for Toxic Substances and Disease Registry (2000). Toxicological profile for toluene. US Department of Health and Human Services, Public Health Service, Agency for Toxic Substances and Disease Registry, Atlanta, Georgia.

1071. Agency for Toxic Substances and Disease Registry (1997). Toxicological profile for trichloroethylene. US Department of Health and Human Services, Public Health Service, Agency for Toxic Substances and Disease Registry, Atlanta, Georgia.

1072. Haupt, R. (1977). [Acute symptomatic psychosis in vitamin A intoxication (author's translation)]. *Nervenarzt* **48**: 91–95. PMID 840348.

1073. Restak, R. M. (1972). Pseudotumor cerebri, psychosis, and hypervitaminosis A. *Journal of Nervous and Mental Disease* **155**: 72–75. PMID 4260849.

1074. O'Donnell, J. (2004). Polar hysteria: an expression of hypervitaminosis A. *American Journal of Therapeutics* **11**: 507–516. PMID 15543093.

1075. Rodahl, K. & Moore, T. (1943). The vitamin A content and toxicity of bear and seal liver. *Biochemical Journal* **37**: 166–168. PMID 16747610.

1076. Eledrisi, M. S., McKinney, K. & Shanti, M. S. (2009). Vitamin A toxicity. URL: http://emedicine.medscape.com/article/126104-overview. Accessed 8 November 2009.
1077. Agency for Toxic Substances and Disease Registry (1997). Toxicological profile for white phosphorus. US Department of Health and Human Services, Public Health Service, Agency for Toxic Substances and Disease Registry, Atlanta, Georgia.
1078. Stores, G. (2007). Clinical diagnosis and misdiagnosis of sleep disorders. *Journal of Neurology, Neurosurgery and Psychiatry* **78**: 1293–1297. PMID 18024690.
1079. Ohayon, M. M. (2000). Prevalence of hallucinations and their pathological associations in the general population. *Psychiatry Research* **97**: 153–164. PMID 11166087.
1080. Connelly, K. P. (2008). Sleep disorder: night terrors. eMedicine. URL: http://emedicine.medscape.com/article/914360-overview. Accessed 16 June 2009.
1081. Wright, J. B. (1993). Mania following sleep deprivation. *British Journal of Psychiatry* **163**: 679–680. PMID 8298841.
1082. Babkoff, H., Sing, H. C., Thorne, D. R., Genser, S. G. & Hegge, F. W. (1989). Perceptual distortions and hallucinations reported during the course of sleep deprivation. *Perceptual and Motor Skills* **68**: 787–798. PMID 2748294.
1083. Sharafkhaneh, A., Giray, N., Richardson, P., Young, T. & Hirshkowitz, M. (2005). Association of psychiatric disorders and sleep apnea in a large cohort. *Sleep* **28**: 1405–1411. PMID 16335330.
1084. Karanti, A. & Landen, M. (2007). Treatment refractory psychosis remitted upon treatment with continuous positive airway pressure: a case report. *Psychopharmacology Bulletin* **40**: 113–117. PMID 17285102.
1085. Downey, R., Gold, P. M. & Wickramasinghe, H. (2006). Obstructive sleep apnea. eMedicine. URL: http://www.emedicine.com/med/topic163.htm. Accessed 18 April 2008.
1086. Fayyaz, J. & Lessnau, K. (2009). Hypoventilation syndromes. eMedicine. URL: http://emedicine.medscape.com/article/304381-overview. Accessed 15 November 2009.
1087. Vourdas, A., Shneerson, J. M., Gregory, C. A., Smith, I. E., King, M. A., Morrish, E. & McKenna, P. J. (2002). Narcolepsy and psychopathology: is there an association? *Sleep Medicine* **3**: 353–360. PMID 14592199.
1088. Baker, M. J. & Benbadis, S. R. (2007). Narcolepsy. eMedicine. URL: http://www.emedicine.com/neuro/topic522.htm. Accessed 18 April 2008.
1089. Sharma, S. (2007). Primary hypersomnia. eMedicine. URL: http://www.emedicine.com/med/topic3129.htm. Accessed 18 April 2008.
1090. Cochen, V., Arnulf, I., Demeret, S., Neulat, M. L., Gourlet, V., Drouot, X., Moutereau, S., Derenne, J. P., Similowski, T., Willer, J. C., Pierrot-Deseilligny, C. & Bolgert, F. (2005). Vivid dreams, hallucinations, psychosis and REM sleep in Guillain–Barre syndrome. *Brain* **128**: 2535–2545. PMID 16000335.
1091. Appelberg, B., Katila, H. & Rimon, R. (2002). REM sleep and prolactin in patients with non-affective psychoses. *Psychoneuroendocrinology* **27**: 661–669. PMID 12084659.
1092. Poulin, J., Daoust, A. M., Forest, G., Stip, E. & Godbout, R. (2003). Sleep architecture and its clinical correlates in first episode and neuroleptic-naive patients with schizophrenia. *Schizophrenia Research* **62**: 147–153. PMID 12765755.
1093. Merabet, L. B., Maguire, D., Warde, A., Alterescu, K., Stickgold, R. & Pascual-Leone, A. (2004). Visual hallucinations during prolonged blindfolding in sighted subjects. *Journal of Neuro-Ophthalmology* **24**: 109–113. PMID 15179062.
1094. Casey, D. A. & Wandzilak, T. (1988). Senile macular degeneration and psychosis. *Journal of Geriatric Psychiatry and Neurology* **1**: 108–109. PMID 3252878.

1095. Miller, T. C. & Crosby, T. W. (1979). Musical hallucinations in a deaf elderly patient. *Annals of Neurology* **5**: 301–302. PMID 443762.
1096. Howard, R., Almeida, O. & Levy, R. (1994). Phenomenology, demography and diagnosis in late paraphrenia. *Psychological Medicine* **24**: 397–410. PMID 8084935.
1097. Pasquini, F. & Cole, M. G. (1997). Idiopathic musical hallucinations in the elderly. *Journal of Geriatric Psychiatry and Neurology* **10**: 11–14. PMID 9100153.
1098. Berrios, G. E. (1990). Musical hallucinations. A historical and clinical study. *British Journal of Psychiatry* **156**: 188–194. PMID 2180526.
1099. Wu, C. Y. & Chiu, C. C. (2006). Usher syndrome with psychotic symptoms: two cases in the same family. *Psychiatry and Clinical Neurosciences* **60**: 626–628. PMID 16958948.
1100. Teunisse, R. J., Cruysberg, J. R., Hoefnagels, W. H., Verbeek, A. L. & Zitman, F. G. (1996). Visual hallucinations in psychologically normal people: Charles Bonnet's syndrome. *Lancet* **347**: 794–797. PMID 8622335.
1101. Teunisse, R. J., Cruysberg, J. R., Verbeek, A. & Zitman, F. G. (1995). The Charles Bonnet syndrome: a large prospective study in The Netherlands. A study of the prevalence of the Charles Bonnet syndrome and associated factors in 500 patients attending the University Department of Ophthalmology at Nijmegen. *British Journal of Psychiatry* **166**: 254–257. PMID 7728372.
1102. Grassian, S. (1983). Psychopathological effects of solitary confinement. *American Journal of Psychiatry* **140**: 1450–1454. PMID 6624990.
1103. Lilly, J. C. (1956). Mental effects of reduction of ordinary levels of physical stimuli on intact, healthy persons. *Psychiatric Research Reports* **30**: 1–9; discussion, 10–28. PMID 13359559.
1104. Wexler, D., Mendelson, J., Leiderman, P. H. & Solomon, P. (1958). Sensory deprivation; a technique for studying psychiatric aspects of stress. *American Medical Association Archives of Neurology and Psychiatry* **79**: 225–233. PMID 13497369.
1105. Leff, J. P. (1968). Perceptual phenomena and personality in sensory deprivation. *British Journal of Psychiatry* **114**: 1499–1508. PMID 5717931.
1106. Bexton, W. H., Heron, W. & Scott, R. H. (1954). Effects of decreased variation in the sensory environment. *Canadian Journal of Psychology* **8**: 70–76. PMID 13160864.
1107. Heron, W., Doane, B. K. & Scott, T. H. (1956). Visual disturbances after prolonged perceptual isolation. *Canadian Journal of Psychology* **10**: 13–18. PMID 13293922.
1108. US Central Intelligence Agency (1963). KUBARK counterintelligence interrogation. The National Security Archive, The George Washington University, Washington, DC. URL: http://www.gwu.edu/~nsarchiv/NSAEBB/NSAEBB122/index.htm. Accessed 4 April 2008.
1109. Ghezzi, A. & Zaffaroni, M. (2001). Neurological manifestations of gastrointestinal disorders, with particular reference to the differential diagnosis of multiple sclerosis. *Neurological Sciences* **22** Suppl 2: S117–122. PMID 11794474.
1110. Ludvigsson, J. F., Osby, U., Ekbom, A. & Montgomery, S. M. (2007). Coeliac disease and risk of schizophrenia and other psychosis: a general population cohort study. *Scandinavian Journal of Gastroenterology* **42**: 179–185. PMID 17327937.
1111. Eaton, W. W., Byrne, M., Ewald, H., Mors, O., Chen, C. Y., Agerbo, E. & Mortensen, P. B. (2006). Association of schizophrenia and autoimmune diseases: linkage of Danish national registers. *American Journal of Psychiatry* **163**: 521–528. PMID 16513876.
1112. West, J., Logan, R. F., Hubbard, R. B. & Card, T. R. (2006). Risk of schizophrenia in people with coeliac disease, ulcerative colitis and Crohn's disease: a general population-based study. *Alimentary Pharmacology and Therapeutics* **23**: 71–74. PMID 16393282.

1113. Campbell, E. B. & Foley, S. (2004). Coeliac disease and schizophrenia: data do not support hypothesis. *British Medical Journal* **328**: 1017; author reply 1017. PMID 15105338.
1114. Cascella, N. G., Kryszak, D., Bhatti, B., Gregory, P., Kelly, D. L., McEvoy, J. P., Fasano, A. & Eaton, W. W. (2009). Prevalence of celiac disease and gluten sensitivity in the United States Clinical Antipsychotic Trials of Intervention Effectiveness study population. *Schizophrenia Bulletin* [ePub ahead of print]. PMID 19494248.
1115. Kalaydjian, A. E., Eaton, W., Cascella, N. & Fasano, A. (2006). The gluten connection: the association between schizophrenia and celiac disease. *Acta Psychiatrica Scandinavica* **113**: 82–90. PMID 16423158.
1116. Wei, J. & Hemmings, G. P. (2005). Gene, gut and schizophrenia: the meeting point for the gene-environment interaction in developing schizophrenia. *Medical Hypotheses* **64**: 547–552. PMID 15617864.
1117. Rothschild, B. M. (2008). Hypereosinophilic syndrome. eMedicine. URL: http://www.emedicine.com/ped/topic1069.htm. Accessed 12 October 2008.
1118. Weller, P. F. & Bubley, G. J. (1994). The idiopathic hypereosinophilic syndrome. *Blood* **83**: 2759–2779. PMID 8180373.
1119. Roufosse, F., Goldman, M. & Cogan, E. (2004). Idiopathic hypereosinophilic syndrome. Orphanet encyclopedia. URL: http://www.orpha.net/data/patho/GB/uk-IdiopHypereosinophSyndr.pdf. Accessed 21 July 2010.
1120. de Deus-Silva, L., de Souza Queiroz, L., de Araújo Zanardi, V., Ghizoni, E., de Costa Pereira, H., Malveira, G. L., Pirani, C., Jr., Damasceno, B. P. & Cendes, F. (2003). Hypertrophic pachymeningitis: case report. *Arquivos de Neuro-Psiquiatria* **61**: 107–111. PMID 12715031.
1121. Masson, C., Henin, D., Hauw, J. J., Rey, A., Raverdy, P. & Masson, M. (1993). Cranial pachymeningitis of unknown origin: a study of seven cases. *Neurology* **43**: 1329–1334. PMID 8327133.
1122. Loganovsky, K. N. & Loganovskaja, T. K. (2000). Schizophrenia spectrum disorders in persons exposed to ionizing radiation as a result of the Chernobyl accident. *Schizophrenia Bulletin* **26**: 751–773. PMID 11087010.
1123. Agency for Toxic Substances and Disease Registry (1999). Toxicological profile for ionizing radiation. US Department of Health and Human Services, Public Health Service, Agency for Toxic Substances and Disease Registry, Atlanta, Georgia.
1124. Bruinvels, J. & Pepplinkhuizen, L. (1984). Impaired glycine-serine conversion and increased plasma taurine levels in episodic psychotic patients with psychedelic symptoms. *Journal of Psychiatric Research* **18**: 307–318. PMID 6436485.
1125. Fekkes, D., Pepplinkhuizen, L., Verheij, R. & Bruinvels, J. (1994). Abnormal plasma levels of serine, methionine, and taurine in transient acute polymorphic psychosis. *Psychiatry Research* **51**: 11–18. PMID 8197268.
1126. Sharma, G. K. & Prisant, L. M. (2007). Atrial myxoma. eMedicine. URL: http://emedicine.medscape.com/article/151362-overview. Accessed 15 May 2009.
1127. Ekinci, E. I. & Donnan, G. A. (2004). Neurological manifestations of cardiac myxoma: a review of the literature and report of cases. *Internal Medicine Journal* **34**: 243–249. PMID 15151670.
1128. Saravay, S. M. & Gupta, A. K. (1998). Atrial myxoma with psychiatric presentation. *Psychosomatics* **39**: 453–455. PMID 9775704.
1129. Boza, R. A. & Liggett, S. B. (1981). Pseudohallucinations: radio reception through shrapnel fragments. *American Journal of Psychiatry* **138**: 1263–1264. PMID 7270748.
1130. Bush, G., Fink, M., Petrides, G., Dowling, F. & Francis, A. (1996). Catatonia. I. Rating scale and standardized examination. *Acta Psychiatrica Scandinavica* **93**: 129–136. PMID 8686483.
1131. Braunig, P., Kruger, S., Shugar, G., Hoffler, J. & Borner, I. (2000). The

catatonia rating scale I – development, reliability, and use. *Comprehensive Psychiatry* **41**: 147–158. PMID 10741894.

1132. Taylor, M. A. & Fink, M. (2003). Catatonia in psychiatric classification: a home of its own. *American Journal of Psychiatry* **160**: 1233–1241. PMID 12832234.

1133. Costall, B. & Olley, J. E. (1971). Cholinergic- and neuroleptic-induced catalepsy: modification by lesions in the caudate-putamen. *Neuropharmacology* **10**: 297–306. PMID 5104497.

1134. Tonkonogy, J., Sholevar, D. P. & Sholevar, E. H. (2006). Neuroleptic malignant syndrome. eMedicine. URL: http://www.emedicine.com/med/topic2614.htm. Accessed 9 December 2008.

1135. Stefan, M., Travis, M. & Murray, R. M. (2002). *An Atlas of Schizophrenia*. London: Parthenon.

1136. World Health Organization (2007). World Health Organization: ICD-10: International Statistical Classification of Diseases and Related Health Problems, 10th Revision, Version for 2007. URL: http://www.who.int/classifications/apps/icd/icd10online/. Accessed 14 December 2007.

1137. Rohricht, F. & Priebe, S. (2002). Do cenesthesias and body image aberration characterize a subgroup in schizophrenia? *Acta Psychiatrica Scandinavica* **105**: 276–282. PMID 11942932.

1138. Goldner, E. M., Hsu, L., Waraich, P. & Somers, J. M. (2002). Prevalence and incidence studies of schizophrenic disorders: a systematic review of the literature. *Canadian Journal of Psychiatry* **47**: 833–843. PMID 12500753.

1139. Kessler, R. C., Angermeyer, M., Anthony, J. C., De Graaf, R., Demyttenaere, K., Gasquet, I., De Girolamo, G., Gluzman, S., Gureje, O., Haro, J. M., Kawakami, N., Karam, A., Levinson, D., Medina Mora, M. E., Oakley Browne, M. A., Posada-Villa, J., Stein, D. J., Aguilar-Gaxiola, S., Alonso, J., Lee, S., Heeringa, S., Pennell, B. E., Berglund, P., Gruber, M. J., Petukhova, M., Chatterji, S. & Ustün, T.B. (2007). Lifetime prevalence and age-of-onset distributions of mental disorders in the World Health Organization's World Mental Health Survey Initiative. *World Psychiatry* **6**: 168–176. PMID 18188442.

1140. Lewis, D. A. & Lieberman, J. A. (2000). Catching up on schizophrenia: natural history and neurobiology. *Neuron* **28**: 325–334. PMID 11144342.

1141. Lieberman, J. A., Drake, R. E., Sederer, L. I., Belger, A., Keefe, R., Perkins, D. & Stroup, S. (2008). Science and recovery in schizophrenia. *Psychiatric Services* **59**: 487–496. PMID 18451003.

1142. Bora, E., Yucel, M. & Pantelis, C. (2010). Cognitive impairment in schizophrenia and affective psychoses: implications for DSM-V criteria and beyond. *Schizophrenia Bulletin* **36**: 36–42. PMID 19776206.

1143. Sams-Dodd, F., Lipska, B. K. & Weinberger, D. R. (1997). Neonatal lesions of the rat ventral hippocampus result in hyperlocomotion and deficits in social behaviour in adulthood. *Psychopharmacology* **132**: 303–310. PMID 9292631.

1144. Niwa, M., Kamiya, A., Murai, R., Kubo, K., Gruber, A. J., Tomita, K., Lu, L., Tomisato, S., Jaaro-Peled, H., Seshadri, S., Hiyama, H., Huang, B., Kohda, K., Noda, Y., O'Donnell, P., Nakajima, K., Sawa, A. & Nabeshima, T. (2010). Knockdown of DISC1 by in utero gene transfer disturbs postnatal dopaminergic maturation in the frontal cortex and leads to adult behavioral deficits. *Neuron* **65**: 480–489. PMID 20188653.

1145. Doody, G. A., Johnstone, E. C., Sanderson, T. L., Owens, D. G. & Muir, W. J. (1998). 'Pfropfschizophrenie' revisited. Schizophrenia in people with mild learning disability. *British Journal of Psychiatry* **173**: 145–153. PMID 9850227.

1146. Rapoport, J. L., Addington, A. M., Frangou, S. & Psych, M. R. (2005). The neurodevelopmental model of schizophrenia: update 2005. *Molecular Psychiatry* **10**: 434–449. PMID 15700048.

1147. Rehn, A. E. & Rees, S. M. (2005). Investigating the neurodevelopmental hypothesis of schizophrenia. *Clinical and Experimental Pharmacology and Physiology* **32**: 687–696. PMID 16173923.

1148. Toyota, T., Yoshitsugu, K., Ebihara, M., Yamada, K., Ohba, H., Fukasawa, M., Minabe, Y., Nakamura, K., Sekine, Y., Takei, N., Suzuki, K., Itokawa, M., Meerabux, J. M., Iwayama-Shigeno, Y., Tomaru, Y., Shimizu, H., Hattori, E., Mori, N. & Yoshikawa, T. (2004). Association between schizophrenia with ocular misalignment and polyalanine length variation in PMX2B. *Human Molecular Genetics* **13**: 551–561. PMID 14709596.

1149. Khashan, A. S., Abel, K. M., McNamee, R., Pedersen, M. G., Webb, R. T., Baker, P. N., Kenny, L. C. & Mortensen, P. B. (2008). Higher risk of offspring schizophrenia following antenatal maternal exposure to severe adverse life events. *Archives of General Psychiatry* **65**: 146–152. PMID 18250252.

1150. St Clair, D., Xu, M., Wang, P., Yu, Y., Fang, Y., Zhang, F., Zheng, X., Gu, N., Feng, G., Sham, P. & He, L. (2005). Rates of adult schizophrenia following prenatal exposure to the Chinese famine of 1959–1961. *Journal of the American Medical Association* **294**: 557–562. PMID 16077049.

1151. Kirov, G., Rujescu, D., Ingason, A., Collier, D. A., O'Donovan, M. C. & Owen, M. J. (2009). Neurexin 1 (NRXN1) deletions in schizophrenia. *Schizophrenia Bulletin* **35**: 851–854. PMID 19675094.

1152. Hall, J., Romaniuk, L., McIntosh, A. M., Steele, J. D., Johnstone, E. C. & Lawrie, S. M. (2009). Associative learning and the genetics of schizophrenia. *Trends in Neurosciences* **32**: 359–336. PMID 19427043.

1153. Walsh, T., McClellan, J. M., McCarthy, S. E., Addington, A. M., Pierce, S. B., Cooper, G. M., Nord, A. S., Kusenda, M., Malhotra, D., Bhandari, A., Stray, S. M., Rippey, C. F., Roccanova, P., Makarov, V., Lakshmi, B., Findling, R. L., Sikich, L., Stromberg, T., Merriman, B., Gogtay, N., Butler, P., Eckstrand, K., Noory, L., Gochman, P., Long, R., Chen, Z., Davis, S., Baker, C., Eichler, E. E., Meltzer, P. S., Nelson, S. F., Singleton, A. B., Lee, M. K., Rapoport, J. L., King, M. C. & Sebat, J. (2008). Rare structural variants disrupt multiple genes in neurodevelopmental pathways in schizophrenia. *Science* **320**: 539–543. PMID 18369103.

1154. Buchanan, R. W. & Heinrichs, D. W. (1989). The Neurological Evaluation Scale (NES): a structured instrument for the assessment of neurological signs in schizophrenia. *Psychiatry Research* **27**: 335–350. PMID 2710870.

1155. Kaczorowski, J. A., Barrantes-Vidal, N. & Kwapil, T. R. (2009). Neurological soft signs in psychometrically identified schizotypy. *Schizophrenia Research* **115**: 293–302. PMID 19651490.

1156. Hui, C. L., Wong, G. H., Chiu, C. P., Lam, M. M. & Chen, E. Y. (2009). Potential endophenotype for schizophrenia: neurological soft signs. *Annals of the Academy of Medicine, Singapore* **38**: 408–413. PMID 19521640.

1157. Conus, P., Abdel-Baki, A., Harrigan, S., Lambert, M. & McGorry, P. D. (2004). Schneiderian first rank symptoms predict poor outcome within first episode manic psychosis. *Journal of Affective Disorders* **81**: 259–268. PMID 15337330.

1158. Negash, A., Kebede, D., Alem, A., Melaku, Z., Deyessa, N., Shibire, T., Fekadu, A., Fekadu, D., Jacobsson, L. & Kullgren, G. (2004). Neurological soft signs in bipolar I disorder patients. *Journal of Affective Disorders* **80**: 221–230. PMID 15207935.

1159. Goswami, U., Gulrajani, C., Varma, A., Sharma, A., Ferrier, I. N., Young, A. H. & Moore, P. B. (2007). Soft neurological signs do not increase with age in euthymic bipolar subjects. *Journal of Affective Disorders* **103**: 99–103. PMID 17367868.

1160. Whitty, P., Clarke, M., McTigue, O., Browne, S., Gervin, M., Kamali, M., Lane, A., Kinsella, A., Waddington, J., Larkin, C. & O'Callaghan, E. (2006).

Diagnostic specificity and predictors of neurological soft signs in schizophrenia, bipolar disorder and other psychoses over the first 4 years of illness. *Schizophrenia Research* **86**: 110–117. PMID 16765029.

1161. Goswami, U., Sharma, A., Khastigir, U., Ferrier, I. N., Young, A. H., Gallagher, P., Thompson, J. M. & Moore, P. B. (2006). Neuropsychological dysfunction, soft neurological signs and social disability in euthymic patients with bipolar disorder. *British Journal of Psychiatry* **188**: 366–373. PMID 16582064.

1162. Perala, J., Suvisaari, J., Saarni, S. I., Kuoppasalmi, K., Isometsa, E., Pirkola, S., Partonen, T., Tuulio-Henriksson, A., Hintikka, J., Kieseppa, T., Harkanen, T., Koskinen, S. & Lonnqvist, J. (2007). Lifetime prevalence of psychotic and bipolar I disorders in a general population. *Archives of General Psychiatry* **64**: 19–28. PMID 17199051.

1163. Maj, M., Pirozzi, R., Magliano, L., Fiorillo, A. & Bartoli, L. (2007). Phenomenology and prognostic significance of delusions in major depressive disorder: a 10-year prospective follow-up study. *Journal of Clinical Psychiatry* **68**: 1411–1417. PMID 17915981.

1164. Tandon, R. & Greden, J. F. (1987). Schneiderian first rank symptoms: reconfirmation of high specificity for schizophrenia. *Acta Psychiatrica Scandinavica* **75**: 392–396. PMID 2884810.

1165. Wolkowitz, O. M., Burke, H., Epel, E. S. & Reus, V. I. (2009). Glucocorticoids. Mood, memory, and mechanisms. *Annals of the New York Academy of Sciences* **1179**: 19–40. PMID 19906230.

1166. Malhi, G. S., Green, M., Fagiolini, A., Peselow, E. D. & Kumari, V. (2008). Schizoaffective disorder: diagnostic issues and future recommendations. *Bipolar Disorders* **10**: 215–230. PMID 18199238.

1167. Kolakowska, T., Williams, A. O., Jambor, K. & Ardern, M. (1985). Schizophrenia with good and poor outcome. III: Neurological 'soft' signs, cognitive impairment and their clinical significance. *British Journal of Psychiatry* **146**: 348–357. PMID 4016437.

1168. Siever, L. J., Silverman, J. M., Horvath, T. B., Klar, H., Coccaro, E., Keefe, R. S., Pinkham, L., Rinaldi, P., Mohs, R. C. & Davis, K. L. (1990). Increased morbid risk for schizophrenia-related disorders in relatives of schizotypal personality disordered patients. *Archives of General Psychiatry* **47**: 634–640. PMID 2360857.

1169. Kraepelin, E. (1913). *Psychiatrie: Ein Lehrbuch für Studierende und Ärzte [8. vollständig umgearbeitete Auflage] [Vol. III]*, J.A. Barth, Leibzig.

1170. Roth, M. & Morrissey, J. D. (1952). Problems in the diagnosis and classification of mental disorder in old age; with a study of case material. *Journal of Mental Science* **98**: 66–80. PMID 14898208.

1171. Roth, M. (1955). The natural history of mental disorder in old age. *Journal of Mental Science* **101**: 281–301. PMID 13243044.

1172. Sato, A. & Ihda, S. (2002). Paraphrenia and late paraphrenia. *Psychogeriatrics* **2**: 20–25.

1173. Phillips, K. A. (2004). Psychosis in body dysmorphic disorder. *Journal of Psychiatric Research* **38**: 63–72. PMID 14690771.

1174. Pillmann, F., Haring, A., Balzuweit, S., Bloink, R. & Marneros, A. (2003). Bouffee delirante and ICD-10 acute and transient psychoses: a comparative study. *Australian and New Zealand Journal of Psychiatry* **37**: 327–333. PMID 12780472.

1175. Johnson-Sabine, E. C., Mann, A. H., Jacoby, R. J., Wood, K. H., Peron-Magnan, P., Olie, J. P. & Deniker, P. (1983). Bouffee delirante: an examination of its current status. *Psychological Medicine* **13**: 771–778. PMID 6665093.

1176. Chabrol, H. (2003). Chronic hallucinatory psychosis, bouffee delirante, and the classification of psychosis in French psychiatry. *Current Psychiatry Reports* **5**: 187–191. PMID 12773270.

1177. Kleist, K. (1928). Über zykloide, paranoide und epileptoide Psychosen und über die Frage der Degenerationspsychosen. *Schweizer*

Archiv für Neurologie und Psychiatrie **23**: 3–37.
1178. Perris, C. (1988). The concept of cycloid psychotic disorder. *Psychiatric Developments* **6**: 37–56. PMID 3050983.
1179. Peralta, V., Cuesta, M. J. & Zandio, M. (2007). Cycloid psychosis: an examination of the validity of the concept. *Current Psychiatry Reports* **9**: 184–192. PMID 17521513.
1180. Meduna, L. J. (1950). *Oneirophrenia: The confusional state*. Champaign-Urbana, IL: University of Illinois Press.
1181. Scharfetter, C., Nusperli, M. & Hurwitz, E. (1979). [The 'schizophrenic reaction' – a follow-up study after 20 years (author's translation)]. *Archiv fur Psychiatrie und Nervenkrankheiten* **226**: 347–368. PMID 454148.
1182. van der Hart, O., Witztum, E. & Friedman, B. (1993). From hysterical psychosis to reactive dissociative psychosis. *Journal of Traumatic Stress* **6**: 43–64.
1183. Casey, P. & Kelly, B. (2007). *Fish's Clinical Psychopathology: Signs and symptoms in psychiatry*. Third edition. London: Gaskell.
1184. Bottas, A., Cooke, R. G. & Richter, M. A. (2005). Comorbidity and pathophysiology of obsessive-compulsive disorder in schizophrenia: is there evidence for a schizo-obsessive subtype of schizophrenia? *Journal of Psychiatry and Neuroscience* **30**: 187–193. PMID 15944743.
1185. Eisen, J. L. & Rasmussen, S. A. (1993). Obsessive compulsive disorder with psychotic features. *Journal of Clinical Psychiatry* **54**: 373–379. PMID 8262879.
1186. Klemperer, F. (1996). Compulsions developing into command hallucinations. *Psychopathology* **29**: 249–251. PMID 8865357.
1187. Sevincok, L., Akoglu, A. & Arslantas, H. (2006). Schizo-obsessive and obsessive-compulsive disorder: comparison of clinical characteristics and neurological soft signs. *Psychiatry Research* **145**: 241–248. PMID 17070933.
1188. Kayahan, B., Ozturk, O., Veznedaroglu, B. & Eraslan, D. (2005). Obsessive-compulsive symptoms in schizophrenia: prevalance and clinical correlates. *Psychiatry and Clinical Neurosciences* **59**: 291–295. PMID 15896222.
1189. Ganesan, V., Kumar, T. C. & Khanna, S. (2001). Obsessive-compulsive disorder and psychosis. *Canadian Journal of Psychiatry* **46**: 750–754. PMID 11692979.
1190. Poyurovsky, M., Fuchs, C. & Weizman, A. (1999). Obsessive-compulsive disorder in patients with first-episode schizophrenia. *American Journal of Psychiatry* **156**: 1998–2000. PMID 10588421.
1191. Dowling, F. G., Pato, M. T. & Pato, C. N. (1995). Comorbidity of obsessive-compulsive and psychotic symptoms: a review. *Harvard Review of Psychiatry* **3**: 75–83. PMID 9384932.
1192. Guz, H. & Aygun, D. (2004). Neurological soft signs in obsessive-compulsive disorder. *Neurology India* **52**: 72–75. PMID 15069243.
1193. Bolton, D., Gibb, W., Lees, A., Raven, P., Gray, J. A., Chen, E. & Shafran, R. (1998). Neurological soft signs in obsessive compulsive disorder: standardised assessment and comparison with schizophrenia. *Behavioural Neurology* **11**: 197–204. PMID 11568420.
1194. Galynker, I., Ieronimo, C., Perez-Acquino, A., Lee, Y. & Winston, A. (1996). Panic attacks with psychotic features. *Journal of Clinical Psychiatry* **57**: 402–406. PMID 9746448.
1195. Goodwin, R. & Davidson, L. (2002). Panic attacks in psychosis. *Acta Psychiatrica Scandinavica* **105**: 14–19. PMID 12086220.
1196. Goodwin, R. D., Fergusson, D. M. & Horwood, L. J. (2004). Panic attacks and psychoticism. *American Journal of Psychiatry* **161**: 88–92. PMID 14702255.
1197. Sareen, J., Cox, B. J., Goodwin, R. D. & Asmundsen, G. J. G. (2005). Co-occurrence of posttraumatic stress disorder with positive psychotic symptoms in a nationally representative sample. *Journal of Traumatic Stress* **18**: 313–322. PMID 16281228.

1198. Butler, R. W., Mueser, K. T., Sprock, J. & Braff, D. L. (1996). Positive symptoms of psychosis in posttraumatic stress disorder. *Biological Psychiatry* **39**: 839–844. PMID 9172704.

1199. Hudson, J. I., Pope, H. G., Jr. & Jonas, J. M. (1984). Psychosis in anorexia nervosa and bulimia. *British Journal of Psychiatry* **145**: 420–423. PMID 6435712.

1200. Miotto, P., Pollini, B., Restaneo, A., Favaretto, G., Sisti, D., Rocchi, M. B. & Preti, A. (2010). Symptoms of psychosis in anorexia and bulimia nervosa. *Psychiatry Research* **175**: 237–243. PMID 20022383.

1201. Links, P. S., Steiner, M. & Mitton, J. (1989). Characteristics of psychosis in borderline personality disorder. *Psychopathology* **22**: 188–193. PMID 2798708.

1202. Pope, H. G., Jr., Jonas, J. M., Hudson, J. I., Cohen, B. M. & Tohen, M. (1985). An empirical study of psychosis in borderline personality disorder. *American Journal of Psychiatry* **142**: 1285–1290. PMID 4061687.

1203. Miller, F. T., Abrams, T., Dulit, R. & Fyer, M. (1993). Psychotic symptoms in patients with borderline personality disorder and concurrent axis I disorder. *Hospital and Community Psychiatry* **44**: 59–61. PMID 8436363.

1204. Howard, R., Rabins, P. V., Seeman, M. V. & Jeste, D. V. (2000). Late-onset schizophrenia and very-late-onset schizophrenia-like psychosis: an international consensus. The International Late-Onset Schizophrenia Group. *American Journal of Psychiatry* **157**: 172–178. PMID 10671383.

1205. Jeste, D. V., Paulsen, J. S. & Harris, M. J. (1995). Late-onset schizophrenia and other related psychosis. In *Psychopharmacology: The Fourth Generation of Progress* (Bloom, F. E. & Kupfer, D. J., Eds.). New York/Nashville, TN: Raven Press/American College of Neuropsychopharmacology.

1206. Bleuler, E. (1911). *Dementia praecox oder Gruppe der Schizophrenien.* Leipzig/Wien: Franz Deuticke.

1207. Ostling, S., Palsson, S. P. & Skoog, I. (2007). The incidence of first-onset psychotic symptoms and paranoid ideation in a representative population sample followed from age 70–90 years. Relation to mortality and later development of dementia. *International Journal of Geriatric Psychiatry* **22**: 520–528. PMID 17117394.

1208. Ostling, S., Borjesson-Hanson, A. & Skoog, I. (2007). Psychotic symptoms and paranoid ideation in a population-based sample of 95-year-olds. *American Journal of Geriatric Psychiatry* **15**: 999–1004. PMID 18056818.

1209. Livingston, G., Kitchen, G., Manela, M., Katona, C. & Copeland, J. (2001). Persecutory symptoms and perceptual disturbance in a community sample of older people: the Islington study. *International Journal of Geriatric Psychiatry* **16**: 462–468. PMID 11376461.

1210. Matson, J. L. & Nebel-Schwalm, M. S. (2007). Comorbid psychopathology with autism spectrum disorder in children: an overview. *Research in Developmental Disabilities* **28**: 341–352. PMID 16765022.

1211. Schneider, D., Szetela, B. R. & Daly, R. C. (2006). Ganser syndrome. eMedicine. URL: http://www.emedicine.com/med/topic840.htm. Accessed 20 April 2008.

1212. Olson, P. R., Suddeth, J. A., Peterson, P. J. & Egelhoff, C. (1985). Hallucinations of widowhood. *Journal of the American Geriatrics Society* **33**: 543–547. PMID 4020000.

1213. Dewi Rees, W. (1971). The hallucinations of widowhood. *British Medical Journal* **4**: 37–41. PMID 5096884.

1214. Johns, L. C., Cannon, M., Singleton, N., Murray, R. M., Farrell, M., Brugha, T., Bebbington, P., Jenkins, R. & Meltzer, H. (2004). Prevalence and correlates of self-reported psychotic symptoms in the British population. *British Journal of Psychiatry* **185**: 298–305. PMID 15458989.

1215. Bartels-Velthuis, A. A., Jenner, J. A., van de Willige, G., van Os, J. & Wiersma, D. (2010). Prevalence and correlates of auditory vocal hallucinations in middle childhood. *British Journal of Psychiatry* **196**: 41–46. PMID 20044659.

1216. Loewy, R. L., Johnson, J. K. & Cannon, T. D. (2007). Self-report of attenuated psychotic experiences in a college population. *Schizophrenia Research* **93**: 144–151. PMID 17459662.
1217. Hanssen, M. S., Bijl, R. V., Vollebergh, W. & van Os, J. (2003). Self-reported psychotic experiences in the general population: a valid screening tool for DSM-III-R psychotic disorders? *Acta Psychiatrica Scandinavica* **107**: 369–377. PMID 12752033.
1218. Kendler, K. S., Gallagher, T. J., Abelson, J. M. & Kessler, R. C. (1996). Lifetime prevalence, demographic risk factors, and diagnostic validity of nonaffective psychosis as assessed in a US community sample. The National Comorbidity Survey. *Archives of General Psychiatry* **53**: 1022–1031. PMID 8911225.
1219. Raine, A. (1991). The SPQ: a scale for the assessment of schizotypal personality based on DSM-III-R criteria. *Schizophrenia Bulletin* **17**: 555–564. PMID 1805349.
1220. Bentall, R. P. & Slade, P. D. (1985). Reliability of a scale measuring disposition towards hallucination: a brief report. *Personality and Individual Differences* **6**: 527–529.
1221. Laroi, F., Marczewski, P. & Van der Linden, M. (2004). Further evidence of the multi-dimensionality of hallucinatory predisposition: factor structure of a modified version of the Launay–Slade Hallucinations Scale in a normal sample. *European Psychiatry* **19**: 15–20. PMID 14969776.
1222. van Os, J., Linscott, R. J., Myin-Germeys, I., Delespaul, P. & Krabbendam, L. (2009). A systematic review and meta-analysis of the psychosis continuum: evidence for a psychosis proneness-persistence-impairment model of psychotic disorder. *Psychological Medicine* **39**: 179–195. PMID 18606047.
1223. Berrios, G. E. & Dening, T. R. (1996). Pseudohallucinations: a conceptual history. *Psychological Medicine* **26**: 753–763. PMID 8817710.
1224. van der Zwaard, R. & Polak, M. A. (2001). Pseudohallucinations: a pseudoconcept? A review of the validity of the concept, related to associate symptomatology. *Comprehensive Psychiatry* **42**: 42–50. PMID 11154715.
1225. Copolov, D., Trauer, T. & Mackinnon, A. (2004). On the non-significance of internal versus external auditory hallucinations. *Schizophrenia Research* **69**: 1–6. PMID 15145464.
1226. Beauchamp, M. C., Lecomte, T., Lecomte, C., Leclerc, C. & Corbiere, M. (2006). Do people with a first episode of psychosis differ in personality profiles? *Schizophrenia Research* **85**: 162–167. PMID 16679000.
1227. Ortet, G., Ibáñez, M. I., Moro, M., Silva, F. & Boyle, G. J. (1999). Psychometric appraisal of Eysenck's revised Psychoticism scale: a cross-cultural study. *Personality and Individual Differences* **27**: 1209–1219.
1228. Chapman, J. P., Chapman, L. J. & Kwapil, T. R. (1994). Does the Eysenck psychoticism scale predict psychosis? A ten year longitudinal study. *Personality and Individual Differences* **17**: 369–375.
1229. Ciarrochi, J. & Heaven, P. C. L. (2007). Longitudinal examination of the impact of Eysenck's psychoticism dimension on emotional well-being in teenagers. *Personality and Individual Differences* **42**: 597–608.
1230. Morrison, A. P., Frame, L. & Larkin, W. (2003). Relationships between trauma and psychosis: a review and integration. *British Journal of Clinical Psychology* **42**: 331–353. PMID 14633411.
1231. Fisher, H., Morgan, C., Dazzan, P., Craig, T. K., Morgan, K., Hutchinson, G., Jones, P. B., Doody, G. A., Pariante, C., McGuffin, P., Murray, R. M., Leff, J. & Fearon, P. (2009). Gender differences in the association between childhood abuse and psychosis. *British Journal of Psychiatry* **194**: 319–325. PMID 19336782.
1232. Janssen, I., Krabbendam, L., Bak, M., Hanssen, M., Vollebergh, W., de Graaf, R. & van Os, J. (2004). Childhood abuse as a risk factor for psychotic experiences. *Acta Psychiatrica Scandinavica* **109**: 38–45. PMID 14674957.

1233. Steel, C., Marzillier, S., Fearon, P. & Ruddle, A. (2009). Childhood abuse and schizotypal personality. *Social Psychiatry and Psychiatric Epidemiology*. PMID 19333529.

1234. Lincoln, T. M., Peter, N., Schafer, M. & Moritz, S. (2008). Impact of stress on paranoia: an experimental investigation of moderators and mediators. *Psychological Medicine* **40**: 1–11. PMID 18940024.

1235. van Winkel, R., Stefanis, N. C. & Myin-Germeys, I. (2008). Psychosocial stress and psychosis. A review of the neurobiological mechanisms and the evidence for gene-stress interaction. *Schizophrenia Bulletin* **34**: 1095–1105. PMID 18718885.

1236. Møller, P. & Husby, R. (2000). The initial prodrome in schizophrenia: searching for naturalistic core dimensions of experience and behavior. *Schizophrenia Bulletin* **26**: 217–232. PMID 10755683.

1237. Harvey, P. D. (2009). When does cognitive decline occur in the period prior to the first episode of schizophrenia? *Psychiatry (Edgmont)* **6**: 12–14. PMID 19724764.

1238. Yung, A. R., Stanford, C., Cosgrave, E., Killackey, E., Phillips, L., Nelson, B. & McGorry, P. D. (2006). Testing the Ultra High Risk (prodromal) criteria for the prediction of psychosis in a clinical sample of young people. *Schizophrenia Research* **84**: 57–66. PMID 16630707.

1239. Yung, A. R., Yuen, H. P., McGorry, P. D., Phillips, L. J., Kelly, D., Dell ' Olio, M., Francey, S. M., Cosgrave, E. M., Killackey, E., Stanford, C., Godfrey, K. & Buckby, J. (2005). Mapping the onset of psychosis: the Comprehensive Assessment of At-Risk Mental States. *Australian and New Zealand Journal of Psychiatry* **39**: 964–971. PMID 16343296.

1240. Jaffe, M. E. & Sharma, K. K. (1998). Malingering uncommon psychiatric symptoms among defendants charged under California's "three strikes and you're out" law. *Journal of Forensic Sciences* **43**: 549–555. PMID 9608690.

1241. Bhatara, V., Alshari, M. G., Warhol, P., McMillin, J. M. & Bhatara, A. (2004). Coexistent hypothyroidism, psychosis, and severe obsessions in an adolescent: a 10-year follow-up. *Journal of Child and Adolescent Psychopharmacology* **14**: 315–323. PMID 15319028.

1242. Hitchcock, C. (2010). Probabilistic Causation. The Stanford Encyclopedia of Philosophy. URL: http://plato.stanford.edu/archives/sum2010/entries/causation-probabilistic/. Accessed 22 July 2010.

1243. Weed, D. L. (1997). On the use of causal criteria. *International Journal of Epidemiology* **26**: 1137–1141. PMID 9447391.

1244. Hill, A. B. (1965). The environment and disease: association or causation? *Proceedings of the Royal Society of Medicine* **58**: 295–300. PMID 14283879.

1245. Gunduz-Bruce, H., McMeniman, M., Robinson, D. G., Woerner, M. G., Kane, J. M., Schooler, N. R. & Lieberman, J. A. (2005). Duration of untreated psychosis and time to treatment response for delusions and hallucinations. *American Journal of Psychiatry* **162**: 1966–1969. PMID 16199847.

1246. Ryder, R. E. J., Mir, M. A. & Freeman, E. A. (2003). *An Aid to the MRCP PACES.* Third edition. Oxford: Blackwell.

1247. Hodkinson, H. M. (1972). Evaluation of a mental test score for assessment of mental impairment in the elderly. *Age and Ageing* **1**: 233–238. PMID 4669880.

1248. Folstein, M. F., Folstein, S. E. & McHugh, P. R. (1975). "Mini-mental state". A practical method for grading the cognitive state of patients for the clinician. *Journal of Psychiatric Research* **12**: 189–198. PMID 1202204.

1249. Mioshi, E., Dawson, K., Mitchell, J., Arnold, R. & Hodges, J. R. (2006). The Addenbrooke's Cognitive Examination Revised (ACE-R): a brief cognitive test battery for dementia screening. *International Journal of Geriatric Psychiatry* **21**: 1078–1085. PMID 16977673.

1250. Kay, S. R., Fiszbein, A. & Opler, L. A. (1987). The positive and negative syndrome scale (PANSS) for schizophrenia. *Schizophrenia Bulletin* **13**: 261–276. PMID 3616518.

1251. Andreasen, N. C., Arndt, S., Miller, D., Flaum, M. & Nopoulos, P. (1995). Correlational studies of the Scale for the Assessment of Negative Symptoms and the Scale for the Assessment of Positive Symptoms: an overview and update. *Psychopathology* **28**: 7–17. PMID 7871123.

1252. Overall, J. E. & Gorham, D. R. (1962). The brief psychiatric rating scale. *Psychological Reports* **10**: 799–812.

1253. Ffytche, D. (2004). Visual hallucination and illusion disorders: a clinical guide. *Advances in Clinical Neuroscience and Rehabilitation* **4**: 16–18.

1254. Wing, J. K., Cooper, J. E. & Sartorius, N. (1974). *Measurement and Classification of Psychiatric Symptoms: An instruction manual for the PSE and Catego Program.* Cambridge: Cambridge University Press.

1255. Intercollegiate Stroke Working Party (2008). National clinical guideline for stroke. Third edition. London: Royal College of Physicians. URL: http://www.library.nhs.uk/stroke/ViewResource.aspx?resID=291241.

1256. Byrne, P. (2007). Managing the acute psychotic episode. *British Medical Journal* **334**: 686–692. PMID 17395949.

1257. Shefrin, A., Puddester, D., Greenham, S., Bisnaire, L. & Gandy, H. (2006). What investigations are ordered in patients with first-episode psychosis? *Jefferson Journal of Psychiatry* **20**: 4–12.

1258. Jubran, A. (1999). Pulse oximetry. *Critical Care* **3**: R11–R17. PMID 11094477.

1259. Moyle, J. T. (1996). Uses and abuses of pulse oximetry. *Archives of Disease in Childhood* **74**: 77–80. PMID 8660057.

1260. Hanning, C. D. & Alexander-Williams, J. M. (1995). Pulse oximetry: a practical review. *British Medical Journal* **311**: 367–370. PMID 7640545.

1261. St John, A., Boyd, J. C., Lowes, A. J. & Price, C. P. (2006). The use of urinary dipstick tests to exclude urinary tract infection: a systematic review of the literature. *American Journal of Clinical Pathology* **126**: 428–436. PMID 16880133.

1262. Armstrong, L. E. (2007). Assessing hydration status: the elusive gold standard. *Journal of the American College of Nutrition* **26**: 575S-584S. PMID 17921468.

1263. Pepys, M. B. & Hirschfield, G. M. (2003). C-reactive protein: a critical update. *Journal of Clinical Investigation* **111**: 1805–1812. PMID 12813013.

1264. Goode, D. J. & Meltzer, H. Y. (1976). Effects of isometric exercise on serum creatine phosphokinase activity. *Archives of General Psychiatry* **33**: 1207–1211. PMID 971030.

1265. Hermesh, H., Manor, I., Shiloh, R., Aizenberg, D., Benjamini, Y., Munitz, H. & Weizman, A. (2002). High serum creatinine kinase level: possible risk factor for neuroleptic malignant syndrome. *Journal of Clinical Psychopharmacology* **22**: 252–256. PMID 12006894.

1266. Manor, I., Hermesh, H., Valevski, A., Benjamin, Y., Munitz, H. & Weizman, A. (1998). Recurrence pattern of serum creatine phosphokinase levels in repeated acute psychosis. *Biological Psychiatry* **43**: 288–292. PMID 9513739.

1267. Meltzer, H. Y., Ross-Stanton, J. & Schlessinger, S. (1980). Mean serum creatine kinase activity in patients with functional psychoses. *Archives of General Psychiatry* **37**: 650–655. PMID 7387337.

1268. Graham, K. A. & Perkins, D. O. (2010). Assessment of psychosis. BMJ Best Practice. URL: http://bestpractice.bmj.com/best-practice/monograph/1066/overview/summary.html. Accessed 8 July 2010.

1269. Lehman, A. F., Lieberman, J. A., Dixon, L. B., McGlashan, T. H., Miller, A. L., Perkins, D. O. & Kreyenbuhl, J. (2004). Practice guideline for the treatment of patients with schizophrenia. Second edition. Arlington, VA: American Psychiatric Association (APA Practice Guidelines; Work Group On Schizophrenia).

1270. Dixon, L., Perkins, D. & Calmes, C. (2009). Guideline watch (September 2009): Practice guideline for the treatment of patients with schizophrenia. Arlington, VA: American Psychiatric Association (APA Practice Guidelines).

1271. Salokangas, R. K., Helminen, M., Koivisto, A. M., Rantanen, H., Oja, H., Pirkola, S., Wahlbeck, K. & Joukamaa, M. (2010). Incidence of hospitalised schizophrenia in Finland since 1980: decreasing and increasing again. *Social Psychiatry and Psychiatric Epidemiology* [Epub ahead of print]. PMID 20306013.

1272. UK National Institute for Health and Clinical Excellence (2008). Structural neuroimaging in first-episode psychosis: NICE technology appraisal guidance 136. United Kingdom National Institute for Health and Clinical Excellence. URL: http://www.nice.org.uk/TA136. Accessed 18 March 2008.

1273. Dean, K. & Murray, R. (2008). *Lectures in Schizophrenia: volume 1.* London: Current Medicine Group.

1274. Weinberger, D. R. (1984). Brain disease and psychiatric illness: when should a psychiatrist order a CAT scan? *American Journal of Psychiatry* **141**: 1521–1527. PMID 6439055.

1275. Clinical Research Network Coordinating Centre (2010). Industry costing template. UK National Institute for Health Research. URL: http://www.ukcrn.org.uk/index/industry/costing.html. Accessed 16 April 2010.

1276. University College London Hospitals NHS Foundation Trust (2010). Provider to provider services 2010–2011 tariff. URL: http://www.uclh.nhs.uk/NR/rdonlyres/24221693–4DDF-4149-B315-F92CB4C81152/106200/FINAL201011P2PTariff.pdf. Accessed 27 April 2010.

1277. Dodgson, G., Crebbin, K., Mitford, E., Brabban, A. & Paxton, R. (2008). Early intervention in psychosis service and psychiatric admissions. *The Psychiatrist* **32**: 413–416.

1278. Curtis, L. (2009). Unit costs of health & social care. University of Kent Personal Social Services Research Unit, Canterbury. URL: http://www.pssru.ac.uk/pdf/uc/uc2009/uc2009.pdf.

1279. World Health Organization (2006). Definition and diagnosis of diabetes mellitus and intermediate hyperglycemia: report of a WHO/IDF consultation. Geneva: World Health Organization.

1280. Inoue, S. (2010). Leukocytosis. eMedicine. URL: http://emedicine.medscape.com/article/956278-overview. Accessed 21 July 2010.

1281. Liss, M., Zeger, E., Lucey, D. R. & Kogulan, P. (2009). Eosinophilia. eMedicine. URL: http://emedicine.medscape.com/article/199879-overview. Accessed 21 July 2010.

1282. Godwin, J. E. & Braden, C. D. (2009). Neutropenia. eMedicine. URL: http://emedicine.medscape.com/article/204821-overview. Accessed 21 July 2010.

1283. Buckley, R. H. (2000). Primary immunodeficiency diseases due to defects in lymphocytes. *New England Journal of Medicine* **343**: 1313–1324. PMID 11058677.

1284. Zaiden, R. & Rana, F. (2010). Asssesment of anaemia. BMJ Best Practice. URL: http://bestpractice.bmj.com/best-practice/monograph/93/overview.html. Accessed 21 July 2010.

1285. Conrad, M. E. (2009). Anemia. eMedicine. URL: http://emedicine.medscape.com/article/198475-overview. Accessed 21 July 2010.

1286. Besa, E. C. & Woermann, U. (2009). Polycythemia, secondary. eMedicine. URL: http://emedicine.medscape.com/article/205039-overview. Accessed 21 July 2010.

1287. Krishnan, K., Smith, S. J. & Vardhana, H. G. (2009). Thrombocytosis, secondary. eMedicine. URL: http://emedicine.medscape.com/article/206811-overview. Accessed 21 July 2010.

1288. Thiagarajan, P. (2009). Platelet disorders. eMedicine. URL: http://emedicine.medscape.com/article/201722-overview. Accessed 21 July 2010.

1289. Limdi, J. K. & Hyde, G. M. (2003). Evaluation of abnormal liver function tests. *Postgraduate Medical Journal* **79**: 307–312. PMID 12840117.

1290. Barkhof, F. & Scheltens, P. (2002). Imaging of white matter lesions. *Cerebrovascular Diseases* **13** Suppl 2: 21–30. PMID 11901239.

1291. Kastrup, O., Wanke, I. & Maschke, M. (2005). Neuroimaging of infections. *NeuroRx* **2**: 324–332. PMID 15897953.

1292. Teodorczuk, A., Firbank, M. J., Pantoni, L., Poggesi, A., Erkinjuntti, T., Wallin, A., Wahlund, L. O., Scheltens, P., Waldemar, G., Schrotter, G., Ferro, J. M., Chabriat, H., Bazner, H., Visser, M., Inzitari, D. & O'Brien, J. T. (2010). Relationship between baseline white-matter changes and development of late-life depressive symptoms: 3-year results from the LADIS study. *Psychological Medicine* **40**: 603–610. PMID 19671212.

1293. Scaletta, T. (2010). Subdural hematoma. eMedicine. URL: http://emedicine.medscape.com/article/828005-overview. Accessed 22 July 2010.

1294. Meagher, R. J. & Young, W. F. (2009). Subdural hematoma. eMedicine. URL: http://emedicine.medscape.com/article/1137207-overview. Accessed 22 July 2001.

1295. Ramachandran, T. S. & Ramachandran, A. (2009). Prion-related diseases. eMedicine. URL: http://emedicine.medscape.com/article/1168941-overview. Accessed 21 July 2010.

1296. Fadare, O. & Hart, H. J. (2004). Anti-Ri antibodies associated with short-term memory deficits and a mature cystic teratoma of the ovary. *International Seminars in Surgical Oncology* **1**: 11. PMID 15537431.

1297. McGuffin, P., Farmer, A. & Harvey, I. (1991). A polydiagnostic application of operational criteria in studies of psychotic illness. Development and reliability of the OPCRIT system. *Archives of General Psychiatry* **48**: 764–770. PMID 1883262.

1298. Oyebode, F. (2008). *Sims' Symptoms in the Mind: An Introduction to Descriptive Psychopathology*. Fourth edition. Edinburgh: Saunders, Elsevier.

1299. Pawar, A. V. & Spence, S. A. (2003). Defining thought broadcast. Semi-structured literature review. *British Journal of Psychiatry* **183**: 287–291. PMID 14519605.

1300. Peralta, V. & Cuesta, M. J. (1999). Diagnostic significance of Schneider's first-rank symptoms in schizophrenia. Comparative study between schizophrenic and non-schizophrenic psychotic disorders. *British Journal of Psychiatry* **174**: 243–248. PMID 10448450.

1301. Koran, L. M., Sox, H. C., Jr., Marton, K. I., Moltzen, S., Sox, C. H., Kraemer, H. C., Imai, K., Kelsey, T. G., Rose, T. G., Jr., Levin, L. C. & Chandra, S. (1989). Medical evaluation of psychiatric patients. I. Results in a state mental health system. *Archives of General Psychiatry* **46**: 733–740. PMID 2787623.

1302. Frith, C. (2005). The neural basis of hallucinations and delusions. *Comptes Rendus Biologies* **328**: 169–175. PMID 15771003.

1303. Collerton, D., Perry, E. & McKeith, I. (2005). Why people see things that are not there: a novel Perception and Attention Deficit model for recurrent complex visual hallucinations. *Behavioral and Brain Sciences* **28**: 737–757; discussion 757–794. PMID 16372931.

1304. Grace, A. A. (2010). Dopamine system dysregulation by the ventral subiculum as the common pathophysiological basis for schizophrenia psychosis, psychostimulant abuse, and stress. *Neurotoxicity Research* **18**: 367–376. PMID 20143199.

1305. Mayberg, H. S. (1997). Limbic-cortical dysregulation: a proposed model of depression. *Journal of Neuropsychiatry and Clinical Neurosciences* **9**: 471–481. PMID 9276848.

1306. Fornito, A., Yucel, M. & Pantelis, C. (2009). Reconciling neuroimaging and neuropathological findings in schizophrenia and bipolar disorder. *Current Opinion in Psychiatry* **22**: 312–319. PMID 19365187.

1307. Knable, M. B. & Weinberger, D. R. (1997). Dopamine, the prefrontal cortex and schizophrenia. *Journal of Psychopharmacology* **11**: 123–131. PMID 9208376.

1308. Lowinger, P. (1959). Leprosy and psychosis. *American Journal of Psychiatry* **116**: 32–37. PMID 13661445.

1309. Lowinger, P. (1974). Letter: Follow-up on leprosy and psychosis. *American Journal of Psychiatry* **131**: 607. PMID 4819060.

1310. Aung, T., Kitajima, S., Nomoto, M., En, J., Yonezawa, S., Arikawa, I. & Goto, M. (2007). Mycobacterium leprae in neurons of the medulla oblongata and spinal cord in leprosy. *Journal of Neuropathology and Experimental Neurology* **66**: 284–294. PMID 17413319.

1311. Ponomareff, G. L. (1965). Phenomenology of delusions in a case of leprosy. *American Journal of Psychiatry* **121**: 1211. PMID 14286061.

1312. Perlas, A. P. & Faillace, L. A. (1964). Psychiatric manifestations of carcinoma of the pancreas. *American Journal of Psychiatry* **121**: 182. PMID 14194218.

1313. Casey, D. A. (1991). Pancreatic carcinoma in an elderly woman with an organic affective disorder and AIDS delusion. *Southern Medical Journal* **84**: 97–98. PMID 1986437.

1314. Perry, T. L., Wright, J. M. & Hansen, S. (1983). Hyperasparaginemia in a schizophrenic patient. *Biological Psychiatry* **18**: 89–97. PMID 6830927.

1315. Perry, T. L., Wright, J. M., Hansen, S., Davis, F. F. & Abuchowski, A. (1985). Use of the polyethylene glycol adduct of L-asparaginase for the treatment of hyperasparaginemia in a schizophrenic patient. *Biological Psychiatry* **20**: 1103–1108. PMID 4041512.

1316. Lahera Forteza, G. & Gonzalez Aguado, F. (2007). Psychotic mania after introduction of continuous positive airway pressure (CPAP) in the treatment of obstructive sleep apnoea. *Actas Espanolas de Psiquiatria* **35**: 406–407. PMID 18004679.

1317. Sykut-Cegielska, J., Gradowska, W., Mercimek-Mahmutoglu, S. & Stockler-Ipsiroglu, S. (2004). Biochemical and clinical characteristics of creatine deficiency syndromes. *Acta Biochimica Polonica* **51**: 875–882. PMID 15625559.

1318. Lindor, N. M., Hoffman, A., O'Brien, J. F., Hanson, N. P. & Thompson, J. N. (1994). Sanfilippo syndrome type A in two adult sibs. *American Journal of Medical Genetics* **53**: 241–244. PMID 7856659.

1319. Yamaguchi, K., Sawada, T., Naraki, T., Igata-Yi, R., Shiraki, H., Horii, Y., Ishii, T., Ikeda, K., Asou, N., Okabe, H., Mochizuki, M., Takahashi, K., Yamada, S., Kubo, K., Yashiki, S., Waltrip, R. W., 2nd & Carbone, K. M. (1999). Detection of Borna disease virus-reactive antibodies from patients with psychiatric disorders and from horses by electrochemiluminescence immunoassay. *Clinical and Diagnostic Laboratory Immunology* **6**: 696–700. PMID 10473520.

1320. Miranda, H. C., Nunes, S. O., Calvo, E. S., Suzart, S., Itano, E. N. & Watanabe, M. A. (2006). Detection of Borna disease virus p24 RNA in peripheral blood cells from Brazilian mood and psychotic disorder patients. *Journal of Affective Disorders* **90**: 43–47. PMID 16324750.

1321. Nunes, S. O., Itano, E. N., Amarante, M. K., Reiche, E. M., Miranda, H. C., de Oliveira, C. E., Matsuo, T., Vargas, H. O. & Watanabe, M. A. (2008). RNA from Borna disease virus in patients with schizophrenia, schizoaffective patients, and in their biological relatives. *Journal of Clinical Laboratory Analysis* **22**: 314–320. PMID 18623121.

1322. Rennick, P. M., Nolan, D. C., Bauer, R. B. & Lerner, A. M. (1973). Neuropsychologic and neurologic follow-up after herpesvirus hominis encephalitis. *Neurology* **23**: 42–47. PMID 4347060.

1323. Nakayama, H., Nakano, Y., Itoh, N., Koike, R., Honma, A., Takahashi, M. & Gotoh, T. (1992). [A case of Castleman's disease with a variable neuropsychiatric symptomatology]. *No To Shinkei (Brain and Nerve)* **44**: 923–928. PMID 1285994.

1324. Greenberg, D. M. & Lee, J. W. (2001). Psychotic manifestations of alcoholism. *Current Psychiatry Reports* **3**: 314–318. PMID 11470038.

1325. Gillberg, C. & Forsell, C. (1984). Childhood psychosis and neurofibromatosis – more than a coincidence? *Journal of Autism and Developmental Disorders* **14**: 1–8. PMID 6423617.

1326. Ramani, S. V. (1981). Psychosis associated with frontal lobe lesions in Schilder's cerebral sclerosis: a case report with CT scan evidence. *Journal of Clinical Psychiatry* **42**: 250–252. PMID 7240108.

1327. Mahr, R. N., Moberg, P. J., Overhauser, J., Strathdee, G., Kamholz, J., Loevner, L. A., Campbell, H., Zackai, E. H., Reber, M. E., Mozley, D. P., Brown, L., Turetsky, B. I. & Shapiro, R. M. (1996). Neuropsychiatry of 18q- syndrome. *American Journal of Medical Genetics* **67**: 172–178. PMID 8723044.

1328. Fisch, G. S. (1993). What is associated with the fragile X syndrome? *American Journal of Medical Genetics* **48**: 112–121. PMID 8362927.

1329. Filho, G. M., Rosa, V. P., Lin, K., Caboclo, L. O., Sakamoto, A. C. & Yacubian, E. M. (2008). Psychiatric comorbidity in epilepsy: a study comparing patients with mesial temporal sclerosis and juvenile myoclonic epilepsy. *Epilepsy & Behavior* **13**: 196–201. PMID 18313989.

1330. Quast, T. M., Sippert, J. D., Sauve, W. M. & Deutsch, S. I. (2005). Comorbid presentation of Kartagener's syndrome and schizophrenia: support of an etiologic hypothesis of anomalous development of cerebral asymmetry? *Schizophrenia Research* **74**: 283–285. PMID 15722007.

1331. Notkin, J. (1952). Psychosomatic implications in a case of Paget's disease with psychosis. *Psychiatric Quarterly* **26**: 307–312. PMID 14920642.

1332. Walton, R. G. (1986). Seizure and mania after high intake of aspartame. *Psychosomatics* **27**: 218–220. PMID 3961094.

1333. Fisch, R. Z. & Lahad, A. (1989). Adverse psychiatric reaction to ketoconazole. *American Journal of Psychiatry* **146**: 939. PMID 2742021.

1334. Sonino, N. & Fava, G. A. (1990). Psychiatric reaction to ketoconazole. *American Journal of Psychiatry* **147**: 677. PMID 2327507.

1335. Navarro, V., Vieta, E. & Gasto, C. (2001). Mannitol-induced acute manic state. *Journal of Clinical Psychiatry* **62**: 126. PMID 11247098.

1336. Labbate, L. A. & Holzgang, A. J. (1989). Manic syndrome after discontinuation of methyldopa. *American Journal of Psychiatry* **146**: 1075–1076. PMID 2750982.

1337. Pushpal, D. & Shamshul, H. N. (2006). Tiagabine withdrawal-emergent mania. *Australian and New Zealand Journal of Psychiatry* **40**: 719. PMID 16866771.

1338. Zisook, S. & Kendler, K. S. (2007). Is bereavement-related depression different than non-bereavement-related depression? *Psychological Medicine* **37**: 779–794. PMID 17306046.

1339. Forty, L., Jones, L., Macgregor, S., Caesar, S., Cooper, C., Hough, A., Dean, L., Dave, S., Farmer, A., McGuffin, P., Brewster, S., Craddock, N. & Jones, I. (2006). Familiality of postpartum depression in unipolar disorder: results of a family study. *American Journal of Psychiatry* **163**: 1549–1553. PMID 16946179.

1340. Whitley, R. J. (1990). Viral encephalitis. *New England Journal of Medicine* **323**: 242–250. PMID 2195341.

1341. Ramírez-Bermúdez, J., Soto-Hernández, J. L., López-Gómez, M., Mendoza-Silva, M., Colin-Piana, R. & Campillo-Serrano, C. (2005). [Frequency of neuropsychiatric signs and symptoms in patients with viral encephalitis.] *Revista de Neurologia* **41**: 140–144. PMID 16047296.

1342. Das, S. K. & Ray, K. (2006). Wilson's disease: an update. *Nature Clinical Practice Neurology* **2**: 482–493. PMID 16932613.

1343. Nanji, A. A. & Denegri, J. (1981). Hypokalaemia in leukaemia. *Postgraduate Medical Journal* **57**: 482–484. PMID 7301694.

1344. Advisory Council on the Misuse of Drugs (2010). Advice on 2-DPMP – 'Ivory Wave' – concerning the Open General Import Licence. URL: http://www.homeoffice.gov.uk/publications/drugs/acmd/advice-ivory-wave/?view=Binary. Accessed 25 November 2010.

1345. Caroff, S. N., Mann, S.C., McCarthy, M., Naser, J., Rynn, M, & Morrison, M. (1998). Acute infectious encephalitis complicated by neuroleptic malignant syndrome. *Journal of Clinical*

Psychopharmacology **18**: 349–351. PMID 9690707.

1346. Amin, S., Singh, S. P., Brewin, J., Jones, P. B., Medley, I. & Harrison, G. (1999). Diagnostic stability of first-episode psychosis. Comparison of ICD-10 and DSM-III-R systems. *British Journal of Psychiatry* **175**: 537–543. PMID 10789350.

1347. Sáez-Fonesca, J.A., Lee, L. & Walker, Z. (2007). Long-term outcome of depressive psuedodementia in the elderly. *Journal of Affective Disorders* **101**: 123–129. PMID 17184844.

1348. Weitzenhoffer, A. M. (1996). Catalepsy tests: what do they tell us? *The International Journal of Clinical and Experimental Hypnosis* **44**: 307–323. PMID 8885530.

Index